北美外科肿瘤临床学会

肝细胞癌、胆管细胞癌和转移性肝癌

Surgical Oncology Clinics of North America: Hepatocellular Cancer, Cholangiocarcinoma, and Metastatic Tumors of the Liver

主　编　［美］劳伦斯 D. 韦格曼（Lawrence D. Wagman）
顾　问　［美］尼古拉斯 J. 彼得雷利（Nicholas J. Petrelli）
主　译　陆骊工

辽宁科学技术出版社
LIAONING SCIENCE AND TECHNOLOGY PUBLISHING HOUSE

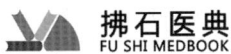
拂石医典
FU SHI MEDBOOK

图书在版编目（CIP）数据

肝细胞癌，胆管细胞癌和转移性肝癌/（美）劳伦斯·韦格曼（Lawrence D. Wagman）主编；陆骊工译.—沈阳：辽宁科学技术出版社，2017.10
ISBN 978-7-5591-0447-2

Ⅰ.①肝… Ⅱ.①劳…②陆… Ⅲ.①肝细胞癌—肿瘤转移—肝癌②胆管肿瘤—肿瘤转移—肝癌 Ⅳ.①R735.7②R735.8

中国版本图书馆CIP数据核字（2017）第244667号

ELSEVIER

Elsevier（Singapore）Pte Ltd.
3 Killiney Road #08-01 Winsland House I, Singapore 239519
Tel：(65) 6349-0200；Fax：(65) 6733-1817

Surgical Oncology Clinics of North America：Hepatocellular Cancer, Cholangiocarcinoma, and Metastatic Tumors of the Liver, 1/E
© 2015 Elsevier Inc. All rights reserved.
ISBN-13：9780323341868

This translation of Surgical Oncology Clinics of North America：Hepatocellular Cancer, Cholangiocarcinoma, and Metastatic Tumors of the Liver [1/E], by Lawrence D. Wagman, was undertaken by Liaoning Science and Technology Publishing House and is published by arrangement with Elsevier（Singapore）Pte Ltd.

Surgical Oncology Clinics of North America：Hepatocellular Cancer, Cholangiocarcinoma, and Metastatic Tumors of the Liver, 1/E by Lawrence D. Wagman 由辽宁科学技术出版社进行翻译，并根据辽宁科学技术出版社与爱思唯尔（新加坡）私人有限公司的协议约定出版。

<肝细胞癌，胆管细胞癌和转移性肝癌>（陆骊工译）
ISBN：978-7-5591-0447-2

Copyright 2017 by Elsevier（Singapore）Pte Ltd.

All rights reserved. No part of this publication may be reproduced or transmitted in any form or by any means, electronic or mechanical, including photocopying, recording, or any information storage and retrieval system, without permission in writing from Elsevier（Singapore）Pte Ltd. Details on how to seek permission, further information about Elsevier's permissions policies and arrangements with organizations such as the Copyright Clearance Center and the Copyright Licensing Agency, can be found at the website：www.elsevier.com/permissions.

This book and the individual contributions contained in it are protected under copyright by the Publisher (other than as may be noted herein).

注 意

本译本由Elsevier（Singapore）Pte Ltd.和辽宁科学技术出版社完成。相关从业及研究人员必须凭借其自身经验和知识对文中描述的信息数据、方法策略、搭配组合、实验操作进行评估和使用。由于医学科学发展迅速，临床诊断和给药剂量尤其需要经过独立验证。在法律允许的最大范围内，爱思唯尔、译文的原文作者、原文编辑及原文内容提供者均不对译文或因产品责任、疏忽或其他操作造成的人身及/或财产承担责任及/或损失担责任，亦不对由于使用文中提到的方法、产品、说明或思想而导致的人身及/或财产伤害及/或损失担责任。

Printed in China by Liaoning Science and Technology Publishing House under special arrangement with Elsevier（Singapore）Pte Ltd. This edition is authorized for sale in the People's Republic of China only, excluding Hong Kong SAR, Macau SAR and Taiwan. Unauthorized export of this edition is a violation of the contract.

版权所有　侵权必究

出版发行：辽宁科学技术出版社
　　　　　北京拂石医典图书有限公司
　　　　　地址：北京海淀区车公庄西路华通大厦B座15层
联系电话：010-88019650/024-23284376
传　　真：010-88019377
E-mail：fushichuanmei@mail.lnpgc.com.cn
印　刷　者：北京时尚印佳彩色印刷有限公司
经　销　者：各地新华书店

幅面尺寸：185mm×260mm
字　　数：337千字　　　　　　印　张：13.75
出版时间：2018年1月第1版　　印刷时间：2018年1月第1次印刷

责任编辑：李俊卿　　　　　　　责任校对：梁晓洁
封面设计：永诚天地　　　　　　封面制作：永诚天地
版式设计：天地鹏博　　　　　　责任印制：高春雨

如有质量问题，请速与印务部联系　联系电话：010-88019750

定　　价：120.00元

原著编委会

顾问

NICHOLAS J. PETRELLI, MD, FACS
Bank of America Endowed Medical Director, Helen F. Graham Cancer Center &Research Institute, Christiana Care Health System, Newark, Delaware; Professor of Surgery, Thomas Jefferson University, Philadelphia, Pennsylvania

主编

LAWRENCE D. WAGMAN, MD, FACS
Executive Medical Director and Director, Liver, Bile Duct and Pancreas Tumor Program, The Center for Cancer Prevention and Treatment, St Joseph Hospital, Orange, California

编者

KEVIN G. BILLINGSLEY, MD
Chief, Division of Surgical Oncology; Professor, Department of Surgery, Oregon Health and Science University, Portland, Oregon

MARIA A. CASSERA, BSc
Research Fellow, Providence Cancer Center, Providence Portland Medical Center, Portland, Oregon

CLIFFORD S. CHO, MD, FACS
Associate Professor; Chief, Section of Surgical Oncology, Department of Surgery, University of Wisconsin School of Medicine and Public Health, Madison, Wisconsin

VINCENT CHUNG, MD, FACP
Clinical Associate Professor; Clinical Director Phase 1 Program, Department of Medical Oncology and Therapeutics Research, City of Hope, Duarte, California

ARAM N. DEMIRJIAN, MD
Assistant Professor, Department of Surgery, University of California – Irvine, Orange, California

KATHRYN J. FOWLER, MD
Assistant Professor of Radiology, Washington University, St Louis, Missouri

T. CLARK GAMBLIN, MD, MS
Division of Surgical Oncology, Department of Surgery, Medical College of Wisconsin, Milwaukee, Wisconsin

PAUL D. HANSEN, MD, FACS
Medical Director, Surgical Oncology; Medical Co – Director, Liver and Pancreas Surgery, Providence Cancer Center, Providence Portland Medical Center, Portland, Oregon

MATTHEW F. KALADY, MD
Digestive Disease Institute, Cleveland Clinic Foundation, Cleveland, Ohio

ALOK A. KHORANA, MD
Taussig Cancer Institute, Cleveland Clinic Foundation, Cleveland, Ohio

T. PETER KINGHAM, MD, FACS
Assistant Attending, Department of Surgery, Division of Hepatopancreatobiliary Surgery, Memorial Sloan Kettering Cancer Center, New York, New York

KELLY J. LAFARO, MD, MPH
Postdoctoral Fellow, Department of Surgery, Johns Hopkins Hospital, The Johns Hopkins University School of Medicine, Baltimore, Maryland

JULIE N. LEAL, MD, FRCSC
Department of Surgery, Division of Hepatopancreatobiliary Surgery, Memorial Sloan Kettering Cancer Center, New York, New York

EDWARD W. LEE, MD, PhD
Interventional Radiology, Department of Radiology, University of California – Los Angeles Medical Center, David Geffen School of Medicine, Los Angeles, California

DAVID LINEHAN, MD
Professor of Surgery, Washington University, St Louis, Missouri

DAVID M. LIU, MD
Interventional Radiology, Department of Radiology, University of British Columbia Medical Center, Vancouver, British Columbia, Canada

KAIHONG MI, MD, PhD
Taussig Cancer Institute, Cleveland Clinic Foundation, Cleveland, Ohio

CHRISTOPH W. MICHALSKI, MD
Division of Surgical Oncology, Oregon Health and Science University, Portland, Oregon

JOHN T. MIURA, MD
Division of Surgical Oncology, Medical College of Wisconsin, Milwaukee, Wisconsin

TIMOTHY M. PAWLIK, MD, MPH, PhD, FACS
Professor of Surgery and Oncology; Chief, Division of Surgical Oncology; John L. Cameron Professor of Alimentary Surgery, Department of Surgery, Johns Hopkins Hospital, Baltimore, Maryland

CRISTIANO QUINTINI, MD
Digestive Disease Institute, Cleveland Clinic Foundation, Cleveland, Ohio

MARIA C. RUSSELL, MD
Assistant Professor of Surgery, Emory University Hospital, Atlanta, Georgia

NAEL E. SAAD, MD
Assistant Professor of Interventional Radiology, Washington University, St Louis, Missouri

BASHIR A. TAFTI, MD
Interventional Radiology, Department of Radiology, University of California – Los Angeles Medical Center, David Geffen School of Medicine, Los Angeles, California

AVNESH S. THAKOR, MD, PhD
Interventional Radiology, Department of Radiology, University of British Columbia Medical Center, Vancouver, British Columbia, Canada

RONALD F. WOLF, MD, FACS
Medical Co – Director, Liver and Pancreas Surgery, Providence Cancer Center, Providence Portland Medical Center, Portland, Oregon

翻译委员会

主译 陆骊工

主审 罗鹏飞

译者

李　勇（珠海市人民医院）	彭秀斌（珠海市人民医院）
许卫国（珠海市人民医院）	程光森（珠海市人民医院）
陈加源（珠海市人民医院）	何　旭（珠海市人民医院）
王　勇（珠海市人民医院）	赵　炜（珠海市人民医院）
忻勇杰（珠海市人民医院）	殷　花（珠海市人民医院）
廖少琴（珠海市人民医院）	傅思睿（珠海市人民医院）
占美晓（珠海市人民医院）	郑游冰（珠海市人民医院）
刘　冰（珠海市人民医院）	刘永康（珠海市人民医院）
李忠亮（珠海市人民医院）	向青锋（珠海市人民医院）
冯宇亮（珠海市人民医院）	周紫章（珠海市人民医院）
邱力戈（珠海市人民医院）	李　佳（珠海市人民医院）
苏燕红（珠海市人民医院）	刘少卿（珠海市人民医院）
华胜妮（珠海市人民医院）	全瑛瑶（珠海市人民医院）
刘　羽（珠海市人民医院）	李海量（珠海市人民医院）
李记华（珠海市人民医院）	杨　旸（珠海市人民医院）
肖　静（珠海市人民医院）	王冰寒（珠海市人民医院）
王　坤（珠海市人民医院）	王春岩（珠海市人民医院）
冯星辉（珠海市人民医院）	唐　凯（珠海市人民医院）
马明峰（珠海市人民医院）	

序

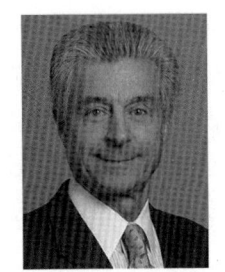

Nicholas J. Petrelli, MD, FACS
Consulting Editor

本书主要讨论肝细胞癌、胆管细胞癌和转移性肝癌。特邀编辑包括 Lawrence D. Wagman，医学博士，来自加利福尼亚洲 Orange，St. Joseph's 医院癌症防治中心的医学执行总监。Wagman 博士在弗吉尼亚医学院完成了普通外科住院医师培训，同时也完成了其在美国卫生部癌症中心外科学组的研究工作。他是一名出色的外科肿瘤学家，擅长肝脏、胆道和胰腺手术。Wagman 博士力主临床试验的进行，他的职业生涯一直致力于制定国家指南和鼓励患者加入国家癌症中心的临床试验。

有人认为肝细胞癌、胆管癌和转移性肝癌的相关信息浩繁，很难整合成 11 章的内容。然而，Wagman 博士及其霍普金斯大学的同事对肝细胞癌的流行病学进行了完善的讨论。David Linehan 博士，来自圣路易斯华盛顿大学及 Siteman 癌症中心肝胆胰及胃肠外科中心的主任，对肝细胞癌、胆管细胞癌和结直肠癌肝转移的影像学表现进行了完善的讨论。其他内容还包括肝切除术和动脉灌注化疗的并发症，以及相关主题。

我希望借此机会感谢 Wagman 博士及其同事对此书的贡献。我希望读者能够分享到本书的更多信息。

Nicholas J. Petrelli, MD, FACS
Helen F. Graham Cancer Center & Research Institute
Christiana Care Health System
4701 Ogletown－Stanton Road, Suite 1213
Newark, DE 19713, USA
E－mail address:
npetrelli@christianacare.org

前 言

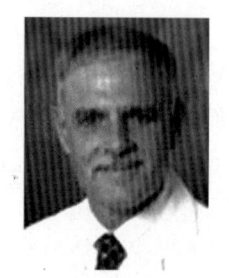

Lawrence D. Wagman, MD, FACS
Editor

北美外科肿瘤学会出版本书的初衷是基于肝脏肿瘤研究的发展和关注度。过去10年，人们对于肝脏肿瘤治疗的研究兴趣与日俱增。相较于20年前对此专题的有限探讨，目前肿瘤学界的每一次会议都对该专题进行讨论，说明目前学界对肝脏肿瘤的关注度有明显上升。为了确定各个章节所涉及领域最权威的新知识，我查阅了最近几年的文献和专题会议，对其中专业化的优秀文献做了整理。

尽管原发性和转移性肝脏肿瘤目前多经多学科会诊，但是多重潜在治疗方法、流程和术式的存在增加了其治疗方案的多样性。肝脏的一些特性会对治疗方案产生较大影响，如其成瘤过程中病毒的作用、双重血供、肝脏药物代谢作用、重要的合成作用、肝功能储备以及最为重要的肝脏独有的细胞再生功能。

本书内容涉及肝脏原发肿瘤（肝细胞癌和胆管细胞癌）以及转移性肿瘤（最常见的是结肠癌转移中最先发生的肝转移）等多个方面。首先从肝细胞癌的流行病学入手，特别介绍了病毒诱导成癌的作用。其后介绍了相关的影像学知识，其中特别突出了扫描方法、造影剂、扫描技术以及癌症特异性的检查方法。背景性介绍对预后和危险因素相关研究做了总结，为后续介绍针对性的干预和治疗方法指明了方向。

其后我们采用抽丝剥茧的方法，细致地对相关手术、影像介入及化疗方法进行了回顾。其中多数章节针对某种特定治疗方法的适应证、预后、危险因素、获益进行了探讨，另有一章专门讨论了肝脏手术的并发症。如此安排旨在使读者按章节阅读后，以简洁的篇幅为其提供最全面的信息。

总而言之，让我首先感谢Petrelli博士邀请我作特邀编辑，也感谢相关作者对其所从事领域的投入。作为特邀编辑，我对本书所涉及内容的简洁性和全面性非常满意。作者在其所给定的范围内依据数据及个人临床经验做出了相关介绍。最后，我要感谢Elsevier的编辑团队，他们参与了本书的策划、构思、校对和成稿工作。

Lawrence D. Wagman, MD, FACS
Bile Duct and Pancreas Tumor Program
The Center for Cancer Prevention and Treatment
St Joseph Hospital
Orange, California 92868, USA
E-mail address:
Lawrence.Wagman@stjoe.org

译者序一

全球癌症调查显示，肝癌的发病率与死亡率分别高居第五位与第二位，而且其发病率还在逐年上升，全世界每年大约有75万新增的肝癌患者，其中半数以上发生在我国。目前，肝癌的治疗方法大致包括手术治疗和非手术治疗，微创介入治疗在肝癌治疗中的地位日趋重要。随着医学科学技术的进步和临床治疗需求的不断增长，肝脏肿瘤的诊疗也得到了迅猛发展，新的器材、新技术不断涌现，系统地对肝脏肿瘤的诊疗技术及新技术新发展进行汇编整理，加强对各级从业人员及研究人员的培训，显得越来越重要。

陆骊工教授长期从事肝脏肿瘤诊疗的研究，在各类良恶性肿瘤，特别是肝癌的微创介入技术的应用方面积累了丰富经验，也是我国肝癌诊疗规范的制定者之一。《肝细胞癌、胆管细胞癌和转移性肝癌，Hepatocallular Cancer, Cholangiocarcinoma, and Metastatic Tumors of Liver》由北美外科肿瘤学会出版，陆骊工教授团队主译。全书内容涵盖了肝脏原发肿瘤以及转移性肿瘤等多个方面，涉及流行病学、发生机制、影像学诊断、癌症特异性检查等，对相关手术治疗、微创介入治疗及化疗方法进行了细致的阐述及循证医学证据汇总，尤其重视最新治疗发展动向及临床试验结果发布，详尽介绍了各项技术的适应证、预后及治疗原则，叙述生动，图文并茂。书中对多学科联合诊疗（MDT）的大力倡导及对循证医学证据的客观分析应用，值得国内同行学习借鉴。

本书具有很强的科学性、系统性和专业性，是肝脏肿瘤诊疗循证医学证据的系统汇编。该书的翻译出版，对于从事肝脏肿瘤诊疗的中青年医师，特别是研究生等初学者具有很高的实际指导作用，对于从事肝癌微创介入诊疗的各级人员来说，是一本十分有益的参考著作，也有助于相关学科的临床医生、研究者加深对新治疗技术的认识。因此，本书的出版将有助于我国肝癌临床治疗整体水平，尤其是微创介入治疗水平的提高，从而促进介入医学事业的发展。

相信本书的出版发行，对促进肝脏肿瘤规范化治疗及临床循证医学思维能力的提升，都将起到积极的推动作用，故乐以为序，推荐此书。

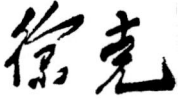

2017年11月

译者序二

原发性肝癌（PLC，以下简称肝癌）是临床上最常见的恶性肿瘤之一，全球发病率逐年增长，发病人数已超过62.6万/年，居于恶性肿瘤的第5位；死亡人数接近60万/年，位居肿瘤相关死亡的第3位。肝癌在我国高发，目前，我国发病人数约占全球的55%；在肿瘤相关死亡中仅次于肺癌，位居第二。可见，肝癌严重威胁我国人民健康和生命。原发性肝癌是一种恶性程度高、浸润和转移性强的癌症，治疗首选手术。然而，多数患者就诊时已是中晚期，只能接受介入、消融、放疗、化疗等非手术治疗。分子靶向药物等新技术新疗法的出现，为这类患者提供了新选择。

由陆骊工教授团队主译的《肝细胞癌、胆管细胞癌和转移性肝癌，*Hepatocallular Cancer, Cholangiocarcinoma, and Metastatic Tumors of Liver*》一书，内容涵盖了肝脏原发肿瘤以及转移性肿瘤等多个方面，对肝脏肿瘤的诊断、手术治疗（肝切除与肝移植）、介入治疗、局部消融治疗、放射治疗、生物治疗、分子靶向治疗、系统化疗等一系列问题的循证医学证据进行了系统汇编，该书既是一本详尽的肝脏肿瘤诊疗参考手册，更是一本不可多得的循证医学证据学习专著。循证医学是介入医学发展不可逾越的阶段。如果说精准医疗代表了医疗发展的未来，那么现阶段建立医学循证，则为介入医学发展奠定了坚实的基础。目前，介入医学的诸多成果需要医学循证支持，而已有循证支持的介入技术将得到大力的推广与发展。以肝动脉栓塞治疗肝癌为例，由于循证基础坚实，几乎在所有关于肝癌的国际指南、治疗标准中，肝动脉栓塞化疗都是标准治疗手段之一，介入治疗也因此成为肝癌治疗的重要手段。因此，有必要不断强调遵循循证医学证据的重要性，尊重循证医学证据的原则，开展更多的介入技术相关的前瞻性多中心、随机研究，通过循证医学的研究方法，进一步推动我国介入医学技术的发展。

相信本书的出版，对提高肝癌多学科规范化综合治疗和研究水平、推动微创介入治疗的学科发展都将起到积极的作用。

欣以为序，推荐本书。

2017年11月

目　录

第一章　肝细胞癌的流行病学研究　　1

　　一、简介 …………………………………………… 1
　　二、发病率 ………………………………………… 2
　　三、致病因素 ……………………………………… 3
　　四、患者因素 ……………………………………… 8
　　五、经济/公共卫生原因 ………………………… 11
　　六、总结 …………………………………………… 11

第二章　肝细胞癌、胆管癌和转移性结肠癌的影像诊断　　17

　　一、简介 …………………………………………… 17
　　二、肝脏影像学检查方法 ………………………… 18
　　三、肝脏肿瘤影像学检查 ………………………… 23
　　四、总结 …………………………………………… 30

第三章　适用于原发性和转移性肝脏恶性肿瘤的预后体系　　38

　　一、简介 …………………………………………… 38
　　二、原发性肝脏恶性肿瘤 ………………………… 39
　　三、总结 …………………………………………… 47

第四章　现代技术在肝脏切除术中的运用　　53

　　一、简介 …………………………………………… 53
　　二、肝脏切除术的适应证 ………………………… 54
　　三、术前功能评估 ………………………………… 55
　　四、肝脏解剖和肝脏切除的术语 ………………… 56
　　五、肝脏手术后的技术考虑和结果 ……………… 57
　　六、体位及设备安装 ……………………………… 57
　　七、切口和牵引 …………………………………… 57

八、术中超声波检查 ·················· 58
　　九、肝脏的游离 ······················ 58
　　十、流入道控制的方法 ················ 59
　　十一、流出道控制的方法 ·············· 60
　　十二、肝实质离断技术 ················ 60
　　十三、具体步骤 ······················ 61

第五章　肝脏切除术并发症　　68

　　一、术后大出血 ······················ 69
　　二、肝脏切除术后静脉血栓形成/栓塞 ···· 71
　　三、肝脏切除术后门静脉、肝动脉血栓形成 ·· 73
　　四、胆漏 ···························· 74
　　五、肝脏切除术后肝衰竭 ·············· 77
　　六、总结 ···························· 80

第六章　肝细胞癌、胆管细胞癌和结肠癌肝转移的消融治疗　　91

　　一、简介 ···························· 91
　　二、消融技术 ························ 92
　　三、患者选择 ························ 95
　　四、消融的途径 ······················ 97
　　五、围手术期准备 ···················· 99
　　六、疗效 ···························· 102

第七章　肝恶性肿瘤的肝动脉灌注化疗方案　　113

　　一、简介 ···························· 113
　　二、技术方面 ························ 115
　　三、处理不同解剖形态的肝动脉 ········ 119
　　四、术后的处理和监测 ················ 121
　　五、并发症 ·························· 121
　　六、行肝动脉灌注化疗患者的临床转归 ·· 126
　　七、肝动脉灌注化疗和原发性肝恶性肿瘤 ·· 132
　　八、肝动脉灌注化疗和非结肠癌肝转移 ·· 133
　　九、总结 ···························· 134

第八章 肝动脉化疗栓塞术治疗原发性肝癌及结肠癌肝转移 141

- 一、简介 ······ 141
- 二、肝动脉化疗栓塞术的准则 ······ 142
- 三、肝细胞癌 ······ 144
- 四、肝内胆管癌 ······ 147
- 五、结直肠癌肝转移 ······ 149
- 六、总结 ······ 150

第九章 Y-90 选择性体内放射治疗 158

- 一、简介 ······ 158
- 二、临床应用 ······ 163
- 三、并发症 ······ 169
- 四、总结 ······ 170

第十章 肝细胞癌和胆管癌的系统性治疗 177

- 一、概述 ······ 177
- 二、肝细胞癌 ······ 178
- 三、胆管癌 ······ 184
- 四、小结 ······ 186

第十一章 全身治疗结合手术治疗转移性结肠癌 188

- 一、简介 ······ 188
- 二、全身疗法治疗转移性结直肠癌 ······ 189
- 三、维持方案 ······ 195
- 四、可能治愈的晚期结直肠癌 ······ 195
- 五、原发性肿瘤切除术的作用 ······ 196
- 六、小结和未来的发展方向 ······ 197

第一章 肝细胞癌的流行病学研究

Kelly J. Lafaro, MD, MPH[a], Aram N. Demirjian, MD[b],
Timothy M. Pawlik, MD, MPH, PhD[c*]

【关键词】

肝细胞癌;慢性肝病;肝硬化;乙型肝炎;丙型肝炎;发病率;危险因素;黄曲霉素

要点

- 肝细胞癌(HCC)是世界范围内的常见癌症,其每年的新发人数和死亡人数大致相等。
- 多数 HCC 是由慢性肝病引起,而后者的病因包括乙肝病毒、丙肝病毒以及长期酗酒。
- 详细了解可能的致病因素及发病机制有助于提高 HCC 的筛查、预防、早期诊断和治疗水平。

一、简介

世界范围内,原发性肝癌的发病率在各型癌症中排名第五,致死率排名第二。2008 年新发病人数达到 74.9 万例,同时 69.5 万例患者死亡。据估计,2012 年新发病例超过 78.2 万例[1]。HCC 是原发性肝癌中最常见的病理类型,占全部原发性肝癌的 85%~90%。HCC 的发生来源于肝细胞,这意味着肝实质细胞也可以发展为 HCC。

经费来源:无(Dr T. M. Pawlik, Dr K. J. Lafaro); Speaker's Bureau - Bayer, Speaker's Bureau - Aptalis (Dr A. N. Demirjian).

版权问题:无。

[a] Department of Surgery, Johns Hopkins Hospital, The Johns Hopkins University School of Medicine, 600 North Wolfe Street, Blalock 688, Baltimore, MD 21287, USA; [b] Department of Surgery, University of California - Irvine, 333 City Boulevard West, Suite 1205, Orange, CA 92868, USA; [c] Division of Surgical Oncology, Department of Surgery, Johns Hopkins Hospital, 600 North Wolfe Street, Blalock 688, Baltimore, MD 21287, USA

* Corresponding author.

E - mail address:tpawlik1@jhmi.edu

肝癌患者的预后较差(患病后死亡率达95%)。因此详细了解可能的致病因素及发病机制对HCC患者的早期筛查、确诊、预后至关重要。多数HCC起源于慢性肝病,而慢性肝病的发病率在地域、性别及其他因素方面具有明显差异性,近年来已经可以对其中一些致病因素进行干预。

二、发病率

HCC的发病率具有地域差异性。80%患病人群位于撒哈拉以南的非洲地区和东亚。据统计,中国的患者占世界患者总数的50%。相对而言,南北美洲以及欧洲HCC的发病率相对较低。这种差异可能由多重特异因素造成的。

1. 亚洲

2008年,中国HCC患者超过全球患病人数的一半,男性发病率达37.4/10万,女性达13.7/10万。蒙古和韩国HCC的发病率同样较高,分别为99/10万和49/10万。以中国为代表的高HCC发病率是由HBV高感染率导致的。而HBV的感染主要由母婴垂直传播引起[2,3]。80年代引入的乙肝疫苗的广泛使用为HBV的控制带来了希望,从而有助于减少HCC的发生。台湾一项随访20年的研究表明,乙肝病毒表面抗体(HBsAg)血清阳性率由10%~17%下降为0.7%~1.7%[4]。这些研究同时表明台湾6~19岁儿童HCC发病率有所下降(6~9岁儿童发病率由0.51/10万下降为0.15/10万;10~14岁儿童由0.6/10万下降为0.19/10万;15~19岁儿童由0.52/10万下降为0.16/10万)[4]。

日本的HCC发病率也较高,为40/10万。与其他亚洲国家以HBV感染为主要病因有所不同,日本的HCC主要由丙肝病毒(HCV)引起,占到全部病例的80%[5]。日本的HCV流行主要出现在二战后,这一现象是由静脉注射药物和输血造成的,其感染率在70年代上升较为明显[5,6]。据估计,2015年日本HCV感染人数已达到最高峰。日本因HCV诱发的HCC病例数是欧洲和美国的2倍,日本和欧美的5年累积发病率分别为30%和17%[7]。其发病率可能是由于日本有1b这种HCV基因类型,1b可以降低抗病毒药物的疗效,与之相对,1a这种欧美国家人群的主要基因型则无此功能[8]。

2. 非洲

非洲的首例HCC报道见于1879年[9]。尽管由于非洲农村地区缺乏有效的医疗保障和筛查,其HCC发病率可能被低估,但是HCC依然是非洲黑种人的主要致死因素。在非洲国家中,莫桑比克HCC发病率最高,年发病率为41.2/10万。多数患者是在农村地区。约60%的人群伴发了肝硬化。非洲白种人发病率较低。慢性HBV感染是非洲HCC发病的主要因素,其传播主要是在儿童时期由亲属传染,这一点与亚洲的垂直传播不同(图1-1)。

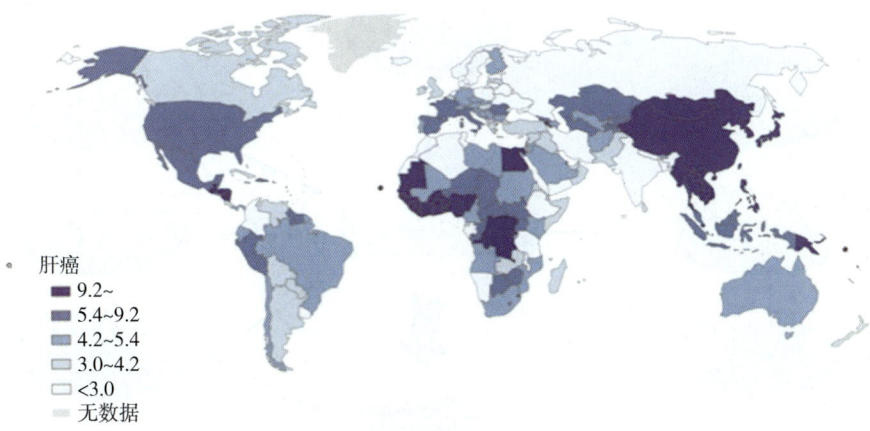

图 1-1 肝细胞癌年龄标化发病率地图

[引自 Ferlay J, Shin H, Bray F, et al. GLOBOCAN 2008 v2.0, Cancer incidence and mortality worldwide: IARC Cancer-Base No. 10. Lyon (France): International Agency for Research on Cancer; 2010.]

3. 欧洲和美国

尽管美国的整体发病率要比世界其他地区低，但同 1975 年相比，2005 年发病率增加了 3 倍，由 1.6/10 万增长至 4.9/10 万[10]。尽管其原因是多样的，但最可能是由于 60 年代和 70 年代未经检测的血制品的输入和静脉注射药物的使用。鉴于美国 HCV 高发感染时期为 20 世纪 80 年代，而 HCV 发展到 HCC 需要 20～40 年，所以未来十年美国 HCC 发病率将持续上升。而美国 HCC 发病也主要与 HCV 相关，HBV 引起的 HCC 仅占 10%～15%，这是由于多数美国人已接种 HBV 疫苗[11]。美国 HCC 确诊的平均年龄是 65 岁，74% 的患者是男性。种族分布：48% 为白种人，13% 为非洲裔美国人，15% 为西班牙裔，24% 为亚洲人和其他人种[5]。HCC 发病率最高的是位于亚太的岛屿居民（11.7/10 万），最低的是白种人（3.9/10 万）[10]。

与美国相比，欧洲的 HCC 发病率稍高（2～4 倍）。地中海国家（意大利、西班牙和希腊）的发病率为 10/10 万至 20/10 万。同时这些国家慢性 HCV 感染也占欧洲 HCV 总感染率的 2/3[12]。中欧国家的 HCC 发病性别差异最为明显，其男/女 HCC 发病的比例高于 4:1[1]。

三、致病因素

肝癌是一种复杂的遗传异质性肿瘤，需要多基因和表观遗传改变以及数个信号通路的参与，所包含的通路有 p53、Ras、MAPK、JAK/STAT、Wnt/β-catenin 和 hedgehog[13,14]。HCC 的诱因有多种，包括 HBV、HCV、酗酒、肥胖、黄曲霉素以及地区因素（图 1-2）。

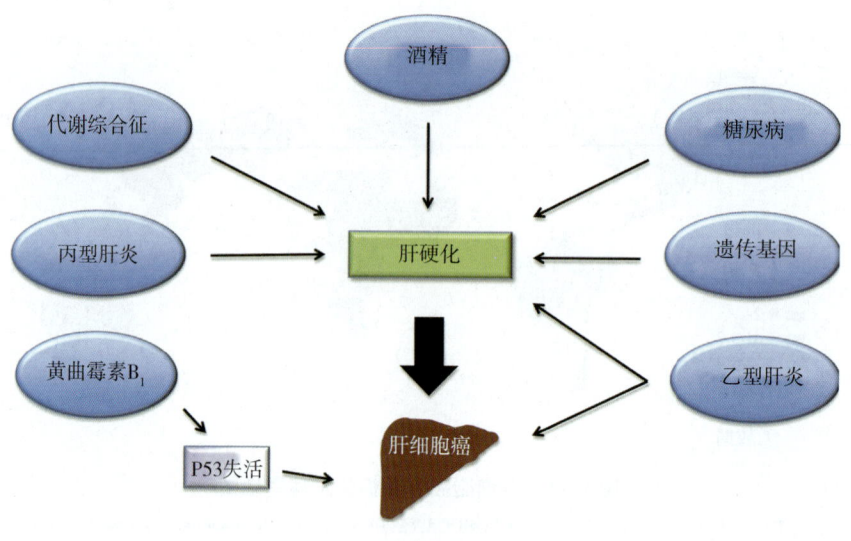

图 1-2　肝细胞癌的致病因素

1. HBV

HBV 是一种由 DNA 编码结构和可复制蛋白的环状 DNA 病毒。HBV 与 HCC 之间的关系最早是由 Beasely 及其同事在台湾 HBsAg 阳性患者中发现的[15]。血清 HBsAg 是 HBV 感染的标志物，在中国，仅 HBV 感染引起的 HCC 就占 HCC 患者总数的 70%，在美国占 41%，在日本占 24%~27%[16]。在亚洲，HBV 的感染多由母婴垂直传播引起，而在非洲，多由少年时期水平传播引起，比如唾液和创伤感染。在低危国家，传播主要为水平型的，传播途径主要是通过静脉药物注射或成年人间的性行为（图 1-3）。

HBV 有 8 个基因类型，分别命名为 A 到 H。各个基因型间有超过 8% 的基因差异。A 型主要见于撒哈拉以南的非洲、西亚和东欧。B 型主要见于日本和东亚。C 型可导致严重肝病，且与 HCC 关系更为密切，主要见于中国、韩国、日本、东南亚以及几个南太平洋岛国。D 型广泛分布于东欧、北非、地中海、俄罗斯、中东、印度和北极地区。E 型主要见于西非。F 型和 H 型主要见于中南美洲。其中关于 C 型的研究较为全面。大量研究证实，携带 C 型人群患肝纤维化及 HCC 的概率更大[17-21]。

和其他危险因素不同，HBV 会同时增加伴或不伴肝硬化患者的 HCC 风险。当伴发肝硬化时，HBV 感染会导致伴有纤维化和肝细胞再生的慢性炎症，这和其他影响因素的影响一致。而 HBV 也可直接通过病毒特异性感染方式诱导继发性肝癌。HBV 是一种具有编码序列和复制蛋白能力的 DNA 环状病毒，可以调控 DNA 复制转录。这种病毒入侵肝细胞后，病毒的信使 RNA 会翻译合成病毒蛋白，同时病毒 DNA 也会插入到宿主细胞的 DNA 序列中。这一过程从多个角度促进了肝癌的发生，包括加速肝脏细胞周期[22]和因病毒 DNA 插入过程导致的不稳定性[23]，它还会插入到编码促癌蛋白的基因序列中[24,25]。此外，HBV 的高表达会导致大鼠的恶性癌变[26]。当 HBV 病毒定量 >13 pg/ml 时，其导致肝癌的可能性会增加[27-29]。

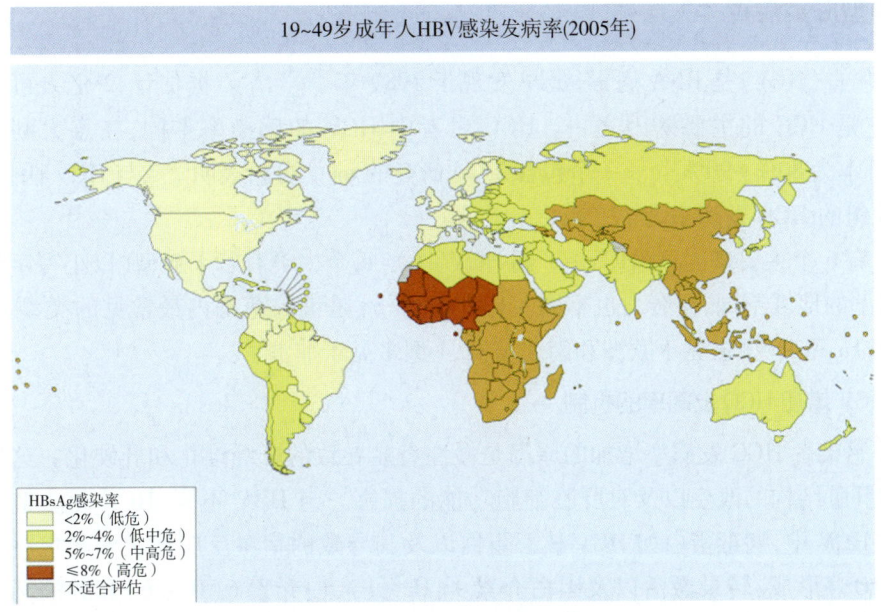

图 1-3 慢性 HBV 感染流行图

(引自 Ott J, Stevens G, Groeger J, et al. Global epidemiology of hepatitis B virus infection: new estimates of age – specific HBsAg seroprevalence and endemicity. Vaccine 2012;30(12):2215; with permission.)

疫苗是防治 HBV 感染的最有效方法,也是第一个可以有效降低癌症发生的方法。尽管有 5%~10% 的人群因 HBV 表面抗体低于 10U/ml 而导致疫苗无效,但是使用疫苗后 HBV 的感染率的确有明显的降低。根据一项 20 年的随访研究表明,在台湾,HBV 水平传播和围产期垂直传播的概率相当,使用 HBV 疫苗后 HBsAg 血清阳性由 10%~17% 降低为 0.7%~1.7%[4]。这项研究同时表明,6~19 岁的儿童 HCC 发病率有所下降(发病率 6~9 岁儿童由 0.51/10 万下降为 0.15/10 万;10~14 岁儿童由 0.6/10 万下降为 0.19/10 万;15~19 岁儿童由 0.52/10 万下降为 0.16/10 万)[4]。但像非洲等国家,疫苗并不是常规注射项。

HBV 致 HCC 机制与其他诱因不同,因为它的致癌作用不以肝硬化为前提。实际上其他 HCC 诱因通常都和肝硬化有关,且肝硬化是其致癌的前提。

2. 肝硬化

肝硬化,即慢性肝损伤中纤维条索附近的组织性再生结节,是 HCC 的一大诱因[30]。除了 HCC,肝硬化的其他并发症包括门静脉高压,伴或不伴出血的静脉曲张以及腹水。尸检显示,意大利和日本 80%~90% 的 HCC 患者有肝硬化[31]。一份欧洲的研究表明,因肝脏原因致死的肝硬化患者中,54%[32]~70%[33] 的患者是因 HCC 死亡。不考虑潜在因素,肝硬化患者的 HCC 发病率在增加。但是,不同的致病因素其危害程度不同:HCV > HBV > 血色素沉着病。肝硬化的分期也会对发生 HCC 的风险产生影响[7,34]。

3. 丙型肝炎病毒

丙肝病毒（HCV）是 RNA 病毒，最早发现于 1989 年[10,35,36]。据估计，2 亿人可能感染了 HCV[6]，它是 HCC 的主要诱因之一。HCC 患者中 HCV 的感染率不同，在意大利为 44%~66%，在日本为 80%~90%[6]。一个包含 21 项研究的 meta 分析表明[37]，与 HCV 阴性组相比，HCV 阳性组的 HCC 发病率高 17 倍。

HCV 有 6 个主要基因型（HCV-1 到 HCV-6），每个大类有若干亚型（以小写字母区分）。这些基因型的地域不同，侵袭力也不同。1 型（a 和 b）是世界范围内最常见的类型。1b 型多见于亚洲，1a 和 1b 型多见于欧洲和南北美洲，4 型多见于非洲[38]。

（1）HCV 增加 HCC 发病率的机制

HCV 感染者 HCC 发病率增加的原因是慢性炎症导致的肝纤维化和肝硬化。这种慢性炎症会导致肝脏结构的改变以及对肝脏细胞功能的损害。与 HBV 不同，HCV 无法整合到宿主体内。在 HCV 中，病毒蛋白如 HCV 核心蛋白以及其导致的宿主反应涉及到凋亡、信号转导、活性氧（ROS）形成、转录激活以及因白介素 1（IL-1）、白介素 6（IL-6）和肿瘤坏死因子 α（TNF-α）上调导致的免疫改变，使得 HCC 发生率上升。

HCV 感染 25~30 年后，肝硬化的发病率在 12%~35%[5,39]。慢性 HCV 感染是肝硬化的首要病因，也是南北美洲、欧洲、澳洲和日本进行肝移植的最常见指征[38,40]。在肝硬化形成过程中，环境因素，如受到感染时的年龄[41]、酒精摄入量（每天>40~50g）、男性、肥胖、谷丙转氨酶增高以及 HBV 和 HCV 的合并感染[42,43]可能比 HCV 基因型或病毒入侵更为关键[39]。

（2）抗 HCV 治疗对 HCC 发病率的影响

与其他病毒感染不同，HCV 的抗病毒治疗可以消除病毒感染，达到抗病毒治疗后持续的病毒学应答（SVR）以及 HCV RNA 阴性。SVR 可以使 HCC 相关以及肝脏相关的致死率下降 54%[44,45]。最近的一项 meta 分析表明，无应答患者的 HCC 年发病率为 1.67%（95% CI，1.15%~2.42%），而 SVR 患者仅为 0.33%（95% CI，0.22%~0.5%）[46]。

4. 酒精

酒精的过量摄入与多种疾病相关，8%~20% 的慢性酗酒会发展为肝硬化[47]。国际癌症研究协会（IARC）在 1988 年提出了摄入酒精和 HCC 的因果关系[48]，并从此将含酒精的饮料定为致癌物。酒精和 HCC 之间的因果关系后来经多项研究证实，其比值比（OR）介于 2.4~7.0[37,49]。慢性酗酒（>80g/d）超过 10 年可使 HCC 发病率上升 5 倍[37,50]。密歇根大学的研究者证明了摄入酒精 1500g-年（60g/d，>25 年）可使 HCC 发病率上升 6 倍（OR:5.7;95% CI 2.4~13.7）[51]。在一项 1992—2006 年间的欧洲关于癌症和营养的前瞻性研究中，4 409 809 例患者的数据表明，大量酒精摄入（男性>40g/d，女性>20g/d）与肝癌发病相关（OR 1.77; 95% CI: 0.73~4.27）[52]。尽管尚未有酒精肝毒性方面的安全阈值，但一项 meta 分析表明，HCC 和酒精摄入的相对危险比（RR）分别为 25g/d:1.19（95% CI 1.12~1.27）[53]；50g/d:1.40（95% CI 1.25~1.56）；100g/d:1.81（95% CI 1.50~2.19）。

相对而言,停止酒精摄入可以降低肝癌的发病危险。一项 meta 分析表明,在停止酒精摄入后,HCC 的发病风险每年下降 6%~7%。另一项研究表明,酒精摄入停止 23 年后,HCC 发病率会回到无酒精影响的水平,而这一过程与肝硬化状态无关[54]。

(1) 酒精致 HCC 发生的机制

酒精在肝脏代谢,其过程是酒精被氧化成为乙醛,进而转化为乙酸盐。这种转化被多重酶通路催化,包括酒精脱氢酶、细胞色素 P4502E1 和过氧化氢酶。在动物实验中,酒精导致肝脏损伤从而诱发 HCC 的机制被认为有两个独立的阶段。首先,因酒精代谢而导致的酒精脂肪肝可诱发肝硬化。氧化代谢过量的还原型烟酰胺腺嘌呤二核苷酸(NADH),导致 NADH/NAD$^+$ 比例增加,从而诱发脂肪氧化障碍,促进脂肪生成[47]。第二个致癌机制是肝脏代谢酒精过程中,会在肝细胞内产生 ROS 以及其他自由基。这一过程会导致 NADH 增加,而后者可以为线粒体电子传递链提供电子,从而导致缺乏 1 个电子的超氧化物形成以及抗氧化剂的消耗[47,55,56]。

(2) 酒精和其他危险因素的联合作用

酒精可协同原发性慢性肝病致 HCC 的发生,慢性肝病可由 HCV、HBV、脂肪肝、烟草和肥胖导致[37,49,57]。Poynard 及其同事[41]在其关于 HCV 患者肝纤维化自然进程的研究中发现,日摄入酒精超过 50g 是导致肝纤维化的三大因素之一。另一项回顾性队列研究[58]证实,与单纯酒精性肝硬化相比,HCV 和酒精共同导致肝硬化的患者 HCC 发病率有所增加[危险比(HR)为 11.2;95% CI:2.3~55.0]。有人认为,HCV 和酒精共同诱发的 HCC 患者在生物学表现上可能不同于单纯 HCV 导致的 HCC 患者。一项针对 HCV 阳性 HCC 患者肝切除标本的研究[59]表明,无酒精摄入的患者高分化 HCC 出现概率[19/42(45%)]远高于高酒精(>86g/d)摄入者[2/42(5%),$P<0.0001$]。相对应的是,单独由 HCV 感染诱导的 HCC 患者无瘤生存率高于由 HCV 和酒精共同诱导的 HCC 患者。

一项包括 210 例美国患者的前瞻性病例对照研究表明[51],摄入酒精超过 1500g - 年者患 HCC 风险上升了 6 倍;吸烟超过 20 包 - 年者患 HCC 风险上升 5 倍;体重指数[BMI,体重(kg) 除以身高(m)的平方]超过 30 者患 HCC 风险上升 4 倍。对应的协同指数分别为:酒精与烟草 3.3、烟草与肥胖 2.9、酒精与肥胖 2.5。

5. 黄曲霉素

黄曲霉素是一种由黄曲霉菌和寄生曲霉菌生成的真菌毒素,它可以污染谷物、豆类、坚果、玉米和花生。此外,当产奶动物食用被黄曲霉素污染的饲料后会产出含黄曲霉毒素 M1 的奶制品。乳制品中含黄曲霉素较高的国家包括莫桑比克、越南、中国和印度,因为这些国家的气候比较潮湿温暖,有助于黄曲霉菌的生长。黄曲霉素被国际癌症研究组织定义为肝脏致癌物[60]。一项 2010 年的风险评估[61]研究表明,世界范围内黄曲霉素和 4.6%~28.2% 的 HCC 相关。共有 4 种黄曲霉素:B1、B2、G1 和 G2。黄曲霉素 B1(AFB1)被证明是这 4 种中致癌性最强的。根据 2006 年的一项测试[1]显示,世界范围内共有 5500 万人暴露在不可控的黄曲霉素环境中。AFB1 会代谢成为活性中间体 AFB1 外式 -8,9 - 环氧化物,后者可以结合到 DNA 中。肿瘤抑癌基因 p53 的 249 号密码子中发现了黄曲霉素的记号,在黄曲霉素富集环境下,

30%~60%的患者会发生 G>T 的颠倒错位[62-64]。

AFB1 与慢性 HBV 感染以及酒精有协同致癌的作用。中国的一项回顾性研究[65]显示，尿液中检测出 AFB1 代谢物的患者 HCC 发病风险增加了 4 倍，而那些同时存在 AFB1 尿液排泄产物和 HBV 阳性者 HCC 的发病风险增加了 60 倍。

四、患者因素

1. 代谢综合征

尽管世界范围内，大多数 HCC 与肝炎病毒以及酒精性肝病相关，但是 5%~20% 的患者是 HBV 和 HCV 双阴性的。非酒精性肝病(NAFLD)以及通过穿刺证实的更为严重的非酒精性脂肪性肝炎(NASH)的特点是无酗酒或未知原因的肝病史，它们已经成为欧美国家人群患隐匿性慢性肝病的主要原因。代谢综合征在肝脏上表现为 NAFLD，这些代谢症状包括高血压、胰岛素抵抗、向心性肥胖和血脂异常。90%肥胖患者有不同程度的脂肪肝，而且肝脂肪变性的程度和 BMI 相关[66]。NASH 可见于 1%~3% 的日本成年人、6% 的西方国家成年人[67-69]。

有多项证据表明，NASH 和 NAFLD 可导致肝硬化和 HCC，最近一项基于 SEER(流行病学和预后)的数据研究表明代谢综合征和 HCC 之间存在关联(HR 2.13；95% CI 1.96~2.31)[70]。同时，丹麦和瑞典的一项队列研究显示，与正常男性相比，肥胖男性更容易患 HCC[71,72]。

有关 NASH 自然病史和预后的数据比较少。有一项日本的队列研究[73]显示，137 例 NASH 患者(肝脏穿刺证实)发生了纤维化，其 HCC 5 年累积发病率为 7.6%。在一项稍大型的研究中，Ascha 和他的同事[74]发现，NASH 导致肝硬化的患者中 HCC 的年累积发病率为 2.6%。而这种累积发病率在 HCV 导致的肝硬化患者中为 4%。同时发现肥胖 HCC 患者死亡率更高。一项持续 16 年的美国前瞻性队列研究表明，与正常人群相比，BMI 为 35~40 的患者比 BMI 正常者 HCC 的死亡率高 5 倍[75]。而现在，这项研究显得更加重要，因为全球，尤其是美国，肥胖发生率都在上升，而这种上升会导致 HCC 发病率上升(图 1-4)。

代谢综合征致 HCC 发病率上升机制：NASH 相关的肝硬化导致肝癌的概率低于 HCV 相关肝硬化致肝癌的概率。胰岛素抵抗和脂肪肝病会导致肝脏的炎症性和血管性改变。脂肪组织会产生促炎症细胞因子 TNF-α 和 IL-6，在机体肥胖状态下，两种炎症因子均存在调控紊乱。这些细胞因子是炎症引起癌变的重要启动子[76]。此外，与其他多种 HCC 诱因一样，NASH 和 NAFLD 会促进肝硬化转化为 HCC。

2. 2 型糖尿病

作为一种代谢综合征，胰岛素抵抗被发现会引起 HCC，其原因极有可能和肝脏炎症性和血管性改变相关。有人研究了与糖尿病(DM)相关的 HCC 风险。与肥胖类似，较大比例(>70%)的 DM 患者患有不同程度的脂肪肝[66]。尽管有一些小的研究持有不同意见[77]，但是 DM 整体上讲是与 HCC 发病率相关的。El-Serag 及其同事[78]进行了一项纵向调查，它包

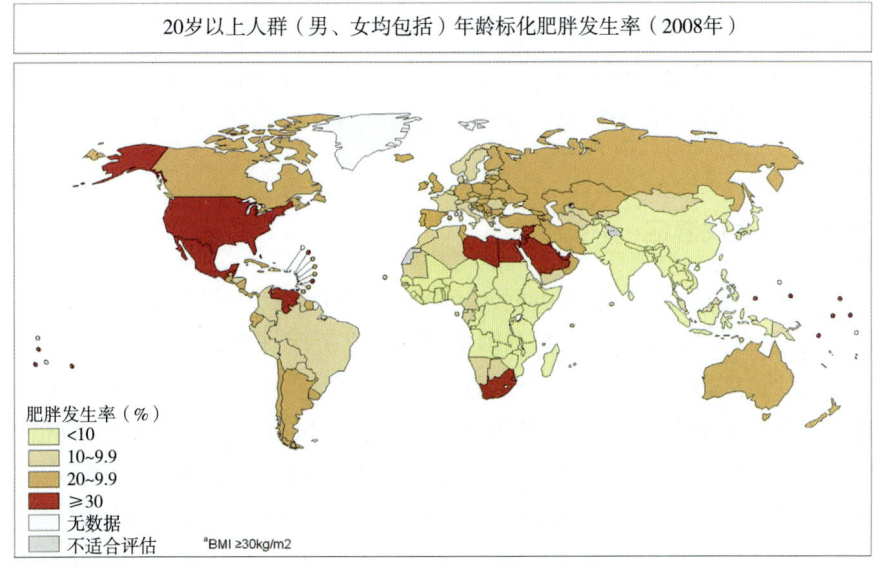

图 1-4 全球肥胖发病率地图

(引自 World Health Organization. World: prevalence of obesity, ages 20+, age standardized: both sexes, 2008. 2011. Available at: http://www.who.int/gho/ncd/risk_factors/obesity_text/en/. Accessed February 10, 2014.)

含了 173 643 例 DM 患者以及 650 620 例无 DM 者(98% 为男性),用以说明 DM 和 HCC 之间的关系。这些研究表明,DM 导致慢性非酒精性肝病的 HR 为 1.98 (95% CI 1.88~2.09),而导致 HCC 的 HR 为 2.16(95% CI 1.86~2.52)。一项美国的病例对照研究[79]对比了 420 例 HCC 患者和 1104 例正常人,结果表明,DM 会通过一种时间依赖性模式增加 HCC 的风险(矫正后 OR 4.2; 95% CI 3.0~5.9)。与患有糖尿病 2~5 年的患者相比,患有糖尿病 6~10 年的患者校正后的 OR 值估计为 1.8(95% CI:0.8~4.1),而这一数字在 10 年以上者为 2.2(95% CI:1.2~4.8)。一项中国的回顾性病例对照研究[80]以逐步推进的线性回归方程证明了糖尿病患者罹患 HCC 风险(OR 2.35;95% CI:1.36~4.05)。Polesel 及其同事[81]在意大利进行了一项包含 185 例 HCC 患者的病例对照研究,结果显示,DM 会增加无 HBV 或 HCV 感染患者的 HCC 发病风险(OR 3.5;95% CI 1.3~9.2)。尽管这些研究中多数都是小样本研究,但是 Wang 和他的同事[82]最近进行的一项 meta 分析入选了 25 个队列研究来分析 DM 和 HCC 之间的关系。研究者认为,与无 DM 个体相比,DM 和 HCC 发病率风险增加相关(HR 2.01;95% CI 1.61~2.51),且会导致 HCC 患者死亡率增加(HR 1.56;95% CI 1.30~1.87)。因此,DM 被认为是导致慢性肝病进展和诱发 HCC 的危险因素。

糖尿病致 HCC 发病率上升的机制是,DM 会通过胰岛素抵抗和高胰岛素血症导致肝细胞损害[83,84]。高胰岛素血症会通过炎症、细胞增殖和抑制凋亡导致 HCC。除此之外,胰岛素水平增加可以抑制肝脏分泌胰岛素生长因子结合蛋白-1,从而提高胰岛素生长因子-1 的生物利用度,同时促细胞增殖和抑制细胞凋亡[85]。胰岛素同时被证明与氧化效应增加以及 ROS 产生相关,这两者都可以导致 DNA 突变[86]。

当以口服降糖胰岛素增敏剂二甲双胍来治疗 DM 后,HCC 的发病风险有所下降。Donadon 及其同事[87]通过一项多变量分析证明,与磺脲类或胰岛素相比,二甲双胍治疗可有效降低 HCC 的风险(OR 0.15;95% CI 0.04 ~ 0.50;P = 0.005)。这些研究者同时发现,以胰岛素或其他降糖口服药如磺脲类治疗 DM 时,胰岛素分泌会增加,而后者会导致高胰岛素血症,进而增加 HCC 发病风险[87]。

3. 遗传性血色素沉着症

遗传性血色素沉着症(hereditary hemochromatosis,HH)是一种常染色体隐性遗传基因介导的遗传疾病,它由 6 号染色体上 HFE 基因单纯的错义突变(C282Y 和 H63D)引发。这种疾病以胃肠道对铁的过度摄取为特点,会导致铁超载。一项包含 1847 例瑞典 HH 患者和其 5973 例一级亲属的人群对照研究[88]显示,HH 患者罹患肝癌的风险比正常人群高 20 倍(标准化风险比 21;95% CI 16 ~ 22)。一项美国国家卫生统计局的大型研究表明,与正常人相比,HH 患者罹患肝癌的风险高达 23 倍[比例风险因素(PMR)22.5;95% CI 20.6 ~ 24.6][89]。HH 导致的铁超载可以通过产生氧自由基和细胞因子,如肿瘤生长因子 β,从而促进肝纤维化[90]。

4. 烟草

多项研究内容与烟草和 HCC 的发生相关,但是其结果却不一致。一项日本的前瞻性队列研究[91]包含了 4050 例 40 岁以上、平均吸烟超过 9 年的男性,其结果显示与不吸烟者相比,吸烟者原发性肝癌的风险上升 3 倍,且此风险增加和吸烟剂量无关。2005 年韩国一项研究[92]随访了 733 134 例男性 4 年,尽管这项研究并未考虑肝炎状态,但它发现已戒烟者 HCC 的 RR 为 1.53(95% CI 1.30 ~ 1.79),未戒烟者为 1.50(95% CI 1.29 ~ 1.74)。密歇根一项前瞻性病例对照研究[51]包含了 210 例 HCC 患者,其结果显示,吸烟超过 20 包 - 年者 HCC 风险超过肝硬化者(OR 4.9;95% CI 2.2 ~ 10.6)和无基础肝病者(OR 63.7;95% CI 16.7 ~ 144.2)。但是,美国一项以筛选后的癌症病例对照数据进行的研究[93]显示,当前吸烟者肝癌发病风险无增加。研究者发现,以前吸烟者患原发性肝癌的风险显著增加(1.85;95% CI:1.05 ~ 3.25)。这项研究的结果可能说明烟草致癌的作用是时间依赖性的。同时有研究表明,吸烟、饮酒和肥胖对于 HCC 的风险有协同作用[51]。

尽管吸烟和 HCC 之间的关联尚未明确,但是研究证实吸烟的 HCC 患者死亡率会增加。2004 年韩国一项研究证实,男性持续的吸烟状态会增加 HCC 的死亡率(RR 1.4;95% CI 1.3 ~ 1.6)[94]。台湾一项包含 12 008 例男性的前瞻性研究显示,烟草与 HCV 抗体阳性存在协同作用,但这种协同作用不具有统计学意义[95]。

5. 性别

在几乎所有国家中,男性患 HCC 风险都超过女性,其中欧洲的差异最高(> 4∶1)[2]。在暴露于致病因素时,男女性患病几率的确有差异。男性更容易感染 HBV、酗酒和吸烟。但是,这些差异也可能由其他因素引起。伦敦早期一项包含 613 例肝硬化患者的研究[96]显示,男性性征是肝硬化进展到 HCC 的重要因素。Yuan 及其同事[97]证实睾酮水平与 HCC 患病风险存在关联,从而说明男性 HCC 潜在高风险。此外,小鼠 HCC 模型同样证实雄性小鼠比雌性容易诱发肝癌。IL-6 是一种与肝脏感染和炎症反应密切相关的细胞因子,也与肝癌发病相关。Naugler 及其同事[98]在小鼠模型上证明雌性大量分泌的雌激素可以抑制 IL-6 的产生并抑制肝脏患癌。

五、经济/公共卫生原因

从 HCV 感染发展至 HCC 需要 20~40 年,所以西方国家 HCC 负担可能会在未来几年随着 HCV 阳性婴儿潮而上升。考虑到 HCV 及其他前文提及的因素,预计 2000—2020 年,美国代偿性肝硬化和肝癌患者将增加 80% 以上[99]。美国 1998 年用于 HCC 的费用据估计达到 9.88 亿美金,其中 9.78 亿美金属于直接花费,1000 万美金属于间接花费,这些间接花费包括因住院、门诊医疗和过早死亡造成的经济损失。直接花费尚可细分为 8900 万门诊花费、5.48 亿住院花费、1.39 亿就诊费用和 8000 万药物费用[100]。随着新型药物用于治疗 HCV 和 HCC,这些花费会持续上升。HCC 对美国和世界其他高发国家的经济和社会已造成沉重的负担。

六、总结

HCC 是世界范围内高发的癌症,其每年新增病例和死亡病例大致相等。多种致病因素可以导致 HCC 的发生,而多数 HCC 发展于慢性肝病之后。虽然西方国家中,非酒精性脂肪肝导致的 HCC 比例在上升,但是 HCC 最主要的致病因素仍然是 HBV、HCV 以及酗酒。对这些致病因素及其致癌机制的进一步研究,有助于 HCC 的筛查、预防、早期诊断和治疗。

参考文献

[1] Ferlay J, Shin H, Bray F, et al. GLOBOCAN 2008 v2.0, Cancer incidence and mortality worldwide: IARC CancerBase No. 10 [Internet]. Lyon (France): International Agency for Research on Cancer; 2010.

[2] Shariff M, Cox I, Gomaa A, et al. Hepatocellular carcinoma: current trends in worldwide epidemiology, risk factors, diagnosis and therapeutics. Expert Rev Gastroenterol Hepatol 2009;3(4):353-67.

[3] Custer B, Sullivan S, Hazlet T, et al. Global epidemiology of hepatitis B virus. J Clin Gastroenterol 2004;38(10):S158-68.

[4] Chang M, You S, Chen C, et al. Decreased incidence of hepatocellular carcinoma in hepatitis B vaccinees: a 20-year follow-up study. J Natl Cancer Inst 2009;101(19):1348-55.

[5] El-Serag H, Rudolph K. Hepatocellular carcinoma: epidemiology and molecular carcinogenesis. Gastroenterology 2007;132(7):2557-76.

[6] Yoshizawa H. Hepatocellular carcinoma associated with hepatitis C virus infection in Japan: projection to other countries in the foreseeable future. Oncology 2002;62(S1):8-17.

[7] Fattovich G, Stroffolini T, Zagni I, et al. Hepatocellular carcinoma in cirrhosis: incidence and risk factors. Gastroenterology 2004;127(5):35 - S50.

[8] Pellicelli A, Romano M, Stroffolini T, et al. HCV genotype 1a shows a better virologic response to antiviral therapy than HCV genotype 1b. BMC Gastroenterol 2012;12(162):1 - 7.

[9] Kew M. Epidemiology of hepatocellular carcinoma in sub - Saharan Africa. Ann Hepatol 2013;12(2): 173 - 82.

[10] Altekruse S, McGlynn K, Reichman M. Hepatocellular carcinoma incidence, mortality, and survival trends in the United States from 1975 to 2005. J Clin Oncol 2009;27(9):1485 - 91.

[11] Mittal S, El - Serag H. Epidemiology of hepatocellular carcinoma: consider the population. J Clin Gastroenterol 2013;47:S2 - 6.

[12] Bosch F, Ribes J, Cle′ries R, et al. Epidemiology of hepatocellular carcinoma. Clin Liver Dis 2005;9 (2):191 - 211.

[13] Branda M, Wands J. Signal transduction cascades and hepatitis B and C related hepatocellular carcinoma. Hepatology 2006;43(5):891 - 902.

[14] Tsai W, Chung R. Viral hepatocarcinogenesis. Oncogene 2010;29(16):2309 - 24.

[15] Beasley R, Hwang L, Lin C, et al. Hepatocellular carcinoma and hepatitis B virus: a prospective study of 22,707 men in Taiwan. Lancet 1981;2(8256):1129 - 33.

[16] Tabor E. Hepatocellular carcinoma: global epidemiology. Dig Liver Dis 2001;33(2):115 - 7.

[17] McMahon B. The influence of hepatitis B virus genotype and subgenotype on the natural history of chronic hepatitis B. Hepatol Int 2009;3(2):334 - 42.

[18] Chan H, Hui A, Wong M, et al. Genotype C hepatitis B virus infection is associated with an increased risk of hepatocellular carcinoma. Gut 2004;53(10):1494 - 8.

[19] Kao J, Chen P, Lai M, et al. Hepatitis B genotypes correlate with clinical outcomes in patients with chronic hepatitis B. Gastroenterology 2000;118(3):554 - 9.

[20] Lee C, Chen C, Lu S, et al. Prevalence and clinical implications of hepatitis B virus genotypes in southern Taiwan. Scand J Gastroenterol 2003;38(1):95 - 101.

[21] Tangkijvanich P, Mahachai V, Komolmit P, et al. Hepatitis B virus genotypes and hepatocellular carcinoma in Thailand. World J Gastroenterol 2005;11(15):2238 - 43.

[22] Chisari F. Rous - Whipple award lecture. Viruses, immunity, and cancer: lessons from hepatitis B. Am J Pathol 2000;156(4):1117 - 32.

[23] Dandri M, Burda M, Bürkle A, et al. Increase in de novo HBV DNA integrations in response to oxidative DNA damage or inhibition of poly(ADP - ribosyl)ation. Hepatology 2002;35(1):217 - 23.

[24] Bonilla Guerrero R, Roberts L. The role of hepatitis B virus integrations in the pathogenesis of human hepatocellular carcinoma. J Hepatol 2005;42(5):760 - 77.

[25] Ferber M, Montoya D, Yu C, et al. Integrations of the hepatitis B virus (HBV) and human papillomavirus (HPV) into the human telomerase reverse transcriptase (hTERT) gene in liver and cervical cancers. Oncogene 2003;22(24):3813 - 20.

[26] Wu B, Li C, Chen H, et al. Blocking of G1/S transition and cell death in the regenerating liver of hepatitis B virus X protein transgenic mice. Biochem Biophys Res Commun 2006;340(3):916 - 28.

[27] Yang H, Lu S, Liaw Y, et al. Hepatitis B e antigen and the risk of hepatocellular carcinoma. N Engl J

Med 2002;347(3):168 – 74.

[28] Yuen M, Tanaka Y, Fong D, et al. Independent risk factors and predictive score for the development of hepatocellular carcinoma in chronic hepatitis B. J Hepatol 2009;10(1):80 – 8.

[29] Chen C, Yang H, Su J, et al. Risk of hepatocellular carcinoma across a biological gradient of serum hepatitis B virus DNA level. JAMA 2006;295(1):65 – 73.

[30] Simonietti R, Camma C, Fiorello F, et al. Hepatocellular carcinoma. A worldwide problem and the major risk factors. Dig Dis Sci 1991;36:962 – 72.

[31] Tiribelli C, Melato M, Croce L, et al. Prevalence of hepatocellular carcinoma and relation to cirrhosis: comparison of two different cities in the world – Trieste, Italy and China, Japan. Hepatology 1989;10: 998 – 1002.

[32] Sangiovanni A, Del Ninno E, Fasani P, et al. Increased survival of cirrhotic patients with a hepatocellular carcinoma detected during surveillance. Gastroenterology 2004;126:1005 – 14.

[33] Benvegnu L, Gios M, Boccato S, et al. Natural history of compensated viral cirrhosis: a prospective study on the incidence and hierarchy of major complications. Gut 2004;53:744 – 9.

[34] Tsai J, Jeng J, Ho M, et al. Effect of hepatitis C and B virus infection on risk of hepatocellular carcinoma: a prospective study. Br J Cancer 1997;76:968 – 74.

[35] McGlynn K, London W. The global epidemiology of hepatocellular carcinoma: present and future. Clin Liver Dis 2011;15(2):223 – 43.

[36] Choo Q, Kuo G, Weiner A, et al. Isolation of a cDNA clone derived from a bloodborne non – A, non – B viral hepatitis genome. Science 1989;244(4902):359 – 62.

[37] Donato F, Tagger A, Gelatti U, et al. Alcohol and hepatocellular carcinoma: the effect of lifetime intake and hepatitis virus infections in men and women. Am J Epidemiol 2002;155(4):323 – 31.

[38] Zaltron S, Spinetti A, Biasi L, et al. Chronic HCV infection: epidemiological and clinical relevance. BMC Infect Dis 2012;12(Suppl 2):S2 – 7.

[39] Freeman A, Dore G, Law M, et al. Estimating progression to cirrhosis in chronic hepatitis C virus infection. Hepatology 2001;34(4):809 – 16.

[40] Seeff L. Natural history of chronic hepatitis C. Hepatology 2002;36(5 Suppl 1):S35 – 46.

[41] Poynard T, Bedossa P, Opolon P. Natural history of liver fibrosis progression in patients with chronic hepatitis C. The OBSVIRC, METAVIR, CLINIVIR, and DOSVIRC groups. Lancet 1997;349(9055):825 – 32.

[42] Shindo M, Arai K, Sokawa Y, et al. The virological and histological states of antihepatitis C virus – positive subjects with normal liver biochemical values. Hepatology 1995;22(2):418 – 25.

[43] Mathurin P, Moussalli J, Cadranel J, et al. Slow progression rate of fibrosis in hepatitis C virus patients with persistently normal alanine transaminase activity. Hepatology 1998;27(3):868 – 72. 14 Lafaro et al

[44] Backus L, Boothroyd D, Phillips B, et al. A sustained virologic response reduces risk of all – cause mortality in patients with hepatitis C. Clin Gastroenterol Hepatol 2011;9(6):509 – 16.

[45] Singal A, Volk M, Jensen D, et al. A sustained viral response is associated with reduced liver – related morbidity and mortality in patients with hepatitis C virus. Clin Gastroenterol Hepatol 2010;8(3):280 – 8.

[46] Morgan R, Baack B, Smith B, et al. Eradication of hepatitis C virus infection and the development of hepatocellular carcinoma: a meta – analysis of observational studies. Ann Intern Med 2013;158(5 Pt 1):

329 – 37.

[47] Zhu H, Jia Z, Misra H, et al. Oxidative stress and redox signaling mechanisms of alcoholic liver disease: updated experimental and clinical evidence. J Dig Dis 2012;13(3):133 – 42.

[48] IARC Working Group. Alcohol drinking. IARC Monogr Eval Carcinog Risks Hum 1988;44:1 – 378.

[49] Yuan J, Govindarajan S, Arakawa K, et al. Synergism of alcohol, diabetes, and viral hepatitis on the risk of hepatocellular carcinoma in blacks and whites in the US. Cancer 2004;101(5):1009 – 17.

[50] Grewal P, Viswanathen V. Liver cancer and alcohol. Clin Liver Dis 2012;16(4):839 – 50.

[51] Marrero J, Fontana R, Fu S, et al. Alcohol, tobacco and obesity are synergistic risk factors for hepatocellular carcinoma. J Hepatol 2005;42(2):218 – 24.

[52] Trichopoulos D, Bamia C, Lagiou P, et al. Hepatocellular carcinoma risk factors and disease burden in a European cohort: a nested case – control study. J Natl Cancer Inst 2011;103(22):1686 – 95.

[53] Corrao G, Bagnardi V, Zambon A, et al. A meta – analysis of alcohol consumption and the risk of 15 diseases. Prev Med 2004;38(5):613 – 9.

[54] Heckley G, Jarl J, Asamoah B, et al. How the risk of liver cancer changes after alcohol cessation: a review and meta – analysis of the current literature. BMC Cancer 2011;11(446):1 – 10.

[55] Boveris A, Fraga C, Varsavsky A, et al. Increased chemiluminescence and superoxide production in the liver of chronically ethanol – treated rats. Arch Biochem Biophys 1983;227(2):534 – 41.

[56] Kukielka E, Dicker E, Cederbaum A. Increased production of reactive oxygen species by rat liver mitochondria after chronic ethanol treatment. Arch Biochem Biophys 1994;309(2):377 – 86.

[57] Kuper H, Tzonou A, Kaklamani E, et al. Tobacco smoking, alcohol consumption and their interaction in the causation of hepatocellular carcinoma. Int J Cancer 2000;85(4):498 – 502.

[58] Berman K, Tandra S, Vuppalanchi R, et al. Hepatic and extrahepatic cancer in cirrhosis: a longitudinal cohort study. Am J Gastroenterol 2011;106(5):899 – 906.

[59] Kubo S, Kinoshita H, Hirohashi K, et al. High malignancy of hepatocellular carcinoma in alcoholic patients with hepatitis C virus. Surgery 1997;121(4):425 – 9.

[60] IARC Working Group. Aflatoxins. IARC Monogr Eval Carcinog Risks Hum 2002;82:171 – 300.

[61] Liu Y, Wu F. Global burden of aflatoxin – induced hepatocellular carcinoma: a risk assessment. Environ Health Perspect 2010;118(6):818 – 24.

[62] Hsu I, Metcalf R, Sun T, et al. Mutational hotspot in the p53 gene in human hepatocellular carcinomas. Nature 1991;350(6317):427 – 8.

[63] Bressac B, Kew M, Wands J, et al. Selective G to T mutations of p53 gene in hepatocellular carcinoma from southern Africa. Nature 1991;350(6317):429 – 31.

[64] Ozturk M. p53 mutation in hepatocellular carcinoma after aflatoxin exposure. Lancet 1991;338(8779):1356 – 9.

[65] Qian G, Ross R, Yu M, et al. A follow – up study of urinary markers of aflatoxin exposure and liver cancer risk in Shanghai, People's Republic of China. Cancer Epidemiol Biomarkers Prev 1994;3(1):3 – 10.

[66] Neuschwander – Tetri B, Caldwell S. Nonalcoholic steatohepatitis: summary of an AASLD Single Topic Conference. Hepatology 2003;37(5):1202 – 19.

[67] Nishikawa H, Osaki Y. Non – B, non – C hepatocellular carcinoma (review). Int J Oncol 2013;43(5):

1333 - 42.

[68] Tokushige K, Hashimoto E, Horie Y, et al. Hepatocellular carcinoma in Japanese patients with nonalcoholic fatty liver disease, alcoholic liver disease, and chronic liver disease of unknown etiology: report of the nationwide survey. J Gastroenterol 2011;46(10):1230 - 7.

[69] Torres D, Harrison S. Nonalcoholic steatohepatitis and noncirrhotic hepatocellular carcinoma: fertile soil. Semin Liver Dis 2012;32(1):30 - 8.

[70] Welzel T, Graubard B, Zeuzem S, et al. Metabolic syndrome increases the risk of primary liver cancer in the United States: a study in the SEER - Medicare database. Hepatology 2011;54(2):463 - 71.

[71] Wolk A, Gridley G, Svensson M, et al. A prospective study of obesity and cancer risk (Sweden). Cancer Causes Control 2001;12(1):13 - 21.

[72] Attner B, Landin - Olsson M, Lithman T, et al. Cancer among patients with diabetes, obesity and abnormal blood lipids: a population - based register study in Sweden. Cancer Causes Control 2012;23(5): 769 - 77.

[73] Hashimoto E, Yatsuji S, Tobari M, et al. Hepatocellular carcinoma in patients with nonalcoholic steatohepatitis. J Gastroenterol 2009;44(Suppl 19):89 - 95.

[74] Ascha M, Hanouneh I, Lopez R, et al. The incidence and risk factors of hepatocellular carcinoma in patients with nonalcoholic steatohepatitis. Hepatology 2010;51(6):1972 - 8.

[75] Calle E, Rodriguez C, Walker - Thurmond K, et al. Overweight, obesity, and mortality from cancer in a prospectively studied cohort of US adults. N Engl J Med 2003;348(17):1625 - 38.

[76] Shimizu M, Tanaka T, Moriwaki H. Obesity and hepatocellular carcinoma: targeting obesity - related inflammation for chemoprevention of liver carcinogenesis. Semin Immunopathol 2013;35(2):191 - 202.

[77] Tung H, Wang J, Tseng P, et al. Neither diabetes mellitus nor overweight is a risk factor for hepatocellular carcinoma in a dual HBV and HCV endemic area: community cross - sectional and case - control studies. Am J Gastroenterol 2010;105(3):624 - 31.

[78] El - Serag H, Tran T, Everhart J. Diabetes increases the risk of chronic liver disease and hepatocellular carcinoma. Gastroenterology 2004;126(2):460 - 8.

[79] Hassan M, Curley S, Li D, et al. Association of diabetes duration and diabetes treatment with the risk of hepatocellular carcinoma. Cancer 2010;116(8): 1938 - 46.

[80] Zheng Z, Zhang C, Yan J, et al. Diabetes mellitus is associated with hepatocellular carcinoma: a retrospective case - control study in hepatitis endemic area. PLoS One 2013;8(12):e84776.

[81] Polesel J, Zucchetto A, Montella M, et al. The impact of obesity and diabetes mellitus on the risk of hepatocellular carcinoma. Ann Oncol 2009;20(2):353 - 7.

[82] Wang C, Wang X, Gong G, et al. Increased risk of hepatocellular carcinoma in patients with diabetes mellitus: a systematic review and meta - analysis of cohort studies. Int J Cancer 2012;130(7):1639 - 48.

[83] Hassan M, Kaseb A. Hepatocellular carcinoma. In: McMasters K, Vauthey JN, editors. Targeted therapy and multidisciplinary care, vol. 1. New York (NY): Springer; 2011. p. 1 - 19.

[84] Harrison S. Liver disease in patients with diabetes mellitus. J Clin Gastroenterol 2006;40(1):68 - 76.

[85] Alexia C, Fallot G, Lasfer M, et al. An evaluation of the role of insulin - like growth factors (IGF) and of type - I IGF receptor signalling in hepatocarcinogenesis and in the resistance of hepatocarcinoma cells against drug - induced apoptosis. Biochem Pharmacol 2004;68(6):1003 - 15.

[86] Hu W, Feng Z, Eveleigh J, et al. The major lipid peroxidation product, trans-4-hydroxy-2-nonenal, preferentially forms DNA adducts at codon 249 of human p53 gene, a unique mutational hotspot in hepatocellular carcinoma. Carcinogenesis 2002;23(11):1781-9.

[87] Donadon V, Balbi M, Dal Mas M, et al. Metformin and reduced risk of hepatocellular carcinoma in diabetic patients with chronic liver disease. Liver Int 2010;30(5):750-8.

[88] Elmberg M, Hultcrantz R, Ekbom A, et al. Cancer risk in patients with hereditary hemochromatosis and in their first-degree relatives. Gastroenterology 2003;125(6):1733-41.

[89] Yang Q, McDonnell S, Khoury M, et al. Hemochromatosis-associated mortality in the United States from 1979 to 1992: an analysis of multiple-cause mortality data. Ann Intern Med 1998;129(11):946-53.

[90] Lata J. Chronic liver diseases as liver tumor precursors. Dig Dis 2010;28(4-5):596-9.

[91] Mizoue T, Tokui N, Nishisaka K, et al. Prospective study on the relation of cigarette smoking with cancer of the liver and stomach in an endemic region. Int J Epidemiol 2000;29(2):232-7.

[92] Yun Y, Jung K, Bae J, et al. Cigarette smoking and cancer incidence risk in adult men: National Health Insurance Corporation Study. Cancer Detect Prev 2005;29(1):15-24.

[93] Zhu K, Moriarty C, Caplan L, et al. Cigarette smoking and primary liver cancer: a population-based case-control study in US men. Cancer Causes Control 2007;18(3):315-21.

[94] Jee S, Ohrr H, Sull J, et al. Cigarette smoking, alcohol drinking, hepatitis B, and risk for hepatocellular carcinoma in Korea. J Natl Cancer Inst 2004;96(24):1851-6.

[95] Sun C, Wu D, Lin C, et al. Incidence and cofactors of hepatitis C virus-related hepatocellular carcinoma: a prospective study of 12,008 men in Taiwan. Am J Epidemiol 2003;157(8):674-82.

[96] Zaman S, Melia W, Johnson R, et al. Risk factors in development of hepatocellular carcinoma in cirrhosis: prospective study of 613 patients. Lancet 1985;1(8442):1357-60.

[97] Yuan J, Ross R, Stanczyk F, et al. A cohort study of serum testosterone and hepatocellular carcinoma in Shanghai, China. Int J Cancer 1995;63(4):491-3.

[98] Naugler W, Sakurai T, Kim S, et al. Gender disparity in liver cancer due to sex differences in MyD88-dependent IL-6 production. Science 2007;317(5834):121-4.

[99] Davis G, Albright J, Cook S, et al. Projecting future complications of chronic hepatitis C in the United States. Liver Transpl 2003;9(4):331-8.

[100] Sandler R, Everhart J, Donowitz M, et al. The burden of selected digestive diseases in the United States. Gastroenterology 2002;122(5):1500-11.

第二章 肝细胞癌、胆管癌和转移性结直肠癌的影像诊断

Kathryn J. Fowler, MD[a][*], Nael E. Saad, MD[b], David Linehan, MD[c]

【关键词】
肝脏影像;转移性肝肿瘤;肝细胞癌;胆管癌;结直肠癌肝转移

要点

- 影像学取代病理学诊断 HCC。
- 胆管癌的影像学诊断主要是为了确定可切除性。
- MRI 是寻找结直肠癌转移灶最敏感的方法。

一、简介

影像学检查是肝脏疾病或者肿瘤患者管理的重要组成部分,其技术可以为诊疗提供有用信息,必要时还可以为肝脏病灶的病理诊断提供支持。本章概述了最常见的肝脏影像学检查方法及其在 HCC、肝内胆管癌(ICC)和结直肠癌(CRC)肝转移方面的应用。

---

[a] Department of Radiology, Washington University, 510 S. Kingshighway Blvd, St. Louis, MO 63110, USA; [b] Department of Interventional Radiology, Washington University, 510 S. Kingshighway Blvd, St. Louis, MO 63110, USA; [c] Department of Surgery, Washington University, 510 S. Kingshighway Blvd, St. Louis, MO 63110, USA

[*] 通讯作者。
E-mail address: fowlerk@mir.wustl.edu

二、肝脏影像学检查方法

1. 超声

(1) 超声的原理

超声(US)是历史最悠久的影像学检查方法之一。探头(探针)会产生超声波,后者穿透组织的过程中会不同程度地被阻碍并反射回探头。由于组织密度的不同,会产生不同的回声强度(亮度)。在进行经皮超声检查时,可根据感兴趣区域和组织的穿透深度,选择不同频率的换能器(3~5MHz 的低频比高频穿透力强)。由于空气有反射作用,所以需要用凝胶来建立良好的声接触。根据内部回声及血流情况的差异,灰度和多普勒超声已被用于评价肝脏局灶性病变;然而这种方法很难确诊,当经皮超声在某些情况下未能提供明确的诊断时,超声检查可用于指导穿刺活检。

(2) 超声造影

使用造影剂后,US 的诊断准确性有大幅提高。然而时至今日,超声造影(CEUS)的使用在美国仍然受到限制,因为它还未得到美国食品药品监督管理局(FDA)的批准。世界范围内现有 3 种造影剂:SonoVue (Bracco, Milan, Italy)、Definity (Bristol - Myers Squibb, New York, NY, USA)和 Sonazoid (GE Healthcare, Oslo, Norway)。前两种只可用于血管,提供关于血管外有无扩散的病变早期动态信息(这点与 CT 和 MRI 的造影剂不同)。Sonazoid 会被 Kupffer 细胞摄取,其注射 1 小时后进入肝胆管期,和 MRI 中的肝胆管期是相似的,其可用于病灶探测和转移灶随访。CEUS 的主要作用是显示肝脏局灶性病变的表征和局部消融治疗监测[1]。与 CT 和 MRI 相比,CEUS 的主要优点是能够实时增强对比度、肾毒性小、电离辐射减少、费用更低。但是,最新的美国肝病研究学会(AASLD)的指南中撤除了 CEUS 的相关内容,因为它可能造成 ICC 被误诊为 HCC[2]。

2. CT

(1) CT 的原理

CT 是一种快速检查方法,其适应证范围内的诊断准确率很高,在影像科医生和临床医生中都受到广泛的认可。CT 影像的基础设备是电离辐射(X 线)源,电离辐射源绕着患者旋转,探测器与源相对,以测量 X 射线束的衰减程度,最终结果是基于不同的衰减系数(它们阻碍 X 射线束的程度)分配给不同结构的不同衰减值(亮度)的断层扫描图像。大多数软组织有相似的衰减效应,因此,血管内造影剂可用来调高器官、病灶和血管的差异性。

CT 造影剂是以碘为介质的,后者会提高 X 线的吸收和离散,从而导致结构的衰减效应增加(表现为高亮度)。器官的相对强化程度比较复杂,与器官本身灌注率、组织体积、构成和血管弥散相关。早期强化主要由血供和心输出量决定,而后期强化则与血流的稀释作用以及造影剂在细胞外的重新分布更相关[3]。因为碘造影剂不能进入细胞内,所以可以假定它通过扩散或毛细血管交换的方式分布在血管内和细胞外[4]。对造影剂药代动力学的研究会方便我们根据不同的强化模式应用造影剂(稍后会讨论)。

在肝脏中,有明确的增强相,肝实质会遵循一个可预测的模式增强。这些事项包括动脉晚期、门静脉期、平衡期和延迟期[5]。多数肝内的肿瘤(特别是富血供的 HCC)主要由肝动脉供血,而正常肝组织主要由门静脉供血[6-8]。这种血供差异适用于多数病灶:富血供肿瘤的背景强化见于动脉晚期;乏血供肿瘤(多数转移瘤)在门静脉期或平衡期出现强化,而此时动脉期强化的病灶已不可见(图 2-1)。除了更清晰地显示病灶外,造影剂不同时期的不同强化类型也有助于鉴别诊断,有时甚至可以替代病理诊断,如血管瘤(图 2-2)。因此,在评估肝肿瘤时,应进行多期对比的肝脏 CT 检查(表 2-1)[9]。

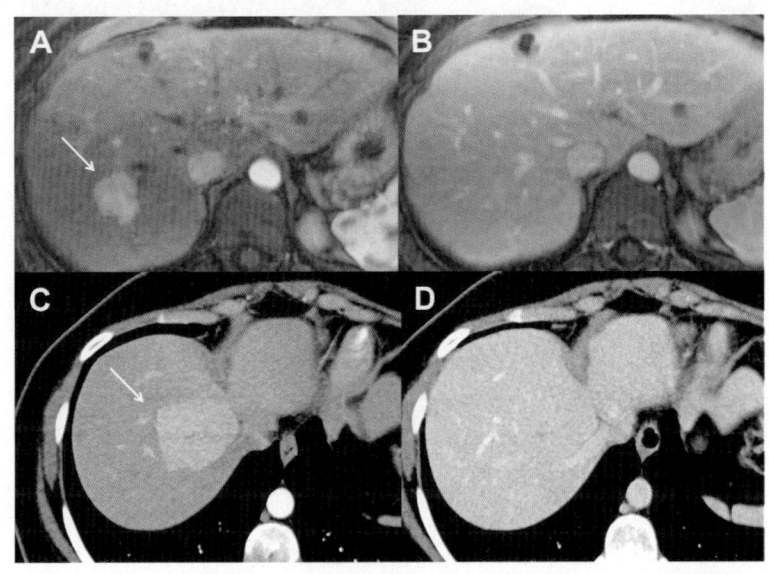

图 2-1 肝脏局灶性结节性增生

箭头所示为 CT 动脉期"快进"现象(A)和静脉期的"快出"现象(B)。这里说明了多期扫描对于病灶定性的重要性。C 为动脉期,D 为门静脉期。另一有肝脏局灶性结节性增生患者动脉期(C)和门静脉期(D)的"快进快出"现象

(2)造影剂的肾毒性

尽管造影剂对于肝脏肿瘤的定性必不可少,但是由于具有肾毒性,应避免用于肾功能不全的患者。美国放射学会定义"造影剂诱导的肾毒性(CIN)"为:未接触其他肾毒性物质时,因近期使用碘造影剂而导致的突发肾损害[10]。不同文献对 CIN 的诊断标准存在争议,因而缺乏关于其发生率、危险因素和诊断的共识。急性肾损伤网建议,当出现肾毒性 48 小时内,如果满足以下任意一项即可诊断为急性肾损伤:血清肌酐水平上升,大于或等于 0.3mg/dl;血清肌酐水平上升大于或等于 50%;持续 6 小时以上,大于或等于 $0.5ml/(kg \cdot h)$ 的尿量减少[11]。鉴于这一标准中肌酐的变化幅度较小,是否可以在临床中使用如此严格的界限尚存在争议。在一项包含 8826 名对比增强 CT 病例的回顾性研究中,碘造影剂的使用被证明是肾小球滤过率(eGFR)小于 $30ml/(min \cdot 1.73m^2)$ 患者肾毒性的危险因素,同时对 eGFR 为 $30 \sim 40ml/(min \cdot 1.73m^2)$ 的患者肾功

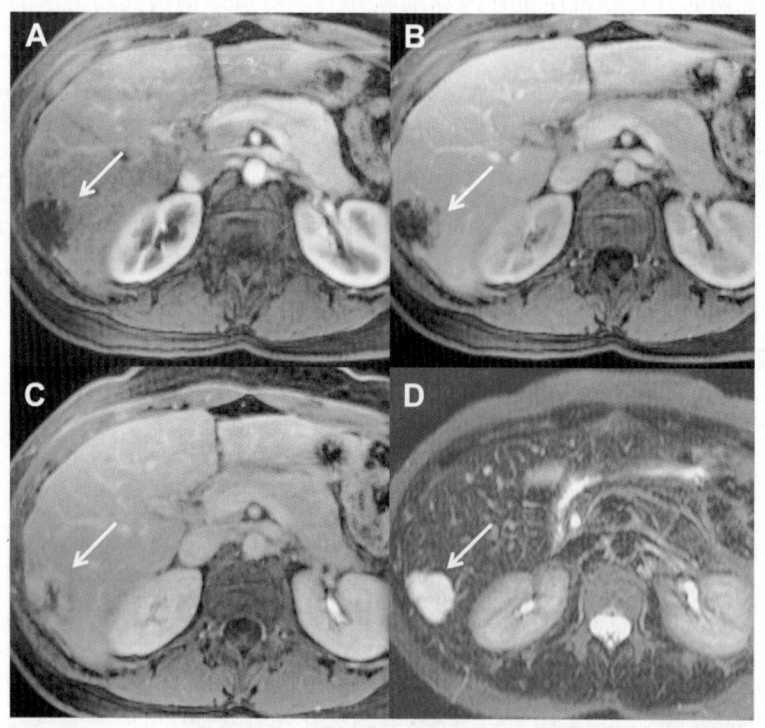

图 2-2 血管瘤的诊断性征象

A. 动脉期，B. 门脉期，C. 延迟期。增强 MRI（A－C）和 T2 加权的脂肪抑制序列（D）显示了血管瘤的诊断性征象（箭头所示）。确诊有赖于多期增强中显示的典型向心性增强

表 2-1 肝脏 CT 标准流程

期相	评价	技术要求
平扫期	提供病灶密度的相关信息（钙化、血供、脂肪） · 病灶定性的最佳选择 · 可用于评价 TACE 术后与碘油/酒精摄取相关的强化	· 多重探头（至少 8 个） · 强力对比剂注射（至少 3ml/s） · 至少 5mm 重建层厚
动脉晚期	全部动脉及部分门静脉强化，肝静脉无强化 · 适用于时间定量（造影剂追踪）	
门静脉期	肝脏实质强化最明显，肝静脉开始强化	
延迟期	造影剂注射＞120 秒，征象有差异	

能有影响[12]。临床危险因素也可能导致造影剂诱导的肾损伤，这些危险因素包括糖尿病、肝脏疾病、慢性肾脏疾病、高血压、低血容量和心衰[13]。对患者这些危险因素的对比管理政策因机构而异，建议对有潜在风险的患者进行筛查。表 2-2 归纳了我们的策略。尽管有大量文献研究了生理盐水、碳酸氢盐和其他方法用于降低肾毒性的可行性，尚无一种方法具有明确优

势,最有效的措施仍是避免在高危患者身上使用造影剂。对于无法进行 CT 增强扫描的患者,可以考虑进行 MRI,后者对于肌酐水平的要求更宽泛,因其使用的钆造影剂不具有肾毒性。

表 2-2　华盛顿大学增强 CT 扫描流程

肾功能	指南
血清 Cr < 1.4	可用造影剂
慢性病程,血清 Cr < 2	可用造影剂
慢性病程未知,血清 Cr > 1.4	计算 eGFR,如果 >30,可用造影剂
血清 Cr 急性升高	尽量避免使用造影剂
血透患者	可用造影剂(目的不在于保持肾功能储备),但建议扫描后安排透析

检查血清 Cr 的指征:
· 适用于全部住院及急症患者;
· 年龄小于 70 岁,Cr 值介于 30~90 是符合要求的
如何避免肾毒性:
· 对于 GFR 升高但需使用造影剂的患者,建议造影前后都进行水化
肾脏病危险因素:
· 家族史,糖尿病,血清蛋白异常综合征,胶原性血管疾病,药物,肾脏手术,长期应用非甾体抗炎药,住院状态

除了 CIN,对碘造影剂的过敏也值得注意。轻微症状(荨麻疹、瘙痒及其他)可以术前用药,如类固醇和抗组胺类药物预防。但是,对于重症患者(喉头水肿、呼吸困难、休克),建议不要使用造影剂。尽管 CT 和 MR 造影剂导致的过敏症状类似,但尚缺乏足够证据证明两者存在交叉致敏性。对于先前有严重 CT 造影剂过敏的患者,可以考虑采用 MRI 检查。

3. MRI

(1) MRI 的原理

MRI 结合引用了强磁场、高频脉冲和弱磁场(渐变),这些成分会导致体内的氢质子被激发并按照共振频率旋转。这种频率信息会被一种复杂的数学方程(傅立叶变换)解码,从而产生图像。图像的明暗程度被称为信号强度,分别以高和低来表示。在肝脏 MRI 的常规检查中会应用几个序列。如此可以得到器官和肿瘤的不同信息。表 2-3 显示了常规的肝脏 MRI 序列[9,14]。

表 2-3 肝脏 MR 检查流程

MR 序列	评价	技术要求
T1WI 化学位移（同反相位，双相梯度回波）	提供肝内及病灶内铁离子和脂肪的相关信息 ·包含脂肪的病灶可能在反相图像中存在信号丢失情况	·磁场强度≥1.5T ·相控线圈加体线圈 ·加压对比剂注射 ·统一的增强前后图像，以利于对比 ·增强后图像层厚≤5mm，其他序列≤8mm ·屏气时间≤20 秒 ·图像分辨率≥128×256
T2 加权（TSE TZ ssFSE） T2 脂肪抑制加权（反转恢复，T2 TSE FS）	液体敏感性序列 病灶的信号强度	
T1 脂肪抑制加权（VIBE，THRIVE，LAVA，GRE）	为增强后强化程度提供增强前基线对照	
动态后增强（VIBE，THRIVE，LAVA，GRE）	和 CT 的动脉期相似	
弥散加权图像	可选但推荐应用 有助于良恶性病灶鉴别 有助于发现转移灶	

和 CT 一样，造影剂通常被用来对肝脏病灶定性改善可视化程度。MR 造影剂含钆元素。钆会与血液中的水分子相互作用从而产生 T1 缩短（表现为高亮信号）。主要的 MR 造影剂是细胞外造影剂，和 CT 造影剂相同，它们会在动脉晚期、门静脉期、平衡/延迟期提供动态增强信息。此外，有 2 种被广泛应用的肝胆管造影剂：钆贝酸二葡甲胺莫迪司（MultiHance，Bracco）和钆塞酸普美显（Eovist, Bayer Healthcare Pharmaceuticals, Whippany, NJ, USA）。接近 4% 的莫迪司会进入胆道，其肝实质的最大强化（肝胆管期）时间出现在注射后约 1 小时。普美显最多会有 50% 进入胆管系统，其肝实质最大强化出现在注射后约 20 分钟。肝细胞对造影剂的摄取被认为主要和肝细胞表面肝特异性多药有机阴离子转运多肽（OATP1B1 和 OATP1B3）的主动转运有关[15-17]。摄取率和诊断可信度可能会因潜在严重肝纤维化、肝硬化和胆汁淤积而降低，因为这几种疾病都会降低转运体的效能[18]。肝胆管造影剂被主要应用于中心性肝脏病灶的定性，且有研究表明普美显可为转移瘤的探测提供额外信息。普美显同时被证明有助于显示胆管结构，原因是它可以大量进入胆管。HCC 中肝胆管造影剂的作用尚存在争议，我们会在后续篇幅对此进行讨论。

MRI 用于肝脏评估的主要优势在于诊断准确率高、分辨率高、非侵入性胆管检查以及无电离辐射。此外，还有一个优点就是钆造影剂无肾毒性。MRI 的主要劣势在于患者适用性。患者不适宜进行 MRI 检查的主要原因有含铁植入设备的使用、幽闭恐惧症、严重腹水以及无法遵循闭气要求。有大量腹水的患者在 MRI 前应先穿刺。此外，为了提高图像质量，患者需具备制动并闭气 15~18 秒的能力。因患者不适造成的身体移位和闭气失败是影响图像质量的主要原因，严重情况下可能导致无法作出诊断。

(2) 肾源性纤维化和 MRI 造影剂

尽管 1977 年肾源性纤维化(NSF)即被当作一种疾病报道,但直到最近才发现它可能与在急性或慢性肾功能不全患者身上使用钆造影剂有关。FDA 在 2006 年首次发布了关于钆用于肾功能衰竭患者的安全性建议,随后在 2010 年进行了钆造影剂的黑框警告。NSF 是一种进行性的皮肤病,在其进展过程中,皮肤增厚、硬化,最终导致关节挛缩。许多 NSF 发生在肾小球滤过率(GFR)<15ml/min 并接受肾透析或腹膜透析的患者身上[19]。美国放射学会建议避免在 GFR<45ml/min 的患者身上使用高危的钆造影剂。多数医院制订了相关政策,强调对于危险患者的筛查,并避免在严重脏器功能不全时使用钆造影剂。表 2-4 讨论了华盛顿大学关于钆造影剂和肾功能不全的政策,以及其他需要在使用 MRI 造影剂时注意的事项。

表 2-4 华盛顿大学增强 MRI 指南

肾功能	指南
GFR>30	可用造影剂
GFR<30	评价患者风险收益比以决定是否用替代检查
透析患者(血液透析或腹膜透析)	不建议使用造影剂

4. PET/CT

PET/CT 检查是将 18-氟脱氧葡萄糖(FDG)经血管注射后,通过 CT 对其在局部组织内的分布进行成像。此过程中 CT 影像不仅提供解剖信息,而且也提供了与 PET 相关的衰减信息,从而允许对不同密度组织(软组织、脂肪和骨)内的吸收进行精确的定量估计。FDG 是一种分布在细胞高葡萄糖代谢区域(如恶性肿瘤)的糖衍生物。但是,炎症存在时糖代谢也会增加,所以有时难以区分炎症和肿瘤。患者受到的辐射由注射的放射制剂和 CT 扫描本身的辐射构成。放射制剂通常由尿液排出体外。但是,体内会被肝脏和肠道大量吸收。肝脏的摄取具有多样性,因此对肝脏病灶的成像可能较为困难,特别是当病灶较小时。PET 影像应用的另一个难题是呼吸影响。为了保证图像数量和质量,PET 检查的时间较长(每个扫描部位 90~120 秒),所以 PET 数据的获得是基于自由呼吸时的影像。受自由呼吸的影响,横膈和肝脏的运动可能导致图像分辨率下降,模糊不清(使内在分辨率由 4mm 下降到 11mm)[20-22]。其结果是小病灶(<1cm)者较难发现。

三、肝脏肿瘤影像学检查

1. 肝细胞癌

HCC 是最常见的肝脏原发恶性肿瘤,它主要起源于慢性肝病。尽管关于影像和实验室检查联合应用于筛查存在争议,但是对高危人群的筛查是必要的,因为 HCC 的早期治疗有较好的生存获益[2,23-26]。图2-3显示了AASLD最新的HCC筛查的诊断指南[2]。

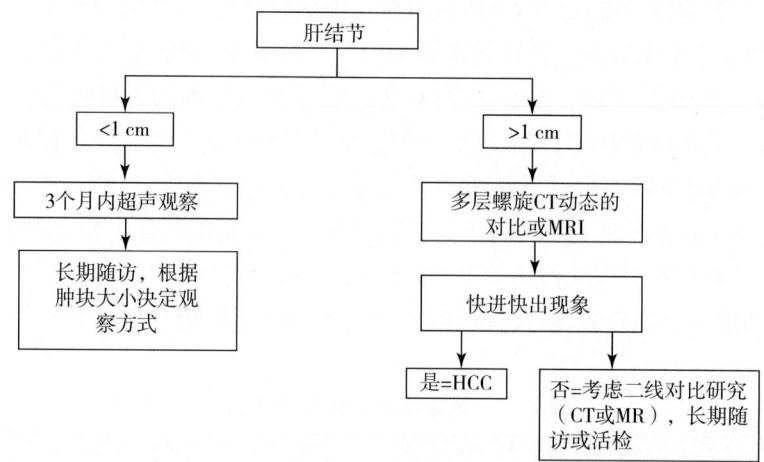

图2-3 AASLD的HCC诊断指南

[Bruix J, Sherman M. Management of hepatocellular carcinoma: an update. Hepatology 2011;53(3):1021.]

HCC有公认的影像学特点,包括快进快出和假包膜(图2-4)。当两者都存在时,HCC的确诊可以不需要病理证实。一些国家和国际组织给出了HCC的影像诊断标准。美国放射学会制定了一套HCC诊断的词典式系统,并命名为肝脏影像报告和数据系统(LI-RADS)[27]。表2-5展示了LI-RADS体系中HCC诊断的主要标准。LI-RADS针对全部危险人群,而不

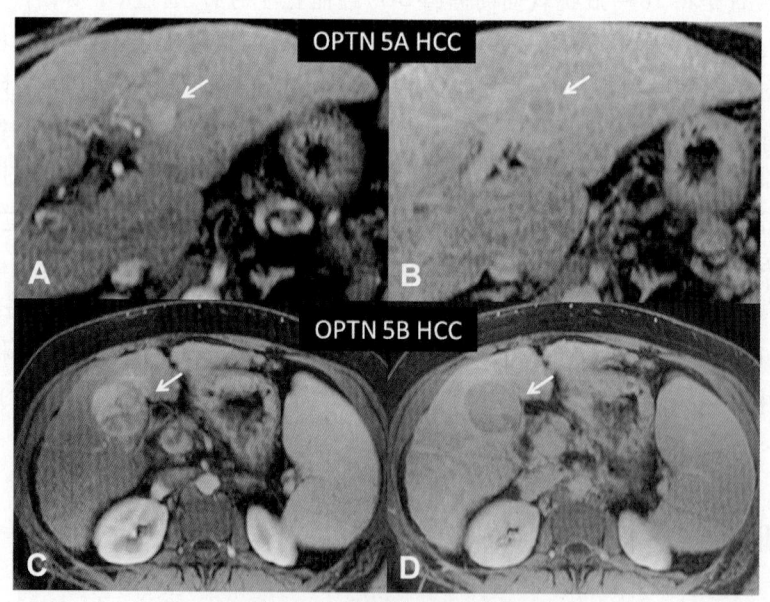

图2-4 典型的HCC征象

A. 动脉期,B. 延迟期,C. 动脉期,D. 延迟期。患者1动脉期和延迟期(A和B)显示1.8cm的病灶,伴有快进快出和包膜征象(箭头所示)。患者2动脉期和延迟期(C和D)显示3cm的病灶,伴有快进快出征象(箭头所示)

仅仅是可进行肝移植的患者。因此，对于那些无法确切诊断的病灶，它提供了一套从明确良性到可能为 HCC 的风险评估量表(表 2-6)。

表 2-5 OPTN 和 LI-RADS 的 HCC 分类。2014 年最新的 LI-RADS 版本采用了 OPTN 增长标准，并统一了 LR-5 和 OPTN5 分类

分类	特点	评价
OPTN 5B	直径 >2cm 且 <5cm 动脉晚期强化 以及下述征象之一： 快进快出、包膜，或 6 个月内增大 >50%[a]	构成肝移植术排除标准
OPTN 5A	直径 ≥1cm 且 <2cm 动脉晚期强化 以下所有征象： 快进快出和包膜	构成 HCC 诊断标准，可适用于肝外转移（如果患者符合 T2 标准）
OPTN 5A-g	直径 ≥1cm 且 <2cm； 动脉晚期强化； 6 个月内增大 >50%[a]	构成 HCC 诊断标准，可适用于肝外转移（如果患者符合 T2 标准）
LI-RADS 5	和 OPTN 5A/B 相同**	尽管未得到 UNOS/OPTN 官方认可用于肝移植，但具有相似性

[a] 可定义增大界值。
** LI-RADS v2014 与 OPTN 病灶增长标准达成了一致。
引自：Wald C, Russo MW, Heimbach JK, et al. New OPTN/UNOS policy for liver transplant allocation: standardization of liver imaging, diagnosis, classification, and reporting of hepatocellular carcinoma. Radiology 2013;266(2):376-82.

表 2-6 U-RADS 定义非 HCC 病灶的标准

LI-RADS 分类	评价	可选诊疗措施
LR-1(确定良性)	可确诊良性肿瘤 ・血管瘤，囊肿，纤维瘤	继续随访
LR-2(可能良性)	倾向良性肿瘤诊断 ・局限性脂肪蓄积，假性肥厚，局限性瘢痕	继续随访
LR-3(中等怀疑 HCC)	影像征象无法鉴别良恶性 ・结节性动静脉瘘，肝硬化结节	结合临床制定个性化随访策略
LR-4(高度怀疑 HCC)	影像征象倾向 HCC 但未达诊断标准	密切随访，并考虑活检或诊断性治疗
LR-M(高度怀疑恶性，但未能确诊是否 HCC)	影像征象显示非 HCC 恶性肿瘤 胆管癌，混合细胞癌	多学科会诊，结合血清标志物，考虑活检

引自 American College of Radiology. Liver imaging reporting and data system version 2013.1. Available at: http://www.acr.org/Quality-Safety/Resources/LIRADS/. Accessed August 2014.

除了 LI-RADS,美国器官捐献网(UNOS)和器官获取网(OPTN)在 2013 年为 HCC 提供了针对性的诊断标准。UNOS/OPTN 历来重视为肿瘤的 T 分级提供指南(符合或不符合米兰标准,T2 分级)[28]。遵循惯例,影像学报告只需证实 HCC 存在而无对说明诊断依据的严格要求。然而,UNOS 数据的回顾性研究对比了影像学报告和病理学报告,其结果表明前者的准确率欠佳,假阳性比例高[29-31]。鉴于准确定性的重要性以及 HCC 患者作为终末期肝病在各方面享受到的优先权,OPTN/UNOS 提出了一套可进行肝移植的 HCC 患者的影像学诊断标准[9]。如果某个病灶在 MRI 或 CT 上符合 HCC 的诊断标准,且患者符合 T2 分级(单个病灶 <5cm 或不超过 3 个 1~3cm 的病灶),则该患者可不经病理诊断在器官排序上获得额外加分。目前,有一项针对 OPTN 分类可接受移植病灶的准确性进行研究的临床试验(ACRIN 6690)。

尽管这些体系高度相似,但 OPTN 体系提供了分类(是否 HCC)的双重标准,因其旨在选择移植候选者并自动给予其额外加分。LI-RADS 针对全部危险人群,因此对临床实践中病灶的定性和风险评估提供了更为全面的指南。

尽管 HCC 有多种影像学和调查量表,CT 和 MRI 之间的选择依然是由医生作出,且无统一标准,而且根据当地影像医生的惯例进行。大量文献指出,MRI 比 CT 有更高的诊断准确性,但是,这些文献中的多数是基于小样本单中心回顾性研究得出的[32-34]。一项基于 15 个比较增强 CT 和 MRI 的 meta 分析指出,与 CT 相比,MRI 敏感性和特异性更好(CT 分别为 91% 和 81%;MRI 分别为 95% 和 93%),特别是对于小肝癌病灶(<2cm)的检测诊断[35]。在一项比较 CT、US 和 MRI 的前瞻性试验中,对于 140 例经病理证实的病变患者而言,动态增强 MRI 准确率高达 83%,而 CT 和 US 分别只有 80% 和 72%(各组间比较 $P<0.001$)[36]。随着肝胆管期扫描的应用,MRI 的准确率提高至 90%。所有检查方法对于小病灶的准确率都较低,特别是对于 <1cm 的病灶。

肝胆造影增强 MRI 在 HCC 诊断中具有重要意义,但也存在争议。大量 HCC 缺乏钆塞酸转运体,因此在肝胆管期显示为低信号。早期 HCC 和小 HCC 在建立丰富血供前表现为肝胆管期的低信号[37,38]。这是其与传统造影剂相比存在优势的机制。但是,钆塞酸增强 MRI 也存在短板。早期 HCC 和肝硬化结节在其中表现较为相似,这可能导致假阳性诊断,且少量 HCC 摄取造影剂并在肝胆管期表现为高信号[39-41]。鉴于这些缺点,且特异性比敏感性更为重要,目前 OPTN 的量表是基于细胞外(传统型)MRI 造影剂给出的。HCC 影像学中肝胆管造影剂的作用是有争议的,不同影像学中心有不同的意见。在我们机构(存在大量移植候选人),肝胆管造影剂不作为常规使用,仅在存在诊断问题时使用。

2. 胆管癌

ICC 起源于胆管上皮细胞,其大体类型有 3 种:胆管周围浸润型、乳头(管内)型和肝内肿块型。美国 ICC 的最常见致癌因素是原发性硬化性胆管炎(PSC);但是,任何慢性炎症状态(如感染、胆石症、病毒性肝炎和胆总管囊肿)都会增加致癌风险[42]。与 HCC 不同,ICC 高危患者的筛查尚缺乏官方指南[43,44]。有人提出以血清 CA19-9 作为诊断依据,当诊断界值定为 100U/ml 时,其敏感性为 53%,阴性预测值为 76%~92%[45]。在一项包含了 230 例 PSC 患者的单中心前瞻性研究中,23 例发展为 ICC,影像和 CA19-9 的结合筛查有效。但是,关于其对生存获益或花费－受益的作用尚缺乏数据[46]。因为缺乏强有力的证据，许多临床医生选择以MRI/MR 胰胆管造影（MRCP）或 US 来作为非侵入性筛查方法。当发现新生狭窄或肿物时，直接内镜逆行胰胆管造影术（ERCP）结合原位刮片甚至荧光染色可用来诊断 ICC[47]。

MRCP 是胆管系统最佳的非侵入性检查方式，它可以鉴别恶性狭窄，并提供胆道和血管受累的分期信息以及肝内肿瘤的准确病变特征。图 2－5 显示的是典型的肝门部巨块状 ICC。外周动脉强化、渐进性中央强化、弥漫性狭窄、胆管阻塞都是 ICC 的典型特征[48,49]。此外，因 ICC 有纤维化基质，所以其在 MRI 上尚有相关的其他表现，如包膜回缩以及 T2 的低信号。尽管这些影像学征象常提示 ICC，但其确诊仍然依赖穿刺病理检查。

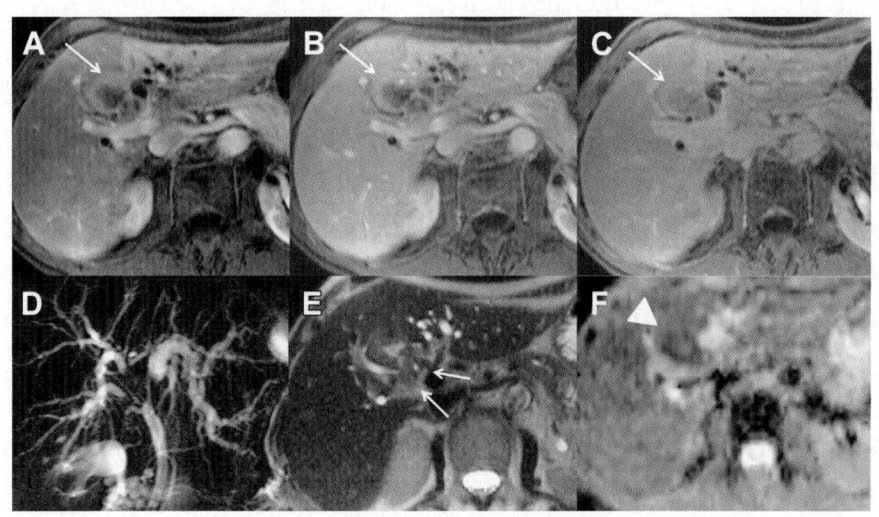

图 2－5　胆管细胞癌

A. 动脉期，B. 门静脉期，C. 延迟期。弥散加权序列（ADC）明确显示该病灶弥散受限，ADC 图像上显示为低信号（箭头所示）。动脉期、门静脉期和延迟期图像显示肝内肿块（箭头）为肝门部胆管细胞癌。MRCP（D）清晰显示右前、后胆管以及左后胆管分支受累。T2 加权（E）显示肝门部胆管的软组织浸润（箭头）。弥散 ADC 图像（F）显示病灶限制弥散（箭头），此为胆管癌特征

ICC 中影像学检查的主要作用是对患者进行分期，从而确定其是否可接受手术切除。ICC 常见于肝门部，根据其对左右肝胆管的侵犯程度尚可依据 Bismuth 分级进行细分[50]。肿瘤和肝动脉以及门静脉的关系也会影响可切除性[51,52]。高质量的 MRI 可提供这些信息，但是当患者体位变动和空间分辨率影响到图像质量时，可采取如薄层增强 CT 或聚焦多普勒/灰阶超声进行辅助检查，以清晰显示血管。MRCP 分级的准确率为 81%～96%，当出现分级错误时，很可能是由于低估了胆管受累的程度[53-58]。CT 对无法切除的阴性预测率较高，达 85%～100%[59-62]。外科干预的目的是达到 R0 切除，因为根据文献报道，当切缘阳性时，切除后的 5 年生存率很低[51]。

尽管如 CT 和 MRCP 等的非侵入性检查一般可以清晰显示胆管系统，但是当患者被植入支架或合并胆道炎症时，对 ICC 的侵袭性很难进行准确估计。在对 ICC 进行干预或支架植入

前建议先进行高质量的影像学检查。当患者有高度胆道狭窄时,可经 ERCP 植入支架。但是向阻塞的胆道注射造影剂可能会导致患者发生胆管炎,因此,超越狭窄部位的造影仅能作为次要选择。如果手术需要对狭窄后部进行检查,当 MRCP 显影不清时,可以考虑经皮肝穿刺胆道造影或支架植入。

除了对原发肿瘤的可切除性进行定性,ICC 的预后因素还包括腹膜侵犯、肝内卫星结节和局部淋巴结。CT 和 MRI 探测淋巴结的敏感性和特异性都有限。PSC 患者通常都有慢性淋巴结肿大,所以淋巴结的大小对转移的预测价值有限。一些研究证实,PET/CT 可改善淋巴结分级并鉴别远处转移,从而导致 17%~30% 患者的治疗措施发生改变[63,64]。在一项包括 123 名被影像诊断为可切除 ICC 患者的研究中,PET/CT 改变了 15.9% 患者的治疗措施,其原因主要是准确检测到局部淋巴结转移(经病理切片证实 PET/CT 为 76%,CT 为 61%)和远处转移(PET/CT 为 88%,CT 为 79%)[65]。PET/CT 有助于排除那些原计划接受切除但实际已处于晚期的患者,但是我们不将其作为常规检查。当存在轻度增大、定性不清的门静脉周围淋巴结时,US 引导下内镜活检可以提供确切诊断。尽管术前检查分辨率较高,但是对于高分级肿瘤(T2 或 T3 病变)患者,分期腹腔镜检查仍然是必要的[66]。较高比例的患者虽经影像评估为可切除,但腹腔镜下的评估最终改变了治疗方案。由于影像检查的进步,这一比例近年来有所下降[67]。

3. 转移性疾病:结直肠癌(CRC)

对局限在肝脏的病灶进行准确分析对治疗至关重要。动态增强 CT 和 MRI 是最常见的肝脏相关检查,两者的敏感性和特异性俱佳(敏感性分别为 73% 和 82%,特异性分别为 97% 和 93%)[68]。图 2-6 显示了一位结直肠癌患者肝脏多发转移。MRI 肝胆管期对病灶的显示最清晰是因为肝脏脂肪变性的存在。在已知为原发性结肠恶性肿瘤时,其对转移的诊断特异性较高。但是,如果是偶然发现的,这种影像学表现就不具有特异性,容易和其他腺癌如 ICC 及其他癌症转移灶相混淆。

文献报道选择合适的 CT 扫描参数、多期增强和多探头 CT 是提高准确性的关键[69,70]。由于缺乏高对比性研究,尚无法确定哪种影像学检查最适宜筛查 CRC 肝转移灶。但是现存的证据显示,当存在肝脂肪变性并结合肝胆管期以及弥散加权图像时,MRI 的准确率较高[71-76]。在一项包含 242 例接受结直肠癌肝转移切除术患者的回顾性研究中,那些术前进行肝胆管 MRI 扫描者术后肝内复发率较低(48% vs 55%,$P=0.04$;接受肝胆管期 MRI 者 n=92,未接受者 n=150),这一数据表明肝胆管期 MRI 可提高分级准确率[75]。MRI 的高昂费用是阻碍其应用的原因之一。但是对于那些因接受化疗而合并肝脂肪变性和准备接受复杂外科手术的患者而言,我们推荐 MRI 检查。对于此类合并肝脂肪变性的患者,它排查转移灶的敏感性较高。当多期 CT 被正确应用时,也可以提供相似信息,因此在其他癌症中心它被用于排查和随访肝转移灶[77]。

CRC 中 PET/CT 的应用较有争议。与增强 CT 或 MRI 相比,其逐个筛查肝转移灶的准确率较低。但是 PET/CT 的价值在于发现妨碍肝切除的肝外转移灶。PET/CT 的发现可导致 8%~10% 患者的治疗措施发生改变[78-80]。但是对于此类情况应谨慎处理,因为 PET 的

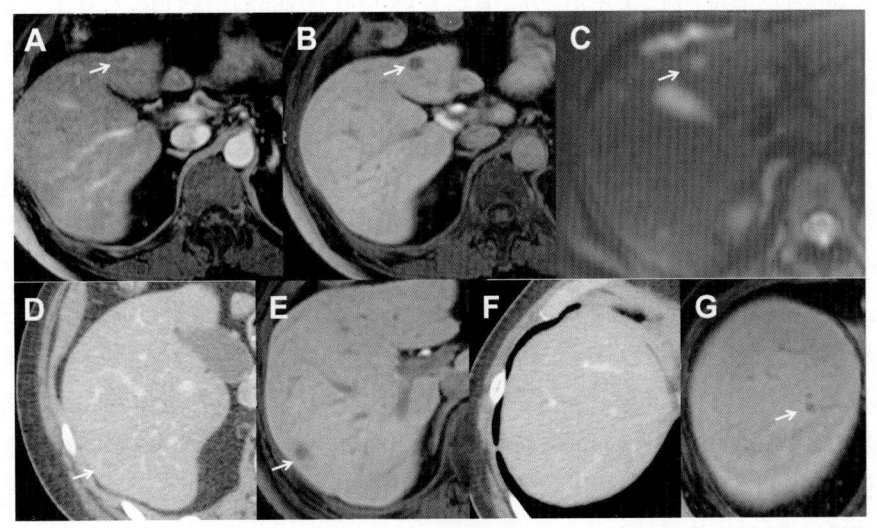

图 2-6 结直肠癌转移灶

动脉期(A)和肝胆管期(B)增强后图像显示转移灶(箭头所示)有早期环形强化并在肝胆管期呈现低密度。该病灶在弥散加权图像上清晰可见(C)。此患者合并肝脂肪变性,对于2个额外转移灶(箭头所示),CT图像(D、F)显影效果有限,而MRI肝胆管期图像显示清晰(E、G)

发现不具有特异性,并可能对最多9%患者的治疗产生消极影响[78]。因为花费高昂且可能出现不明确的结果,将PET/CT作为常规检查可能无法使患者受益。对于选择后的病例,当肝外摄取的可能性与复杂肝切除的风险性相抵消时,PET/CT有助于阻止无效的肝切除。在我们的临床实践中,当存在肝外播散的患者准备接受分步或复杂肝切除时,可行PET/CT检查。

近年来,CRC转移灶影像学检查面临的一个难点是病灶消失,随着系统治疗的改进,这种情况越来越普遍。一些以PET/CT进行的研究证实,最多只有64%的影像学完全缓解与镜检和病理检查的完全缓解存在关联[81-83]。其他研究显示影像学完全缓解和病理反应相关性更差[84,85]。随着影像学检查的敏感性升高,特别是肝胆管MRI的出现,转移灶消失的定义需要重新修订。Kessel及其同事[86]进行的一项meta分析对比了MRI、CT和PET/CT对化疗后转移灶的诊断价值。MRI的敏感性是85.7%,CT为69.9%,PET/CT为51.7%。Auer及其同事[82]进行的一项研究显示,CT显示消失的病灶可在后续MRI上重新出现,术前未行MRI检查会导致术中发现原本被认为消失的病灶的概率增加。最近,Bischof及其同事[87]在其综述中对与病灶消失相关的争议进行讨论。尽管存在治疗方面的争议,但是证据显示,对于化疗后准备接受肝切除的患者,肝胆管增强MRI可能是最佳选择。

4. 术前和消融计划的影像学检查

(1) 评估剩余肝脏的状况

术前检查的目的之一是估计术后肝脏保留(FLR)是否足够及其功能。术前肝功能不足者,约三分之一肝切除术后会出现肝衰竭,这种情况最常见于肝硬化[88-90]。CT和MRI都可以筛查肝脂肪变性,后者对接受半肝切除术患者的 FLR 功能和代偿性肥大有重要的预测作用。对全肝或部分肝脏体积的计算可以上述任何一种形式完成,但最佳时期是门静脉期,因为此时肝动脉和门静脉都能很好地显影。有共识认为肝脏正常患者安全的 FLR 界限为 20%;当存在包括与化疗相关的肝病背景时,FLR 的安全界限无法确切界定,建议保留 30%～40%[91,92]。当患者 FLR 体积为边界值或不足时,可以通过门静脉栓塞(PVE)来诱导剩余肝脏的增生以便于肝切除。尽管多数人认为应以全肝体积为标准计算 FLR 是否足够,但是最近 Shindoh 和同事的研究表明[90],动态增长率(KGR)可以更好地预测术后肝功能是否足够。研究者定义 KGR 为 PVE 后首次肝脏增生除以 PVE 后的天数。他们发现,周 KGR≥2% 可以预防肝并发症和肝功能衰竭相关死亡。所有考虑接受肝切除的患者应有足够的术前肝脏体积,而对于那些 FLR 体积为边界值和/或存在肝病背景者,应以手术诱导肝脏增生。一些研究表明,普美显增强 CT、^{99m}Tc mebrofenin 扫描以及吲哚菁绿清除试验可以为 FLR 提供直接数据。在我们机构,为了明确纤维化或 PVE 和/或肝切除术前功能储备,可以行活检以避免肝衰竭。

(2)消融计划的特殊因素

如果可行手术时,手术切除要优于消融。但当患者存在禁忌证、先前已接受切除或肝功能储备不足时,消融可能是更好的选择。当考虑以局部消融治疗肝脏恶性肿瘤时,需要通过影像学检查明确病灶与胆管、血管、邻近器官(横膈、肠道和皮下组织)的位置关系,也需要测量病灶的大小以明确是否可取得足够的消融边界。CT 和 MRI 都可为明确病灶和周围结构的关系提供足够质量的图像。增强 MRI 显示胆道的效果更好;而且门静脉期图像也可以提供胆道和门脉三联管(与门静脉分支伴行的胆管)的解剖位置关系。热消融技术,如微波和射频消融等可受到热沉效应的阻碍,后者指当病灶靠近大血管时,因热量流失导致的治疗效果降低[93,94]。此效应对射频消融的影响超过对微波消融的影响。对射频技术的选择通常决定于病灶直径、位置、相邻器官和术者的经验。消融前的影像检查应侧重于病灶和周围结构的三维关系,CT 和 MRI 都可以做到这点。图 2-7 显示了消融术后并发症的实例。

四、总结

随着影像技术的进步,外科医生和临床工作者可以选择更多方式来确定肝脏肿瘤的可切除性。对每种影像学检查方法优缺点的了解是必要的。包括诊断性和介入性影像学在内的多学科合作有助于复杂病例的诊断、分期和治疗。

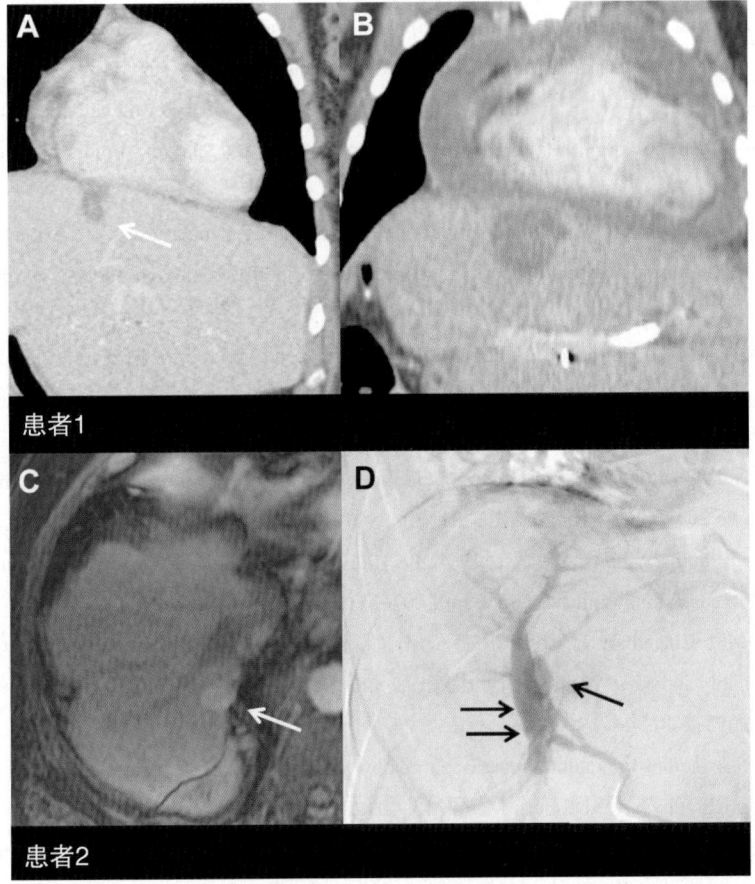

图2-7 消融的并发症

A. 患者1接受2段病灶射频消融[复发性CCA转移（箭头所示）]。B. 由于病灶靠近心脏，导致心包膜受损，心包积血，并需心包穿刺处理。C. 患者2接受冷冻消融术治疗7段HCC（箭头所示）。D. 因肝动脉假性动脉瘤导致胆道出血[血管造影（黑箭头所示）]和胆瘘（双重黑箭头所示），后续以钢圈封堵

参考文献

[1] Claudon M, Dietrich CF, Choi BI, et al. Guidelines and good clinical practice recommendations for contrast enhanced ultrasound (CEUS) in the liver – pdate 2012: a WFUMB – EFSUMB initiative in cooperation with representatives of AFSUMB, AIUM, ASUM, FLAUS and ICUS. Ultraschall Med 2013;34(1): 11 – 29.

[2] Bruix J, Dietrich CF, Choi B, et al. Management of hepatocellular carcinoma: an update. Hepatology 2011;53(3):1020 – 2.

[3] Bae KT. Intravenous contrast medium administration and scan timing at CT: considerations and approaches. Radiology 2010;256(1):32 – 61.

[4] Bae KT, Heiken JP, Brink JA. Aortic and hepatic contrast medium enhancement at CT. Part I. Prediction with a computer model. Radiology 1998; 207(3):647 – 55.

[5] Pomfret EA, Washburn K, Wald C, et al. Report of a national conference on liver allocation in patients with hepatocellular carcinoma in the United States. Liver Transpl 2010;16(3):262-78.

[6] Archer SG, Gray BN. Vascularization of small liver metastases. Br J Surg 1989; 76(6):545-8.

[7] Ackerman NB, Lien WM, Kondi ES, et al. The blood supply of experimental liver metastases. I. The distribution of hepatic artery and portal vein blood to "small" and "large" tumors. Surgery 1969;66(6):1067-72.

[8] Lien WM, Ackerman NB. The blood supply of experimental liver metastases. II. A microcirculatory study of the normal and tumor vessels of the liver with the use of perfused silicone rubber. Surgery 1970;68(2):334-40.

[9] Wald C, Russo MW, Heimbach JK, et al. New OPTN/UNOS policy for liver transplant allocation: standardization of liver imaging, diagnosis, classification, and reporting of hepatocellular carcinoma. Radiology 2013;266(2):376-82.

[10] JSN, JRS and JCS Joint Working Group. Guidelines on the use of iodinated contrast media in patients with kidney disease 2012. Jpn J Radiol 2013;31(8): 546-84.

[11] Mehta RL, Kellum JA, Shah SV, et al. Acute Kidney Injury Network: report of an initiative to improve outcomes in acute kidney injury. Crit Care 2007;11(2):R31.

[12] Davenport MS, Khalatbari S, Cohan RH, et al. Contrast material-induced nephrotoxicity and intravenous low-osmolality iodinated contrast material: risk stratification by using estimated glomerular filtration rate. Radiology 2013;268(3):719-28.

[13] Traub S. Risk factors for radiocontrast nephropathy after emergency department contrast-enhanced computerized tomography. Acad Emerg Med 2013; 20(1):40-5.

[14] Wile GE, Leyendecker JR. Magnetic resonance imaging of the liver: sequence optimization and artifacts. Magn Reson Imaging Clin N Am 2010;18(3): 525-47, xi.

[15] van Montfoort JE, Stieger B, Meijer DK, et al. Hepatic uptake of the magnetic resonance imaging contrast agent gadoxetate by the organic anion transporting polypeptide Oatp1. J Pharmacol Exp Ther 1999;290(1):153-7.

[16] Leonhardt M, Keiser M, Oswald S, et al. Hepatic uptake of the magnetic resonance imaging contrast agent Gd-EOB-DTPA: role of human organic anion transporters. Drug Metab Dispos 2010;38(7):1024-8.

[17] Nassif A, Jia J, Keiser M, et al. Visualization of hepatic uptake transporter function in healthy subjects by using gadoxetic acid-enhanced MR imaging. Radiology 2012;264(3):741-50.

[18] Lee NK, Kim S, Kim GH, et al. Significance of the "delayed hyperintense portal vein sign" in the hepatobiliary phase MRI obtained with Gd-EOB-DTPA. J Magn Reson Imaging 2012;36(3):678-85.

[19] Cowper SE, Rabach M, Girardi M. Clinical and histological findings in nephrogenic systemic fibrosis. Eur J Radiol 2008;66(2):191-9.

[20] Mawlawi O, Townsend DW. Multimodality imaging: an update on PET/CT technology. Eur J Nucl Med Mol Imaging 2009;36(Suppl 1):S15-29.

[21] Alessio AM, Stearns CW, Tong S, et al. Application and evaluation of a measured spatially variant system model for PET image reconstruction. IEEE Trans Med Imaging 2010;29(3):938-49.

[22] Daou D. Respiratory motion handling is mandatory to accomplish the high-resolution PET destiny. Eur J Nucl Med Mol Imaging 2008;35(11):1961-70.

[23] Garcia-Tsao G, Lim JK. Management and treatment of patients with cirrhosis and portal hypertension: recommendations from the Department of Veterans Affairs Hepatitis C Resource Center Program and the National Hepatitis C Program. Am J Gastroenterol 2009;104(7):1802-29.

[24] FerenciP, FriedM, LabrecqueD, et al. WorldGastroenterologyOrganisationGuideline. Hepatocellular carcinoma (HCC): a global perspective. J Gastrointestin Liver Dis 2010;19(3):311-7.

[25] Kudo M, Izumi N, Kokudo N, et al. Management of hepatocellular carcinoma in Japan: Consensus-Based Clinical Practice Guidelines proposed by the Japan Society of Hepatology (JSH) 2010 updated version. Dig Dis 2011;29(3):339-64.

[26] Omata M, Lesmana LA, Tateishi R, et al. Asian Pacific Association for the Study of the Liver consensus recommendations on hepatocellular carcinoma. Hepatol Int 2010;4(2):439-74.

[27] Radiology, A. C. O. Liver Imaging Reporting and Data System (LI-RADS). 2013. Available at: www.acr.org/quality-safety/Resources/LIRADS. Accessed July 1,2013.

[28] Mazzaferro V, Regalia E, Doci R, et al. Liver transplantation for the treatment of small hepatocellular carcinomas in patients with cirrhosis. N Engl J Med 1996;334(11):693-9.

[29] Freeman RB, Mithoefer A, Ruthazer R, et al. Optimizing staging for hepatocellular carcinoma before liver transplantation: a retrospective analysis of the UNOS/OPTN database. Liver Transpl 2006;12(10):1504-11.

[30] Compagnon P, Grandadam S, Lorho R, et al. Liver transplantation for hepatocellular carcinoma without preoperative tumor biopsy. Transplantation 2008;86(8): 1068-76.

[31] Hayashi PH, Trotter JF, Forman L, et al. Impact of pretransplant diagnosis of hepatocellular carcinoma on cadveric liver allocation in the era of MELD. Liver Transpl 2004;10(1):42-8.

[32] Quaia E, De Paoli L, Angileri R, et al. Evidence of diagnostic enhancement pattern in hepatocellular carcinoma nodules </52 cm according to the AASLD/EASL revised criteria. Abdom Imaging 2013;38(6): 1245-53.

[33] Onishi H, Kim T, Imai Y, et al. Hypervascular hepatocellular carcinomas: detection with gadoxetate disodium-enhanced MR imaging and multiphasic multidetector CT. Eur Radiol 2012;22(4):845-54.

[34] Pitton MB, Kloeckner R, Herber S, et al. MRI versus 64-row MDCT for diagnosis of hepatocellular carcinoma. World J Gastroenterol 2009;15(48):6044-51.

[35] Chen L, Zhang L, Bao J, et al. Comparison of MRI with liver-specific contrast agents and multidetector row CT for the detection of hepatocellular carcinoma: a meta-analysis of 15 direct comparative studies. Gut 2013;62(10):1520-1.

[36] Di Martino M, De Filippis G, De Santis A, et al. Hepatocellular carcinoma in cirrhotic patients: prospective comparison of US, CT and MR imaging. Eur Radiol 2013;23(4):887-96.

[37] Rhee H, Kim MJ, Park MS, et al. Differentiation of early hepatocellular carcinoma from benign hepatocellular nodules on gadoxetic acid-enhanced MRI. Br J Radiol 2012;85(1018):e837-44.

[38] Sun HY, Lee JM, Shin CI, et al. Gadoxetic acid-enhanced magnetic resonance imaging for differentiating small hepatocellular carcinomas (< or 52 cm in diameter) from arterial enhancing pseudolesions: special emphasis on hepatobiliary phase imaging. Invest Radiol 2010;45(2):96-103.

[39] Kitao A, Zen Y, Matsui O, et al. Hepatocellular carcinoma: signal intensity at gadoxetic acid-enhanced MR Imaging 束 orrelation with molecular transporters and histopathologic features. Radiology 2010;256

(3):817-26.

[40] Saito K, Kotake F, Ito N, et al. Gd-EOB-DTPA enhanced MRI for hepatocellular carcinoma: quantitative evaluation of tumor enhancement in hepatobiliary phase. Magn Reson Med Sci 2005;4(1):1-9.

[41] Kogita S, Imai Y, Okada M, et al. Gd-EOB-DTPA-enhanced magnetic resonance images of hepatocellular carcinoma: correlation with histological grading and portal blood flow. Eur Radiol 2010;20(10):2405-13.

[42] Yazici C, Niemeyer DJ, Iannitti DA, et al. Hepatocellular carcinoma and cholangiocarcinoma: an update. Expert Rev Gastroenterol Hepatol 2014;8(1):63-82.

[43] Chapman R, Fevery J, Kalloo A, et al. Diagnosis and management of primary sclerosing cholangitis. Hepatology 2010;51(2):660-78.

[44] European Association for the Study of the Liver. EASL Clinical Practice Guidelines: management of cholestatic liver diseases. J Hepatol 2009;51(2):237-67.

[45] Patel AH, Harnois DM, Klee GG, et al. The utility of CA 19-9 in the diagnoses of cholangiocarcinoma in patients without primary sclerosing cholangitis. Am J Gastroenterol 2000;95(1):204-7.

[46] Charatcharoenwitthaya P, Enders FB, Halling KC, et al. Utility of serum tumor markers, imaging, and biliary cytology for detecting cholangiocarcinoma in primary sclerosing cholangitis. Hepatology 2008;48(4):1106-17.

[47] Barr Fritcher EG, Voss JS, Jenkins SM, et al. Primary sclerosing cholangitis with equivocal cytology: fluorescence in situ hybridization and serum CA 19-9 predict risk of malignancy. Cancer Cytopathol 2013;121(12):708-17.

[48] Chung YE, Kim MJ, Park YN, et al. Varying appearances of cholangiocarcinoma: radiologic-pathologic correlation. Radiographics 2009;29(3):683-700.

[49] Maetani Y, Itoh K, Watanabe C, et al. MR imaging of intrahepatic cholangiocarcinomawith pathologic correlation. AJR Am J Roentgenol 2001;176(6):1499-507.

[50] Bismuth H, Corlette MB. Intrahepatic cholangioenteric anastomosis in carcinoma of the hilus of the liver. Surg Gynecol Obstet 1975;140(2):170-8.

[51] Jarnagin WR, Fong Y, DeMatteo RP, et al. Staging, resectability, and outcome in 225 patients with hilar cholangiocarcinoma. Ann Surg 2001;234(4):507-17 [discussion:517-9].

[52] Ruys AT, Busch OR, Rauws EA, et al. Prognostic impact of preoperative imaging parameters on resectability of hilar cholangiocarcinoma. HPB Surg 2013;2013:657309.

[53] Vogl TJ, Schwarz WO, Heller M, et al. Staging of Klatskin tumours (hilar cholangiocarcinomas): comparison of MR cholangiography, MR imaging, and endoscopic retrograde cholangiography. Eur Radiol 2006;16(10):2317-25.

[54] Lopera JE, Soto JA, Munera F. Malignant hilar and perihilar biliary obstruction:use of MR cholangiography to define the extent of biliary ductal involvement and plan percutaneous interventions. Radiology 2001;220(1):90-6.

[55] Zidi SH, Prat F, Le Guen O, et al. Performance characteristics of magnetic resonance cholangiography in the staging of malignant hilar strictures. Gut 2000; 46(1):103-6.

[56] Yeh TS, Jan YY, Tseng JH, et al. Malignant perihilar biliary obstruction: magnetic resonance cholangiopancreatographic findings. Am J Gastroenterol 2000; 95(2):432-40.

[57] Manfredi R, Brizi MG, Masselli G, et al. Malignant biliary hilar stenosis: MR cholangiography compared with direct cholangiography. Radiol Med 2001; 102(1-2):48-54 [in Italian].

[58] Altehoefer C, Ghanem N, Furtwängler A, et al. Breathhold unenhanced and gadolinium-enhanced magnetic resonance tomography and magnetic resonance cholangiography in hilar cholangiocarcinoma. Int J Colorectal Dis 2001; 16(3):188-92.

[59] Lee HY, Kim SH, Lee JM, et al. Preoperative assessment of resectability of hepatic hilar cholangiocarcinoma: combined CT and cholangiography with revised criteria. Radiology 2006;239(1):113-21.

[60] Aloia TA, Charnsangavej C, Faria S, et al. High-resolution computed tomography accurately predicts resectability in hilar cholangiocarcinoma. Am J Surg 2007;193(6):702-6.

[61] Tillich M, Mischinger HJ, Preisegger KH, et al. Multiphasic helical CT in diagnosis and staging of hilar cholangiocarcinoma. AJR Am J Roentgenol 1998; 171(3):651-8.

[62] Cha JH, Han JK, Kim TK, et al. Preoperative evaluation of Klatskin tumor: accuracy of spiral CT in determining vascular invasion as a sign of unresectability. Abdom Imaging 2000;25(5):500-7.

[63] Petrowsky H, Wildbrett P, Husarik DB, et al. Impact of integrated positron emission tomography and computed tomography on staging and management of gallbladder cancer and cholangiocarcinoma. J Hepatol 2006;45(1):43-50.

[64] Anderson CD, Rice MH, Pinson CW, et al. Fluorodeoxyglucose PET imaging in the evaluation of gallbladder carcinoma and cholangiocarcinoma. J Gastrointest Surg 2004;8(1):90-7.

[65] Kim JY, Kim MH, Lee TY, et al. Clinical role of 18F-FDG PET-CT in suspected and potentially operable cholangiocarcinoma: a prospective study compared with conventional imaging. Am J Gastroenterol 2008;103(5):1145-51.

[66] Jarnagin WR, Weber S, Tickoo SK, et al. Combined hepatocellular and cholangiocarcinoma: demographic, clinical, and prognostic factors. Cancer 2002; 94(7):2040-6.

[67] Rotellar F, Pardo F. Laparoscopic staging in hilar cholangiocarcinoma: is it still justified? World J Gastrointest Oncol 2013;5(7):127-31.

[68] Bhattacharjya S, Bhattacharjya T, Baber S, et al. Prospective study of contrastenhanced computed tomography, computed tomography during arterioportography, and magnetic resonance imaging for staging colorectal liver metastases for liver resection. Br J Surg 2004;91(10):1361-9.

[69] Onishi H, Murakami T, Kim T, et al. Hepatic metastases: detection with multidetector row CT, SPIO-enhanced MR imaging, and both techniques combined. Radiology 2006;239(1):131-8.

[70] Numminen K, Isoniemi H, Halavaara J, et al. Preoperative assessment of focal liver lesions: multidetector computed tomography challenges magnetic resonance imaging. Acta Radiol 2005;46(1):9-15.

[71] Kulemann V, Schima W, Tamandl D, et al. Preoperative detection of colorectal liver metastases in fatty liver: MDCT or MRI? Eur J Radiol 2011; 79(2):e1-6.

[72] van Kessel CS, van Leeuwen MS, van den Bosch MA, et al. Accuracy of multislice liver CT and MRI for preoperative assessment of colorectal liver metastases after neoadjuvant chemotherapy. Dig Surg 2011;28(1):36-43.

[73] Koh DM, Collins DJ, Wallace T, et al. Combining diffusion-weighted MRI with Gd-EOB-DTPA-enhanced MRI improves the detection of colorectal liver metastases. Br J Radiol 2012;85(1015):980-9.

[74] Macera A, Lario C, Petracchini M, et al. Staging of colorectal liver metastases after preoperative chemo-

therapy. Diffusion – weighted imaging in combination with Gd – EOB – DTPA MRI sequences increases sensitivity and diagnostic accuracy. Eur Radiol 2013;23(3):739 – 47.

[75] Knowles B, Welsh FK, Chandrakumaran K, et al. Detailed liver – specific imaging prior to pre – operative chemotherapy for colorectal liver metastases reduces intra – hepatic recurrence and the need for a repeat hepatectomy. HPB (Oxford) 2012;14(5):298 – 309.

[76] Hammerstingl R, Huppertz A, Breuer J, et al. Diagnostic efficacy of gadoxetic acid (Primovist) – enhanced MRI and spiral CT for a therapeutic strategy: comparison with intraoperative and histopathologic findings in focal liver lesions. Eur Radiol 2008;18(3):457 – 67.

[77] Shindoh J, Loyer EM, Kopetz S, et al. Optimal morphologic response to preoperative chemotherapy: an alternate outcome end point before resection of hepatic colorectal metastases. J Clin Oncol 2012;30(36): 4566 – 72.

[78] Ramos E, Valls C, Martinez L, et al. Preoperative staging of patients with liver metastases of colorectal carcinoma. Does PET/CT really add something to multidetector CT? Ann Surg Oncol 2011;18(9):2654 – 61.

[79] Briggs RH, Chowdhury FU, Lodge JP, et al. Clinical impact of FDG PET – CT in patients with potentially operable metastatic colorectal cancer. Clin Radiol 2011;66(12):1167 – 74.

[80] Llamas – Elvira JM, Rodríguez – Fernádez A, Gutierrez – Sainz J, et al. Fluorine – 18 fluorodeoxyglucose PET in the preoperative staging of colorectal cancer. Eur J Nucl Med Mol Imaging 2007;34(6):859 – 67.

[81] Tanaka K, Takakura H, Takeda K, et al. Importance of complete pathologic response to prehepatectomy chemotherapy in treating colorectal cancer metastases. Ann Surg 2009;250(6):935 – 42.

[82] Auer RC, White RR, Kemeny NE, et al. Predictors of a true complete response among disappearing liver metastases from colorectal cancer after chemotherapy. Cancer 2010;116(6):1502 – 9.

[83] Elias D, Youssef O, Sideris L, et al. Evolution of missing colorectal liver metastases following inductive chemotherapy and hepatectomy. J Surg Oncol 2004; 86(1):4 – 9.

[84] Benoist S, Brouquet A, Penna C, et al. Complete response of colorectal liver metastases after chemotherapy: does it mean cure? J Clin Oncol 2006;24(24): 3939 – 45.

[85] Tan MC, Linehan DC, Hawkins WG, et al. Chemotherapy – induced normalization of FDG uptake by colorectal liver metastases does not usually indicate complete pathologic response. J Gastrointest Surg 2007;11(9):1112 – 9.

[86] van Kessel CS, Buckens CF, van den Bosch MA, et al. Preoperative imaging of colorectal liver metastases after neoadjuvant chemotherapy: a meta – analysis. Ann Surg Oncol 2012;19(9):2805 – 13.

[87] Bischof DA, Clary BM, Maithel SK, et al. Surgical management of disappearing colorectal liver metastases. Br J Surg 2013;100(11):1414 – 20.

[88] Mullen JT, Ribero D, Reddy SK, et al. Hepatic insufficiency and mortality in 1,059 noncirrhotic patients undergoing major hepatectomy. J Am Coll Surg 2007; 204(5):854 – 62 [discussion: 862 – 4].

[89] Kishi Y, Abdalla EK, Chun YS, et al. Three hundred and one consecutive extended right hepatectomies: evaluation of outcome based on systematic liver volumetry. Ann Surg 2009;250(4):540 – 8.

[90] Shindoh J, Truty MJ, Aloia TA, et al. Kinetic growth rate after portal vein embolization predicts posthepatectomy outcomes: toward zero liver – related mortality in patients with colorectal liver metastases and small future liver remnant. J Am Coll Surg 2013;216(2):201 – 9.

[91] Truty MJ, Vauthey JN. Uses and limitations of portal vein embolization for improving perioperative outcomes in hepatocellular carcinoma. Semin Oncol 2010;37(2):102-9.

[92] Abdalla EK, Barnett CC, Doherty D, et al. Extended hepatectomy in patients with hepatobiliary malignancies with and without preoperative portal vein embolization. Arch Surg 2002;137(6):675-0 [discussion: 680-1].

[93] Lu DS, Yu NC, Raman SS, et al. Radiofrequency ablation of hepatocellular carcinoma: treatment success as defined by histologic examination of the explanted liver. Radiology 2005;234(3):954-0.

[94] Brace CL. Radiofrequency and microwave ablation of the liver, lung, kidney, and bone: what are the differences? Curr Probl Diagn Radiol 2009;38(3):135-3.

第三章　适用于原发性和转移性肝脏恶性肿瘤的预后体系

Clifford S. Cho, MD

【关键词】

预后；肝脏；恶性肿瘤；原发性；转移性

要点

- 传统的肿瘤－淋巴结－转移分期模式无法完美阐释原发性和转移性肝癌的疾病生物学。
- 手术切除影响长期生存，因此在原发性和转移性肝癌中，预后体系需结合解剖学和生物学特征评价可切除性。
- 因存在连续变量，一些研究致力于改善个体肿瘤结局预测列线图，并且某些预后因素相比其他更重要。

一、简介

传统的肿瘤－淋巴结－转移（TNM）分期体系是许多上皮性恶性肿瘤分期的基础，这一基础基于以下两个肿瘤生物学的基本观点。首先，肿瘤是渐进性发展的，其特性为原发性肿瘤对组织浸润的范围加大、解剖学深度加深，区域淋巴结的扩散及远处血行播散。其次，在预后方面，淋巴结转移的重要性超过肿瘤在原发部位的进展，远处转移的严重程度超过肿瘤在原发部位或区域性淋巴结的进展。TNM 分期模式虽已成功应用于多种肿瘤的预后，但其在肝脏恶性肿瘤方面效果有限。其中一个原因是,许多肝脏肿瘤的表现为转移性疾病,使得多数患者被划分为Ⅳ期。而此种分期方法无法反映患者在生存方面的巨大差异。同时,淋巴结转移(通常是衡量上皮恶性肿瘤患者预后的重要因素)在原发性和转移性肝癌中较为罕见,其预后意义也不甚明了。此外,肝癌患者的预后通常取决于手术切除的可行性。所以,实用的预后体系应当包含对病灶部位解剖学(如重要血管的受累)及肿瘤分布(例如多个病灶)的评估。同时,许多肝脏恶性肿瘤继发于肝功能受损的背景下,所以在预后方面评估肝功能受损程度与肿瘤大小、数量等传统肿瘤指标同样重要。为了适应预后变量的多样性和异质性,许多非传统的分期和评分系统被用于肝脏恶性肿瘤患者的预后分级。本文对原发性和转移性肝脏恶性肿瘤患者的预后体系做一概述。

二、原发性肝脏恶性肿瘤

1. 肝细胞癌

(1)概论

肝细胞癌(HCC)是全球致死率排名前列的疾病。因为 HCC 伴随的慢性炎症和慢性肝细胞死亡与再生促进其发生发展,所以慢性病毒性肝炎和长期肝硬化患者罹患 HCC 的危险性更高。同时,这些患者的肝脏拥有癌变的适宜环境,并且容易导致多发肿瘤和切除后复发。肝癌的治疗方法包括全身化疗、肝动脉单纯栓塞、化疗栓塞、选择性内部放疗、无水酒精注射、射频或微波热消融术、切除术以及全肝切除术后原位肝移植。多数情况下,患者无法接受激进的干预措施,因此治疗方法的多样化是必需的[1]。

(2)预后变量

回顾性研究表明,传统的肿瘤指标如大小和数量可以反映疾病的进展和最终的预后。基于肿瘤大小和数量,美国器官共享网络和加州大学旧金山分校所制定的标准对适宜接受肝移植的患者进行筛选[2,3]。因为有研究证实孤立性大肝癌切除术后预后良好,因此肿瘤大小和预后的关系很可能不是线性的[4-8]。在这些特定患者中,肿瘤并没有因体积增大表现出更多的转移性倾向,因此其肿瘤可能是惰性的。区域淋巴结(肝门部胆管和肝周)转移的预后意义依旧不明,虽然淋巴结转移是预后不良的标志,但其发病率比较低[9-12]。虽然肝外转移提示预后不良,但是慢性肝病的致癌特性使肝内复发的危险性高于远处转移[13,14]。

肿瘤血管侵犯是切除术和移植术后高复发性的一个预后变量[13,15-23]。虽然肝门或肝血管等大血管侵犯可以在影像学上得以诊断,但在大多数情况下无法排除切除术和移植术前的微血管侵犯。微血管侵犯对预后的重要影响使得一些研究者建议在移植术前对肝癌行常规穿刺活检[24,25]。一些研究者指出,晚期肿瘤分级、血清 AFP 水平显著升高或巨大肿瘤等预后不良因素可提示微血管侵犯[24,26-29]。

因慢性病毒性肝炎/肝硬化和 HCC 之间存在因果关系,所以这些致癌因素是治疗后复发的重要标志物[13,30-34]。此外,因为晚期肝硬化会限制激进的治疗手段,所以诸如 Child - Pugh[35,36]和 MELD(末期肝病)[37]等评分体系可以定量评价肝功能受损,它们对长期生存和治疗过程中的并发症及死亡的预测作用和传统的肿瘤学指标同等重要。例如,尽管一位左肝存在两个HCC病灶、每个3cm、肝功能良好的患者可以接受治愈性治疗,但是另一位仅有单发的2cm的HCC而肝功能受损的患者却无法接受此类治疗。

若干针对HCC切除后的研究表明,围手术期事件,如出血[22,38]以及术后并发症[39]可能直接影响预期的生存结果。

(3)预测系统

早期的分期系统试图将传统的TNM方案应用于肝癌预后(表3-1)。在结合肿瘤大小、数量、血管侵犯等重要预后变量后,1997美国癌症联合会(AJCC)分期系统通过对这3种变量进行复杂的组合分成了10个T分类[40]。国际肝胆胰协会(IHPBA)部分减少了这种复杂性,其依据3项指标的有无(肿瘤最大直径大于2cm,多发性肿瘤,血管侵犯)设计了一个评分系统,分成了4种T类别[41]。这两个体系在肿瘤大小方面都以肿瘤最大直径2cm为分界点。在认识到以5cm为分界点会有更好的分层效果,Vauthey分期系统出现了[42],这种改良被整合入另一个系统——2002美国癌症联合会(AJCC)分期系统。

表3-1 肝癌分期系统纳入的预后变量

分期系统	不良的预后变量
AJCC系统,第五版[40]	肿瘤大小>2cm 多发性肿瘤 双侧肿瘤 微血管侵犯 重要血管侵犯 肝外侵犯
IHPBA系统[41]	肿瘤大小>2cm 多发性肿瘤 血管侵犯
Vauthey系统[42]	肿瘤大小>5cm 多发性肿瘤 微血管侵犯 重要血管侵犯
AJCC系统,第六版[43]	肿瘤大小>5cm 多发性肿瘤 微血管侵犯 重要血管侵犯
Okuda系统[44]	>50%肝实质受累 腹水 血清白蛋白≤3mg/dl 血清胆红素≥3mg/dl

续表

分期系统	不良的预后变量
BCLC 系统[45]	肿瘤大小>3cm
	肿瘤大小>5cm
	多发性肿瘤
	血管侵犯
	肝外侵犯
	症状
	Child-Pugh 分级
CLIP 系统[46]	多发性肿瘤
	>50%肝实质受累
	AFP≥400ng/ml
	门静脉癌栓
JIS[47]	肿瘤大小>2cm
	多发性肿瘤
	血管侵犯
	Child-Pugh 评分

缩写:AJCC, American Joint Committee on Cancer; BCLC, Barcelona Clinic Liver Cancer; CLIP, Cancer of the Liver Italian Program; IHPBA, International Hepato-Pancreato-Biliary Association; JIS, Japanese Integrated System

这些体系中一个潜在的局限性是它们未能将肝功能损伤作为一个预后或治疗选择的依据。1985 年 Okuda 体系做了结合肿瘤特异性和肝功能特异性变量的尝试。它使用了 4 项指标(肿瘤累及大于 50%肝实质,腹水,血清白蛋白≤3mg/dl,血清胆红素≥3mg/dl)将患者分为 3 期(A 期,0 指标;B 期,1~2 项指标;C 期,3~4 项指标),准确地对生存期进行了预后分级。意大利肝癌方案(CLIP)分期体系利用以 Child-Pugh 评价的肝功能、以形态学评估如肿瘤数量和肝实质累及程度评价的肿瘤负荷、AFP、门静脉癌栓建立了 0~6 分的评价体系。巴塞罗那(BCLC)分期系统于 1999 年首次被提出,也整合了肿瘤负荷和肝功能的因素,同时引入一般健康状态(PS)。因此,BCLC 体系可对患者的治疗策略进行分类[45]。A 类患者大多数疾病负荷小,肝功能完好,一般健康状态好,能够进行肝移植术。B 类患者肝功能和一般健康状态良好,但肿瘤负荷超出移植标准,故此类患者通常接受肝切除术。C 类患者的一般健康状态或疾病负荷使得他们不适合接受切除术或移植术,首选经肝动脉治疗。D 类患者的肝功能、一般健康状态和肿瘤负荷使得他们只能接受支持治疗。BCLC 体系对患者适宜治疗方案进行了分类,而不仅仅只是一种预测方式。将传统肿瘤特异性和肝功能特异性指标整合纳入肝癌预后,日本综合系统(JIS)有其自身优点,它将 IHPBA 分期系统和 Child-Pugh 分级整合为一个简单的评分系统,并对肝癌切除术后的生存期进行分级[47]。

2008 年,MSKCC 对 184 名接受部分肝切除术的肝癌患者进行了研究,以此来验证这些预后体系[22]。像预期一样,大多数体系可对总生存期和无复发生存期进行分级。但是,没有任何一个能够给出个体生存期的准确分级。在分析中,研究者用一致性指数来检测每个体系对随机配对患者的长期生存的预测。当检测一对随机患者时,一致性指数为1.0意味着这个体系预测的生存期有100%的准确性;一致性指数为0.5意味着这个体系预测的生存期有50%的准确性。不同体系的一致性指数介于0.54~0.59,只有2002 AJCC分期体系有大于0.5的95%可信区间,提示其他所有分期系统无法对个体的生存期做出分级。在提高预测个体生存期影响因素的尝试中,研究者用数据生成一个预后列线图,并基于预后因素和生存期的关系给予加权评分。用这种方法,一个整合了患者年龄、术中出血量的估计、无瘤边界、卫星病灶、血管侵犯、肿瘤大小和AFP水平的评分系统被用于评估患者的个体生存期和无复发生存期。同时,这一体系体现了变量在预后价值方面的差异,列线图也便于纳入连续变量(如失血量的估计)。肝癌MSKCC列线图在预测总生存期方面的一致性指数是0.74(95%可信区间,0.68~0.80),在预测无复发生存期方面的一致性指数是0.67(95%可信区间,0.61~0.73),表明其能够提高个体生存期预测准确性。

2. 胆管癌

(1)概述

起源于胆管上皮细胞的胆管癌(CCA)可以表现为肝内或肝门变异(肝外胆管癌本文暂不讨论)。胆管癌与丙型肝炎、慢性胆道寄生虫感染、原发性硬化性胆管炎有关,但胆管癌与HCC不同,因其大多非继发于已知的肝细胞或胆道失调背景下。与HCC类似,胆管癌的最佳治疗方法是手术切除,所以,解剖学因素也与预后相关。胆管癌沿着胆道隐匿性纵向生长的能力使我们要尽可能摘除肿瘤,尤其是肝门胆管癌,其最佳治疗不仅要切除胆道肿瘤,还要切除上游的半个肝脏和邻近的胆管根部。除了纵向生长,胆管癌还可以呈放射状生长,通常从胆道侵犯到邻近的组成门管区的门静脉和肝动脉。解剖区域包括肝门,因胆道靠近门静脉和肝静脉,意味着CCA明显累及双侧重要结构时会导致部分CCA无法切除[1]。

(2)预后变量

像其他上皮恶性肿瘤一样,胆管癌似乎也遵循着局部肿瘤进展的模式,从黏膜内侵犯开始,最终侵犯全层。此外,胆管癌易发生肝门区淋巴结转移[1]。和HCC相似,对接受外科切除术的肝癌患者而言,肿瘤大小和数量是可靠的预后指标。胆管癌发生肝门淋巴结转移的概率高于HCC,并且淋巴结转移是严重预后不良因素。肿瘤内淋巴管浸润可提示淋巴结转移,也是预后不良因素[48-50]。生存期差异也和肿瘤分化程度相关[51,52]。血清肿瘤标志物如糖类抗原19-9(CA19-9)、癌胚抗原(CEA)的显著升高,与预后不良相关[53-55]。与HCC相比,胆管癌更容易发生肝外转移,并且预示着预后不良。胆管癌有沿着胆道系统纵向生长的能力,其微观浸润可超过肉眼可识别区。镜下的无瘤切缘与生存期延长相关[56-60]。

(3)预后体系

①肝内胆管癌:CCA有典型的肿瘤进展、淋巴结转移和远处血行播散方式,使其适用于传统的TNM分期(表3-2)。与HCC的分期系统类似,肝内胆管癌的早期分期体系基于肿瘤大小和数量[61]。2001年,来自东京国家癌症中心医院的Okabayashi及其同事[62]对60例接受CCA切除术的患者进行了研究,证实了在多因素分析中,肝门淋巴结转移、多发性肿瘤、肿瘤

相关症状和任何血管结构的微观或宏观浸润均是预后相关因素。利用这些变量,他们提出一个新的分期体系:Ⅰ期是单个肿瘤、无血管侵犯,Ⅱ期是单个肿瘤但存在血管侵犯,ⅢA 期是多发性肿瘤,ⅢB 期是出现淋巴结转移,Ⅳ期是出现远处转移。这个分期体系能够对总生存率和无复发生存率进行分级,使其最终被纳入 AJCC 分期。AJCC 基于肿瘤数量和血管侵犯的有无,提出了 T 分类系统:T3 定义为肿瘤扩散至肝外组织,T4 为弥漫性浸润、胆管周围浸润[63]。一些研究者提议预后因素应当纳入肿瘤的大小[64,65]。2013 年,Wang 及其同事[55]基于 CEA 水平、CA19-9 水平、血管侵犯、淋巴结转移、肝外转移、肿瘤数量和肿瘤最大直径提出了一个预后列线图。这个列线图使用了与 Cho[22]类似的方法,对 367 名接受部分肝切除术的患者进行了分析。结果表明,这种预后列线图优于 AJCC 第七版分期系统(一致性指数 0.74 vs 0.65)。Hyder 等[66]通过对包含 514 名接受切除术的肝内胆管癌患者的国际性数据进行研究,结合了年龄、血管侵犯、淋巴结转移、肿瘤数量、肿瘤最大直径、肝硬化等预后变量,提出了一个一致性指数为 0.69 的类似预后列线图[66]。

表 3-2 肝内胆管癌分期系统纳入的预后变量

分期系统	不良预后变量
UICC 系统	肿瘤大小 >2cm 多发性肿瘤 双侧肿瘤 微血管侵犯 重要血管侵犯
Okabayashi 系统	多发性肿瘤 血管侵犯

②肝门部胆管癌:基于肿瘤大小进行 T 分期的早期 AJCC 分期系统并不能很好地适用于肝门部胆管癌,因为一些小的但是位置不佳的肿瘤是不可切除的(表 3-3)。1975 年,Bismuth 和 Corlette[67]提出了一个肝门部胆管癌的解剖学分类系统,它可被用于确定手术的路径和可切除性。随后 MSKCC 提出一个纳入邻近血管侵犯的替代性 T 分类系统,基于可切除性对患者进行分级[58]。MSKCC 系统也可对预后进行分级,因为不可行切除术患者的生存期比可行切除术的患者更短[60]。基于对肝门内肿瘤侵犯的解剖学认知,最新的肝门部胆管癌 AJCC 分期系统纳入了 MSKCC 分期体系中的因素以确定 T 分期[63]。Bismuth Corlette 和 MSKCC 系统的一个不同点是前者包含更多信息(如右侧与左侧侵犯对比),以进行解剖学描述和手术规划;Deoliveira[68]最近提出一种类似但更全面的解剖学分类方式,它不但有左右两侧的对比、淋巴结转移和远处转移的对比,还包括肿瘤大小、形态学,潜在肝脏疾病,切除后残余肝脏的预期状况,切除肿瘤时胆管、门静脉及肝动脉的受侵范围。

表 3-3 肝门部胆管癌分期系统纳入的预后变量

分期系统	不良预后变量
MSKCC 系统	单侧肝管侵犯
	同侧肝脏萎缩
	同侧门静脉侵犯
	双侧肝管侵犯
	门静脉主干包绕
AJCC 系统,第七版	肿瘤侵犯超出胆管壁脂肪组织
	肿瘤侵犯邻近的肝实质
	单侧门静脉或肝动脉受累
	主要或双侧门静脉侵犯
	普通肝动脉侵犯
	对侧门静脉侵犯
	对侧肝动脉侵犯
	肿瘤侵犯双侧的二级胆管根部
	区域性淋巴结转移
	腹主动脉旁、腔静脉旁、腹腔动脉或肠系膜动脉淋巴结转移

3. 结直肠癌肝转移

(1) 概述

与其他全身播散性癌症的转归不同,结直肠癌肝转移可经手术切除。肝脏通常是结直肠癌唯一的转移部位。肝脏转移瘤患者的长期随访表明,接受肝转移瘤切除的患者中,接近 1/5 的患者有治愈的可能性[69,70]。此外,过去几十年里转移性结直肠癌的治疗和预后大有进步。这些进步中的少数是基于手术和围术期技术的改善,多数得益于全身化疗技术的进步。这些进步使得外科医生能够对曾经不适合行外科治疗的患者进行治愈性干预,并且使转移性结直肠癌患者比过去存活更长时间。这些治疗措施的进步同时改变了预后变量与长期生存率的关系[71-74]。

(2) 预后变量

在结直肠癌肝转移瘤切除后,四大类因素可影响患者预后。第一个涉及原发肿瘤的特征,反映个体肿瘤生物学特性。有几项分析表明,原发肿瘤的变量,如原发灶横向侵犯(>T3)或淋巴结转移(N1),似乎会对转移性疾病切除术后的预后造成影响[75-79],表明原发灶表现出来的疾病生物学内在本质也会影响转移瘤切除后的预后。第二类因素是疾病进展的速度。多项分析发现,与继发转移相比,同步肝转移提示预后不良,且原发灶和转移灶之间的无病间隔时间与转移瘤切除术后的生存期成反比[75-77,79,80]。第三类因素是肿瘤负荷和/或技术可切除性,还包括肿瘤大小、肿瘤数目、双侧侵犯或血清 CEA 水平等变量[75-79,81]。第四类是全身化疗反应性。早期研究表明,肝转移瘤对新辅助化疗的影像学反应与切除术后预后有关[82-84]。随着全身化疗效果增加(化疗后疾病进展的可能性下降),此类变量对预后的影响也随之改变[85]。许多近期研究表明,对特定药物的反应性预测指标(如 K-ras 基因突变状态对西妥昔单抗的疗效预测)可能是具有重要意义的变量[86-88]。

(3) 预后体系

鉴于结直肠癌肝转移的外科干预日益普及,更加需要一套具体的分期系统,以对依据 Duke、Astler-Collins、AJCC 分期为 D 期或 Ⅳ 期患者的生存进行更好的分级。从 20 世纪 90 年代后期开始,有人通过对接受肝转移瘤切除患者的研究,依据影响预后的因素(原发性肿瘤淋巴结转移;原发性肿瘤与转移性肿瘤的间隔时间;肿瘤数目、大小及解剖学分类;CEA 水平)提出若干分期体系。这些评分体系的简要分析表明,它们存在显著的一致性(表 3-4),表明这些研究者独立地对相同的生物特征进行了分析。其中广泛使用的是风险评分系统(CRS)或 Fong 评分系统(以第一次依据对 MSKCC 研究分析提出该体系的作者命名)[77]。Fong 等确定了 7 个预后变量:切缘阳性,存在肝外疾病,原发性肿瘤淋巴结阳性,原发性与转移性之间的无病间隔时间 <12 个月,多灶性(>1 个)肿瘤,肿瘤最大直径 >5cm,CEA 水平 >200ng/ml。在这些变量中,他们剔除了切缘状态(因为术前并不能准确评估)和肝外疾病(这个指标被认为是肝转移瘤切除术的禁忌证)后,使用剩余 5 个变量来创建 0~5 分的评分体系,将患者分为 6 种预后级别。一些研究验证了这个评分体系,并将其作为对预后进行分级的一种方式[93,94]。

表 3-4 结直肠癌肝转移风险评分系统所纳入的预后变量

研究	不良预后变量
Nordlinger 等,1996[89]	年龄≥60 岁 原发肿瘤侵犯浆膜 原发性淋巴结阳性 无病间隔时间≤2 年 肝转移瘤大小≥5cm 肝转移瘤数目≥4 个 肝切除边缘≤1cm
Iwatsuki 等,1999[90]	无病间隔时间≤30 个月 肝转移瘤大小≥8cm 肝转移瘤数目≥2 个 双侧肝转移瘤 肝切除边缘阳性 肝外转移

续表

研究	不良预后变量
Fong 等,1999[77]	原发性淋巴结阳性 无病间隔时间≤1年 肝转移瘤大小≥5cm 肝转移瘤数目≥1个 CEA>200ng/ml
Nagashima 等,2004[91]	原发肿瘤侵犯浆膜 原发性淋巴结阳性 肝转移瘤大小≥5cm 肝转移瘤数目≥1个 可切除的肝外转移瘤
Rees 等,2008[92]	原发性淋巴结阳性 原发性肿瘤分化良好 原发性肿瘤分化差 CEA 6~60 ng/ml CEA>60 ng/ml 肝转移瘤数目≥3个 肝转移瘤大小 5~10cm 肝转移瘤大小≥10cm 肝切除边缘阳性 肝外转移

2008年,Kattan等[95]重新对MSKCC作了分析,进而以一种列线图对接受肝转移瘤切除术患者的生存期进行预测。CRS对每个变量给予相同权重并将其视为分类变量,5个额外的预后变量被加入到列线图中,并对这些变量进行了加权和整合。针对1998年CRS提出后接受治疗患者的研究表明,MSKCC列线图[整合了患者年龄、性别、原发肿瘤部位(结肠或直肠)、无病间隔时间、CEA水平、肿瘤数目、肿瘤最大直径、双侧切除、肿瘤侵犯超过半个肝脏、原发肿瘤的淋巴结状态]的预后效果更佳(一致性指数 0.688 vs 0.648,$P=0.03$)。

早期已证实,随着更新和更有效的化疗方案出现,结直肠腺瘤肝转移患者的预后已经得到了改善。需要注意的是,这些评分体系,包括MSKCC,大多是基于现代全身化疗应用之前患者资料的。近期的研究表明,随着奥沙利铂、伊立替康和生物制剂如贝伐单抗、西妥昔单抗的出现,有些曾经具有预后价值的因素可能不再具有预后意义。例如,一项近期研究表明,在奥沙利铂和伊立替康出现以前,肝转移瘤切除术后的生存期受原发肿瘤的淋巴结状态影响,但这种影响现已不复存在[96]。一项对德州大学安德森癌症中心肝转移瘤切除术前接受新辅助奥沙利铂或伊立替康化疗患者的研究发现,只有手术切缘状态和对化疗的影像学反应与生存相关,这说明,在现在有效的全身化疗得以应用后,大肠癌肝转移的预后有可能被简化为一个技术问题,即其是否可被完全切除[97]。

三、总结

分期体系的作用在于:①了解癌症预后的巨大差异;②预测癌症患者个体生存。肝脏肿瘤的分期和预后一直富有挑战性,因为原发性和转移性肝癌中反映预后和治疗应答的指标一直在改变。随着我们对这些疾病的理解的进步和发展,相应预测体系也会改变。这些进步包括修改传统的 TNM 分期来适应肝癌独特的生物学特征,也包括采纳一些未能纳入 TNM 方案但与预后密切相关的指标。虽然这些体系能够就患者的预后做出不同的分类,近期列线图的使用可使我们从群体预后转变为个体预后。毫无疑问,这一章节里所讨论的预测系统在将来也会继续得以完善。

参考文献

[1] Cho C, Fong Y. Benign and malignant primary liver neoplasms. In: Zinner MJ, Ashley SW, editors. Maingot's abdominal operations. New York: McGraw-Hill; 2013. p. 927-54.

[2] Mazzaferro V, Regalia E, Doci R, et al. Liver transplantation for the treatment of small hepatocellular carcinomas in patients with cirrhosis. N Engl J Med 1996; 334(11):693-9.

[3] Yao FY, Ferrell L, Bass NM, et al. Liver transplantation for hepatocellular carcinoma: expansion of the tumor size limits does not adversely impact survival. Hepatology 2001;33(6):1394-403.

[4] Lee NH, Chau GY, Lui WY, et al. Surgical treatment and outcome in patients with a hepatocellular carcinoma greater than 10 cm in diameter. Br J Surg 1998;85(12):1654-7.

[5] Regimbeau JM, Farges O, Shen BY, et al. Is surgery for large hepatocellular carcinoma justified? J Hepatol 1999;31(6):1062-8.

[6] Poon RT, Fan ST, Wong J. Selection criteria for hepatic resection in patients with large hepatocellular carcinoma larger than 10 cm in diameter. J Am Coll Surg 2002;194(5):592-602.

[7] Pawlik TM, Poon RT, Abdalla EK, et al. Critical appraisal of the clinical and pathologic predictors of survival after resection of large hepatocellular carcinoma. Arch Surg 2005;140(5):450-7.

[8] Liau KH, Ruo L, Shia J, et al. Outcome of partial hepatectomy for large (>10 cm) hepatocellular carcinoma. Cancer 2005;104(9):1948-55.

[9] Uenishi T, Hirohashi K, Shuto T, et al. The clinical significance of lymph node metastases in patients undergoing surgery for hepatocellular carcinoma. Surg Today 2000;30(10):892-905.

[10] Jaeck D. The significance of hepatic pedicle lymph node metastases in surgical management of colorectal liver metastases and of other liver malignancies. Ann Surg Oncol 2003;10(9):1007-11.

[11] Grobmyer SR, Wang L, Gonen M, et al. Perihepatic lymph node assessment in patients undergoing partial hepatectomy for malignancy. Ann Surg 2006;244(2):260-4.

[12] Xiaohong S, Huikai L, Feng Q, et al. Clinical significance of lymph node metastasis in patients undergoing partial hepatectomy for hepatocellular carcinoma. World J Surg 2010;34(5):1028-33.

[13] Cha C, Fong Y, Jarnagin WR, et al. Predictors and patterns of recurrence after resection of hepatocellular

carcinoma. J Am Coll Surg 2003;197(5):753-8.

[14] Yang Y, Nagano H, Ota H, et al. Patterns and clinicopathologic features of extrahepatic recurrence of hepatocellular carcinoma after curative resection. Surgery 2007;141(2):196-202.

[15] Ringe B, Pichlmayr R, Wittekind C, et al. Surgical treatment of hepatocellular carcinoma: experience with liver resection and transplantation in 198 patients. World J Surg 1991;15(2):270-85.

[16] Chen MF, Hwang TL, Jeng LB, et al. Hepatic resection in 120 patients with hepatocellular carcinoma. Arch Surg 1989;124(9):1025-8.

[17] Vauthey JN, Klimstra D, Francheschi D, et al. Factors affecting long-term outcome after hepatic resection for hepatocellular carcinoma. Am J Surg 1995;169(1):28-34.

[18] Lau H, Fan ST, Ng IO, et al. Long term prognosis after hepatectomy for hepatocellular carcinoma: a survival analysis of 204 consecutive patients. Cancer 1998;83(11):2303-11.

[19] Tsai TJ, Chau GY, Lui WY, et al. Clinical significance of microscopic tumor venous invasion in patients with resectable hepatocellular carcinoma. Surgery 2000;127(6):603-8.

[20] Cho CS, Knechtle SJ, Heisey DM, et al. Analysis of tumor characteristics and survival in liver transplant recipients with incidentally diagnosed hepatocellular carcinoma. J Gastrointest Surg 2001;5(6):594-601.

[21] Shah SA, Cleary SP, Wei AC, et al. Recurrence after liver resection for hepatocellular carcinoma: risk factors, treatment, and outcomes. Surgery 2007;141(3):330-9.

[22] Cho CS, Gonen M, Shia J, et al. A novel prognostic nomogram is more accurate than conventional staging systems for predicting survival after resection of hepatocellular carcinoma. J Am Coll Surg 2008;206(2):281-91.

[23] Sumie S, Kuromatsu R, Okuda K, et al. Microvascular invasion in patients with hepatocellular carcinoma and its predictable clinicopathological factors. Ann Surg Oncol 2008;15(5):1375-82.

[24] Esnaola NF, Lauwers GY, Mirza NQ, et al. Predictors of microvascular invasion in patients with hepatocellular carcinoma who are candidates for orthotopic liver transplantation. J Gastrointest Surg 2002;6(2):224-32.

[25] Tamura S, Kato T, Berho M, et al. Impact of histological grade of hepatocellular carcinoma on the outcome of liver transplantation. Arch Surg 2001;136(1):25-30.

[26] Shijo H, Okazaki M. Prediction of portal vein invasion by hepatocellular carcinoma: a correlation between portal vein tumor thrombus and biochemical test. Jpn J Clin Oncol 1991;21(2):94-9.

[27] Pawlik TM, Delman KA, Vauthey JN, et al. Tumor size predicts vascular invasion and histologic grade: Implications for selection of surgical treatment for hepatocellular carcinoma. Liver Transpl 2005;11(9):1086-92.

[28] Cillo U, Vitale A, Navaglia F, et al. Role of blood AFP mRNA and tumor grade in the preoperative prognostic evaluation of patients with hepatocellular carcinoma. World J Gastroenterol 2005;11(44):6920-5.

[29] Cucchetti A, Piscaglia F, Grigioni AD, et al. Preoperative prediction of hepatocellular carcinoma tumour grade and micro-vascular invasion by means of artificial neural network: a pilot study. J Hepatol 2010;52(6):880-8.

[30] Kubo S, Hirohashi K, Tanaka H, et al. Effect of viral status on recurrence after liver resection for patients with hepatitis B virus-related hepatocellular carcinoma. Cancer 2000;88(5):1016-24.

[31] Ahmad SA, Bilimoria MM, Wang X, et al. Hepatitis B or C virus serology as a prognostic factor in patients

[32] Sasai Y, Yamada T, Tanaka H, et al. Risk of recurrence in a long – term follow – up after surgery in 217 patients with hepatitis B – or hepatitis C – related hepatocellular carcinoma. Ann Surg 2006;244(5):771 – 80.

[33] Bozorgzadeh A, Orloff M, Abt P, et al. Survival outcomes in liver transplantation for hepatocellular carcinoma, comparing impact of hepatitis C versus other etiology of cirrhosis. Liver Transpl 2007;13(6):807 – 13.

[34] Cescon M, Cucchetti A, Grazi GL, et al. Role of hepatitis B virus infection in the prognosis after hepatectomy for hepatocellular carcinoma in patients with cirrhosis: a Western dual – center experience. Arch Surg 2009;144(10): 906 – 13.

[35] Child CG, Turcotte JG. Surgery and portal hypertension. In: Child CG, editor. The liver and portal hypertension. Philadelphia: WB Saunders; 1964. p. 50 – 62.

[36] Pugh RN, Murray – Lyon IM, Dawson JL, et al. Transection of the oesophagus for bleeding oesophageal varices. Br J Surg 1973;60(8):646 – 9.

[37] Kamath PS, Wiesner RH, Malinchoc M, et al. A model to predict survival in patients with end – stage liver disease. Hepatology 2001;33(2):464 – 70.

[38] Katz SC, Shia J, Liau KH, et al. Operative blood loss independently predicts recurrence and survival after resection of hepatocellular carcinoma. Ann Surg 2009;249(4):617 – 23.

[39] Kusano T, Sasaki A, Kai S, et al. Predictors and prognostic significance of operative complications in patients with hepatocellular carcinoma who underwent hepatic resection. Eur J Surg Oncol 2009;35(11): 1179 – 85.

[40] American Joint Committee on Cancer. Liver (including intrahepatic bile ducts). In: Fleming ID, et al, editors. AJCC cancer staging manual. Philadelphia: Lippincott – Raven; 1998. p. 98 – 126.

[41] Makuuchi M, Belghiti J, Belli G, et al. IHPBA concordant classification of primary liver cancer: working group report. J Hepatobiliary Pancreat Surg 2003;10(1):26 – 30.

[42] Vauthey JN, Lauwers GY, Esnaola NF, et al. Simplified staging for hepatocellular carcinoma. J Clin Oncol 2002;20(6):1527 – 36.

[43] American Joint Committee on Cancer. Liver (including intrahepatic bile ducts). In: Greene FL, et al, editors. AJCC cancer staging manual. New York: Springer; 2002. p. 131 – 8.

[44] Okuda K, Ohtsuki T, Obata H. Natural history of hepatocellular carcinoma and prognosis in relation to treatment: study of 850 patients. Cancer 1985;56(4): 918 – 28.

[45] Llovet JM, Bru C, Bruix J. Prognosis of hepatocellular carcinoma: the BCLC staging classification. Semin Liver Dis 1999;19(3):329 – 38.

[46] Prospective validation of the CLIP score: a new prognostic system for patients with cirrhosis and hepatocellular carcinoma. The Cancer of the Liver Italian Program (CLIP) Investigators. Hepatology 2000;31(4):840 – 5.

[47] Kudo M, Chung H, Osaki Y, et al. Prognostic staging system for hepatocellular carcinoma (CLIP score): its value and limitations, and a proposal for a new staging system, the Japan Integrated Staging Score (JIS score). J Gastroenterol 2003;38(3):207 – 15.

[48] Weber SM, Jarnagin WR, Klimstra D, et al. Intrahepatic cholangiocarcinoma: resectability, recurrence pattern, and outcomes. J Am Coll Surg 2001;193(4): 384 – 91.

[49] Uenishi T, Hirohashi K, Kubo S, et al. Clinicopathological factors predicting outcome after resection of mass

- forming cholangiocarcinoma. Br J Surg 2001;88(7):969 – 74.

[50] Suzuki S, Sakaguchi T, Yokoi Y, et al. Clinicopathological prognostic factors and impact of surgical treatment of mass – forming intrahepatic cholangiocarcinoma. World J Surg 2002;26(6):687 – 93.

[51] Shirabe K, Mano Y, Taketomi A, et al. Clinicopathological prognostic factors after hepatectomy for patients with mass – forming intrahepatic cholangiocarcinoma: relevance of the lymphatic invasion index. Ann Surg Oncol 2010;17(7):1816 – 22.

[52] Saxena A, Chua TC, Sarkar A, et al. Clinicopathologic and treatment – related factors influencing recurrence and survival after hepatic resection intrahepatic cholangiocarcinoma: a 19 – year experience from an established Australian hepatobiliary unit. J Gastrointest Surg 2010;14(7):1128 – 38.

[53] Ohtsuka A, Ito H, Kimura F, et al. Results of surgical treatment for intrahepatic cholangiocarcinoma and clinicopathological factors influencing survival. Br J Surg 2002;89(12):1525 – 31.

[54] Cho SY, Park SJ, Kim SH, et al. Survival analysis of intrahepatic cholangiocarcinoma after resection. Ann Surg Oncol 2010;17(7):1823 – 30.

[55] Wang Y, Li J, Xia Y, et al. Prognostic nomogram for intrahepatic cholangiocarcinoma after partial hepatectomy. J Clin Oncol 2013;31(9):1188 – 95.

[56] Cherqui D, Tantawi B, Alon R, et al. Intrahepatic cholangiocarcinoma. Results of aggressive surgical management. Arch Surg 1995;130(10):1073 – 8.

[57] Su H, Tsay SH, Wu CC, et al. Factors influencing postoperative morbidity, mortality, and survival after resection for hilar cholangiocarcinoma. Ann Surg 1996;223(4):384 – 94.

[58] Burke EX, Jarnagin WR, Hochwald SN, et al. Hilar cholangiocarcinoma: patterns of spread, the importance of hepatic resection for curative operation, and a presurgical clinical staging system. Ann Surg 1998;228(3):385 – 94.

[59] Tsao JI, Nimura Y, Kamiya J, et al. Management of hilar cholangiocarcinoma: comparison of an American and a Japanese experience. Ann Surg 2000;232(2):166 – 74.

[60] Jarnagin WR, Fong Y, DeMatteo RP, et al. Staging, resectability, and outcome in 225 patients with hilar cholangiocarcinoma. Ann Surg 2001;234(4):507 – 17.

[61] International Union Against Cancer. TNM classification of malignant tumours. New York: Wiley – Liss; 1997.

[62] Okabayashi T, Yamamoto K, Kosuge T, et al. A new staging system for massforming intrahepatic cholangiocarcinoma: analysis of preoperative and postoperative variables. Cancer 2001;92(9):2374 – 83.

[63] American Joint Committee on Cancer. Liver. In: Edge SB, et al, editors. AJCC Cancer Staging Manual. New York: Springer; 2010. p. 191 – 210.

[64] Nathan H, Aloia TA, Vauthey JN, et al. A proposed staging system for intrahepatic cholangiocarcinoma. Ann Surg Oncol 2009;16(10):14 – 22.

[65] Jiang W, Zeng ZC, Tang ZY, et al. A prognostic scoring system based on clinical features of intrahepatic cholangiocarcinoma: the Fudan score. Ann Oncol 2011;22(7):1644 – 52.

[66] Hyder O, Marques H, Pulitano C, et al. A nomogram to predict long – term survival after resection for intrahepatic cholangiocarcinoma: an Eastern and Western experience. JAMA Surg 2014;149(5):432 – 8.

[67] Bismuth H, Corlette MB. Intrahepatic cholangioenteric anastomosis in carcinoma of the hilus of the liver. Surg Gynecol Obstet 1975;140(2):170 – 8.

[68] Deoliveira ML, Schulick RD, Nimua Y, et al. New staging system and a registry for perihilar cholangiocarcinoma. Hepatology 2011;53(4):1363-71.

[69] Tomlinson JS, Jarnagin WR, DeMatteo RP, et al. Actual 10-year survival after resection of colorectal liver metastases defines cure. J Clin Oncol 2007;25(29):4575-80.

[70] Pulitano C, Castillo F, Aldrighette L, et al. What defined 'cure' after liver resection for colorectal metastases? Results after 10 years of follow-up. HPB (Oxford) 2010;12(4):244-9.

[71] Choti MA, Sitzmann JV, Tiburi MF, et al. Trends in long-term survival following liver resection for hepatic colorectal metastases. Ann Surg 2002;235(6):759-66.

[72] Andres A, Majno PE, Morel P, et al. Improved long-term outcome of surgery for advanced colorectal liver metastases: reasons and implications for management on the basis of a severity score. Ann Surg Oncol 2008;15(1):134-43.

[73] House MG, Ito H, Gonen M, et al. Survival after hepatic resection for metastatic colorectal cancer: trends in outcomes for 1,600 patients during two decades at a single institution. J Am Coll Surg 2010;210(5):752-5.

[74] Vigano L, Russolillo N, Ferrero A, et al. Evolution of long-term outcome of liver resection for colorectal metastases: analysis of actual 5-year survival rates over two decades. Ann Surg Oncol 2012;19(6):2035-44.

[75] Schlag P, Hohenberger P, Herfarth C. Resection of liver metastases in colorectal cancer-competitive analysis of treatment results in synchronous versus metachronous metastases. Eur J Surg Oncol 1990;16(4):360-5.

[76] Scheele J, Stang R, Altendort-Hofmann A, et al. Resection of colorectal liver metastases. World J Surg 1995;19(1):59-71.

[77] Fong Y, Fortner J, Sun RL, et al. Clinical score for predicting recurrence after hepatic resection for metastatic colorectal cancer: analysis of 1001 consecutive cases. Ann Surg 1999;230(3):309-21.

[78] Ambiru S, Miyazaki M, Isono T, et al. Hepatic resection for colorectal metastases: analysis of prognostic factors. Dis Colon Rectum 1999;42(5):632-9.

[79] Yamada H, Kondo S, Okushiba S, et al. Analysis of predictive factors for recurrence after hepatectomy for colorectal liver metastases. World J Surg 2001;25(9):1121-33.

[80] Tsai MS, Su YH, Ho MC, et al. Clinicopathological features and prognosis in resectable synchronous and metachronous colorectal liver metastasis. Ann Surg Oncol 2007;14(2):786-94.

[81] Cady B, Stone MD, McDermott WV Jr, et al. Technical and biological factors in disease-free survival after hepatic resection for colorectal cancer metastases. Arch Surg 1992;127(5):561-8.

[82] Allen PJ, Kemeny N, Jarnagin W, et al. Importance of response to neoadjuvant chemotherapy in patients undergoing resection of synchronous colorectal liver metastases. J Gastrointest Surg 2003;7(1):109-15.

[83] Small RM, Lubezky N, Schmueli E, et al. Response to chemotherapy predicts survival following resection of hepatic colo-rectal metastases in patients treated with neoadjuvant therapy. J Surg Oncol 2009;99(2):93-8.

[84] Broquet A, Abdalla EK, Kopetz S, et al. High survival rate after two-stage resection of advanced colorectal liver metastases: response-based selection and complete resection define outcome. J Clin Oncol 2011;29(8):1083-90.

[85] Gallagher DJ, Zheng J, Capanu M, et al. Response to neoadjuvant chemotherapy does not predict overall survival for patients with synchronous colorectal hepatic metastases. Ann Surg Oncol 2009;16(7):1844 – 51.

[86] Khambata – Ford S, Garrett CR, Meropol NJ, et al. Expression of epiregulin and amphiregulin and K – ras mutation status predict disease control in metastatic colorectal cancer patients treated with cetuximab. J Clin Oncol 2007;25(2):3230 – 7.

[87] Karapetis CS, Khambata – Ford S, Jonker DJ, et al. K – ras mutations and benefit from cetuximab in advanced colorectal cancer. N Engl J Med 2008;359(17): 1757 – 65.

[88] Levi F, Karaboue A, Gorden L, et al. Cetuximab and circadian chronomodulated chemotherapy as salvage treatment for metastatic colorectal cancer (mCRC): safety, efficacy and improved secondary surgical resectability. Cancer Chemother Pharmacol 2011;67(2):339 – 48.

[89] Nordlinger B, Guiguet M, Vaillant JC, et al. Surgical resection of colorectal carcinoma metastases to the liver. A prognostic scoring system to improve case selection, based on 1568 patients. Association Francaise de Chirurgie Cancer 1996; 77(7):1254 – 62.

[90] Iwatsuki S, Dvorchik I, Madariaga JR, et al. Hepatic resection for metastatic colorectal adenocarcinoma: a proposal of a prognostic scoring system. J Am Coll Surg 1999;189(3):291 – 9.

[91] Nagashima I, Takada T, Matsuda K, et al. A new scoring system to classify patients with colorectal liver metastases: proposal of criteria to select candidates for hepatic resection. J Hepatobiliary Pancreat Surg 2004;11 (2):79 – 83.

[92] Rees M, Tekkis PP, Welsh FK, et al. Evaluation of long – term survival after hepatic resection for metastatic colorectal cancer: a multifactorial model of 929 patients. Ann Surg 2008;247(1):125 – 35.

[93] Merkel S, Bialecki D, Meyer T, et al. Comparison of clinical risk scores predicting prognosis after resection of colorectal liver metastases. J Surg Oncol 2009; 100(5):349 – 57.

[94] Rahbari NN, Reissfelder C, Schulze – Bergkamen H, et al. Adjuvant therapy after resection of colorectal liver metastases: the predictive value of the MSKCC clinical risk score in the era of modern chemotherapy. BMC Cancer 2014;14:174.

[95] Kattan MW, Gonen M, Jarnagin WR, et al. A nomogram for predicting diseasespecific survival after hepatic resection for metastatic colorectal cancer. Ann Surg 2008;247(2):282 – 7.

[96] Thomay AA, Nagorney DM, Cohen SJ, et al. Modern chemotherapy mitigates adverse prognostic effect of regional nodal metastases in stage IV colorectal cancer. J Gastrointest Surg 2014;18(1):69 – 74.

[97] Blazer DG 3rd, Kishi Y, Maru DM, et al. Pathologic response to preoperative chemotherapy: a new outcome end point after resection of hepatic colorectal metastases. J Clin Oncol 2008;26(33):5344 – 51.

第四章 现代技术在肝脏切除术中的运用

Christoph W. Michalski, MD[a], Kevin G. Billingsley, MD[b]

【关键词】

肝脏手术;原发性肝肿瘤;肝转移;外科技术

要点

- 大部分肝脏手术可安全进行。
- 制定准确的术前治疗计划是必需的。
- 术中超声促进对肝脏流入道和流出道的管理。
- 低中央静脉压和精确离断对减少出血非常重要。

一、简介

过去20年,肝脏肿瘤外科切除技术已取得很大进步,切除手术适应证也逐步扩大。近年来,肝脏外科手术变得更为安全且肝脏切除手术的数量也有所增加[1-3]。结直肠癌肝转移的多学科治疗模式已扩大了潜在适合肝切除的患者人群。一系列方法的使用促进了复杂切除手术的施行,这些方法包括各种电切设备的使用,以及为了保障术后残肝体积和功能的术前门静脉栓塞。

决定肝切除手术安全的关键因素是术前详细评估,如肝功能的判断和肝脏解剖学的界定。术中管理包括低中心静脉压的麻醉技术以及麻醉师和医生间在手术中的配合交流。肝脏切除

作者无其他声明。

[a] Division of Surgical Oncology, Oregon Health and Science University, 3181 Southwest Sam Jackson Park Road, Portland, OR 97239, USA; [b] Division of Surgical Oncology, Department of Surgery, Oregon Health and Science University, 3181 Southwest Sam Jackson Park Road, Portland, OR 97239, USA

* Corresponding author.

E-mail address:billingk@ohsu.edu

术中涉及的技术包括控制肝脏流入道、控制流出道（肝静脉）和游离肝实质及肝脏内定位。本章节将对以上问题进行详述。

二、肝脏切除术的适应证

尽管大部分外科切除手术主要应用于原发性或转移性肝癌，但在特定情况下也可以进行良性疾病的肝切除术。

1. 良性病变

肝腺瘤是需要进行肝切除的最常见良性病变。这些病灶可能会增大甚至使机体出现疾病反应。同时，这些病灶具有较低的恶变及破裂风险[4]。局灶性结节性增生和血管瘤均是良性病变，患者只有出现明显相关症状时才考虑进行切除。因为局灶性结节性增生是绝对的良性病变，只有在出现性命攸关的症状时才会选择切除。这些症状包括持续性腹痛、餐后饱胀及过早饱腹感等。肝腺瘤易大出血且具有癌变的风险[5]，因此对于病灶直径在5cm以上的患者，特别是停用激素治疗后且病灶没有继续增大者，常推荐肝脏切除。和恶性肿瘤不同的是，切除边缘的距离对患者预后没有决定性作用，且外科医生在评估切除边界时无需严格控制流入道和流出道。

2. 转移性结直肠癌

可切除的转移性结直肠癌是肝切除术最常见的适应证。结直肠癌肝转移患者病灶完全切除术的预后差别较大，主要和以下因素有关：病灶数量、大小、慢性病史及淋巴结侵犯程度等[6-8]。完全切除术后患者远期预后好，5年生存率可达到30%~45%[6,8]。

从肿瘤学角度来看，对患者治疗的最理想目标是清除肝内所有病灶，并达到切缘阴性。因为大多数结直肠癌肝转移患者接受了肝切除术，而这类患者常常涉及多模式治疗，均包含以使用奥沙利铂或伊立替康为主的术前化疗。一项由欧洲癌症研究治疗组织（EORTC）开展的随机研究结果表明，术前奥沙利铂为主的化疗可以改善疾病无进展时间但不能延长总生存期[9,10]。除了可控制疾病进展外，术前化疗可使少数患者的不可切除病灶变得可切除，并诱导有效的肿瘤应答。目前对于外科切除边缘的最佳距离仍存在争议，然而，有证据表明，显微镜下手术切缘阳性同肿瘤复发密切相关。因此，对于所有肝脏切除术，切除依然需要达到显微镜下切缘阴性。许多研究关注到这个问题，虽然争论依然在持续，但目前一致的看法是切缘阴性对预后有利，且阴性切缘需要至少达到1mm。

3. 神经内分泌源性肝转移癌

神经内分泌源性肿瘤，尤其是良性肿瘤，虽然在肝脏内常常是多病灶的，但进展缓慢，手术切除可达到治愈[11]。这些手术常涉及小病灶多重切除手术。当然，也可以采取针对肝脏病灶的非手术形式对患者进行治疗[12]。

4. 非结直肠癌非神经内分泌源性肝转移

目前,支持其他肝转移癌接受切除术的确切数据较少。但对以下各种组织学的肝转移癌实行肝切除术后,病灶远期控制良好,包括肾细胞癌、乳腺癌、肛门癌、黑色素瘤及罕见肺癌等。对这些患者中的大多数,肝切除术不作为标准治疗,且是否进行切除术要根据患者个体情况由多学科联合诊疗团队决定。

5. 肝细胞癌

肝脏切除术是肝细胞癌患者的根治手段。然而,大多数北美肝细胞癌患者由于存在肝硬化和病灶弥漫的情况而不适合手术切除。一般来说,如果未发现其他肝脏疾病且病灶技术上可切除,那么肝脏切除术就是首选,或基于目前的标准,选择肝移植治疗。如果伴随其他肝脏疾病背景,那么治疗模式的选择就取决于疾病的严重程度。因此,这也需要用到巴塞罗那临床肝癌(BCLC)分期体系[13]。BCLC 分期 0 或 A 期患者适合进行肝切除术,而 BCLC 分期 B~D 期患者由于预后较差而不适宜进行外科切除。然而,最近的研究数据表明,肝脏切除术可以帮助治疗一些 BCLC 分期为 B 期的患者[14]。

6. 胆管癌

胆管癌包含 3 种类型:肝内、肝门部和肝外胆管癌。其中肝内和肝门部胆管癌若技术上可切除且未发现有肝外严重病变,可以进行外科切除术。尽管肝内胆管癌手术技术上的难度与肠癌肝转移、肝细胞癌相似,但肝外胆管癌(Klatskin 癌)几乎都需要进行肝脏和部分胆管的切除[15]。原位肝移植尚存在很大争议,目前全世界仅有部分医疗中心会选择使用[16]。肝外胆管癌通常涉及到胆管的胰腺部位,因此手术治疗时还需要进行胰十二指肠切除术。

本文将对患者的选择过程、围术期管理及现代肝脏手术的技术细节进行总体介绍。结直肠癌肝转移由于是肝切除术最常见的指征而受到格外重视,其治疗方案是多学科综合的结果。

三、术前功能评估

残肝大小及功能的术前评估在以下情况十分重要:①对有肝脏疾病背景(如纤维化/肝硬化、化学性肝损伤)的患者进行肝切除术;②对预测术后残肝较小的患者进行扩大肝切除术。右三段切除术(或扩大右肝切除术,包括 4a 和 4b 段切除)是最常见的扩大术式。残肝体积的预测可通过以下方法进行:基于影像学的残肝体积的计算和/或通过 ICG 清除实验对残存肝功能进行评估[17,18]。对于健康的肝脏,大约 30% 的残肝体积即可保留足够的术后肝功能。尽管影像学可以较为准确地预测残肝体积,但还是需要由具有丰富经验的医生评估患者接受扩大切除术的风险,尤其是对于残存肝脏体积不足 30% 的患者。在转移性结直肠癌中,术前长期化疗可能导致与化疗相关的脂肪性肝炎[19]。与化疗相关的治疗过程将影响肝脏再生,这点在扩大切除术时也必须考虑到。通过门静脉栓塞及分期肝切除以增加适合进行扩大肝切除术的患者人数[20-22]。许多病例结果已显示,门静脉栓塞可以增加残肝体积,这也使得原来被认为不可切除的病灶变得可切除[22-24]。

四、肝脏解剖和肝脏切除的术语

Couinaud[25]根据基于门静脉流入道对肝脏进行的分段,进而归纳了现代肝脏手术的解剖学要点。然而,随着肝脏切除术使用频率的上升,其在临床上广泛的使用,以及扩大肝切术的发展,需要更贴近临床实践的分类。2000年,国际肝胆胰协会定义了一个联合分类法(Brisbane分类法)[26]。该分类法定义了3类肝切除术:①左半肝或右半肝切除术;②左三叶或右三叶等包含有三个肝段或三个肝段以上的切除手术被定义为大范围肝切除术;③小范围肝切除被定义为楔形切除或小于等于两个肝段的切除手术。这种综合分类法使得肝脏切除手术的描述变得更加精确,目前在肝脏手术的报告结果中已被广泛采纳。然而,主要的易混淆之处在于肝三叶切除术和肝三区切除术(扩大右或左半肝切除术)。该文规范使用了 Brisbane 术语(表4-1)。

表4-1 肝脏解剖和肝脏切除术 Brisbane 分类和术语

解剖术语	肝脏分段	手术名称
第一级划分		
右半肝或右肝	5~8 段(+/-1 段)	右半肝切除或右肝切除(表明+/-1 段切除)
左半肝或左肝	2~4 段(+/-1 段)	左半肝切除或左肝切除(表明+/-1 段切除)
第二级划分		
右前区	5,8 段	解剖名称加切除名称,如右前区切除
右后区	6,7 段	右后区切除
左内区	4 段	左内区切除,或 4 段切除
左外区	2,3 段	左外区切除,或 2,3 段切除
右半肝加左内区	4~8 段(+/-1 段)	右三区切除,或扩大右半肝切除
左半肝加右前区	2~4 加 5,8 段(+/-1 段)	左三区切除,或扩大左半肝切除
第三级划分		
1~9 段	从 1~9 段中任何一段	段切除
两个相连段	1~9 段中任何两个相连段	两相连段切除

改自 The Terminology Committee of the IHPBA. The Brisbane 2000 terminology of hepatic anatomy and resections. HPB 2000;2: 333-9; with permission.

五、肝脏手术后的技术考虑和结果

相比其他腹部手术，肝脏手术在围手术期甚至手术中死亡的风险依然很高。大出血和术后肝衰竭是导致术后死亡的主要因素。肝切除技术的进步主要依赖于术中更好地使用超声和精细控制肝脏流入及流出道的技术发展。另外，近年来肝血流阻断术和术前对残肝体积、功能更为准确的预测也逐渐得到关注。

每个患者在术中均应对肝脏进行超声检查，以明确肝门部的结构（流入道和肝内胆管分支的间接可视化）、肝静脉（流出道）和肿瘤的位置、浸润范围。为达到这些目的，需要运用有着双功能和能产生血管多普勒效应的高分辨率超声。超声检查也有利于明确肝脏中是否存在一些额外的病灶，特别是对残肝的检查，还将有助于评估肿瘤组织中肝内血管和胆管结构的关系。

一旦明确了解剖结构，建议对右叶和/或左叶进行广泛探查。尽管这会比较耗时，但这样就可以控制流入道和流出道，进而在肝内控制困难时，减少血液流失。实施肝脏离断术时需要用到许多技术和设备，但尚没有一项表现出明显的优越性[27]。较认可的技术[28]包括钳夹离断[29]、切割闭合器断肝[30]、水射流切割[31]和超声刀[32]。尽管超声下的切开技术可能更加耗时，但许多外科医生偏好于它，因为它对肝内组织和血管可精确地区分和控制。

六、体位及设备安装

患者取仰卧位，双臂自然伸开。这种体位为双臂静脉化疗创造途径，且为扩大右侧横向肋下切口提供了便利。当然也有例外，如果外科医生期望使用右侧胸腹切口，因为该切口有时适于右肝巨大肿瘤的患者，那么在这种情况下，理想的体位是以飞机式夹板将其右臂悬挂在头部上面，且轻微提拉胸部以使得胸部充分暴露。

在患者准备好之前，手术灯就应该摆置准确。因为肝脏精确解剖需要术中超声，所以建议术前在外科医生可视的区域放置超声设备。设备摆位安装完成后，整个团队就可以稍作休息。这一过程十分强调外科医生与麻醉医师和护士间的配合，此时还应再次评估肝脏切除术的潜在风险，特别是大出血和血流动力不稳定等。这时候，应考虑到中心静脉压的控制（尤其是在肝血流阻断阶段）和手术室里的血液制剂。

七、切口和牵引

由于切除的幅度和外科医生喜好的不同，开放性肝脏手术的潜在切口是多样的。对于（扩大）肝右叶切除术，通常用中线延伸的右肋下切口。肋下切口位置常在肋边缘以下大约3指，最大扩展至右侧髂嵴线。正中切口扩展到剑突，有时沿着剑突边缘到胸骨，使腔静脉和肝静脉更好地暴露。如果肝脏游离比较困难，可考虑扩展切口到左侧肋下。如果是肝右叶巨大肿瘤，有时需要胸腹联合切口。手术过程中手术区域可通过正中切口延伸至右半腹部及右胸，分开肋下缘且胸部开放于第八或第九肋间。外围隔膜被分开并随后被修补。左肝也常常选择中线延伸至右肋下切口。如果肝左外叶段较大且需要广泛的左侧游离，那么应该采用双侧肋下切口（需或不需要正中延伸）。

在牵引器放好之前，需要分开肝圆韧带和镰状韧带。该技巧可以避免肝包膜和肝实质不必要的撕裂。为了避免对切口的强迫性牵拉，许多自动牵引器都可以迫使伤口的上下端回缩，可用来对切口进行双十字交叉捆绑。一些体壁牵引器使肝脏尽可能地暴露出来，而肝门是可伸缩的。

八、术中超声检查

笔者在所有肝脏切除术中都会用到术中超声和双重超声检查。肝脏游离之后，肝门静脉和肝静脉的解剖结构均需要分析。决定肝门和肝动脉流入肝脏的右边还是左边是最基础的分析，这主要用于肝蒂夹住后切除肝脏的比较。

分析肝静脉解剖结构，尤其要注意肝中静脉，这在许多患者血流阻断时都要精确考虑。肝中静脉较大分支可以通过电凝在肝脏表面进行标记，这主要用于肝实质横切时的早期识别。

肝脏扫描结果显示肿瘤或转移瘤，把这一结果与术前影像学检查相比较，可能会识别出额外的病灶。分辨肿瘤的门静脉和肝静脉的关系，并据此制订手术计划。

九、肝脏的游离

除了表面的楔形切除术，通常必须进行肝脏患侧的游离。对于肝右叶切除术，为了保护残肝，需要对右肝进行游离。而对于肝左叶切除术，为了控制下腔静脉，绝大多数情况下需要全肝游离。

右肝的游离是从肝静脉的解剖位置开始，特别注意不要破坏这些血管。考虑到肝脏回缩至左边，分离右冠状动脉和三角韧带。谨慎操作使腔静脉露出，并使肾上腺与下腔静脉分离。结扎从肾上腺至下腔静脉的小血管。如果下腔静脉充盈完全，此时麻醉医师最主要的任务就是开始降低中心静脉压。如果肝后静脉受到损伤，那么在中心静脉压增加幅度超过 5mmHg 的情况下继续分离肝脏与腔静脉很有可能会导致出血。肝脏进一步向左侧回缩，逐步暴露肝短静脉。此时，在肝血流阻断阶段，最重要的是尽可能多地控制小血管，使之靠近左边，以更好地加强对下腔静脉的控制，尾状叶有时向下腔静脉扩展至右肝，有必要使用吻合器进行分离。根据计划的手术切除范围和术中个体解剖结构差异，切开肝右静脉并用血管环加以控制。在肝脏的头侧方，环绕在下腔静脉的周缘带就在肝静脉下方。这种所谓的静脉韧带可用缝合装置或电外科装置划开。一旦该周缘带被分割，就能充分利用肝右静脉了。

左肝游离的第一步与三角韧带和左肝静脉的腹侧边界的切开相似。左外侧段的游离是通过分开肝胃韧带和左冠状动脉韧带实现的。切开肝左静脉（也可能肝中静脉）并用血管环加以控制。如果尾状叶必须切除的话，那么要实现完全游离，就要从肝脏左右边一步一步来控制下腔静脉的各小静脉分支。

十、流入道控制的方法

在控制肝脏流入道的不同方法中,研究者根据患者的基础疾病和计划手术切除范围使用了两种常规方法。肝脏横切,大多数适用于肝转移瘤和肝内胆管癌肝切除术中;针对肝门部胆管癌和靠近肺门疾病的临床情况,主要进行肝门各个血管的静脉解剖和分离。这两种技术的联合主要用于肝纤维化/肝硬化患者的肝切除手术,其中操作 Pringle 法时,间隔时间要尽可能短[33-35]。

1. 肝内/肝实质流入道的控制

因为切开肝门部时,存在意外损伤胆道的风险,尤其是在断流后的残存肝胆管,因此对于肝转移和肝内胆管癌患者的肝切除手术,门静脉的肝内控制是一种合理的方法。如果术中超声可显示肝左右叶的常规解剖位置和专属流入道的话,横断面将在肝表面划分,而肝实质则朝向门静脉左或右主干支被分割。在断流前没有必要控制肝蒂。运用 Pringle 法来间断控制流入道从而控制出血,沿着横切手术线将肝实质切开,直到探查到肝蒂,并将其从周边切开。根据笔者的经验,在超声下解剖切开可以帮助肝蒂的精确骨架化。

当术中探查到肝蒂,仔细切开并确保不要损伤胆管系统,并行夹闭试验。夹闭试验后重复超声检查以确保残肝有专属的流入道。运用血管吻合器或血管钳和血管缝合技术等分开各自的肝蒂。从肿瘤学的角度考虑,尽可能在条件允许时切开肝蒂亚结构,以防需要进行肝右叶切除术(如右前或右后肝门蒂)。这种方法可安全地识别区分肝门蒂右侧和左侧主干结构。对于肝左叶切除术,在左叶脐裂(确保疾病侵犯到该区域之后)的基础上切开肝门蒂左侧主干结构。此时控制左侧肝蒂保证对左肝解剖区域流入道的完全控制,同时还可以提供安全边界以避免损伤右肝门蒂。这种方法降低了肝门蒂流入道到残存左肝的风险。由于肿瘤边界较小,常常只有较少的空间可用于前肝门蒂和后肝门蒂的分离。在这种情况下,笔者在残端运用 DST 系列 TA45 型吻合器(Coviden 公司,曼斯菲尔德,马萨诸塞州,美国)切断开口端,然后在开口端缝合血管或胆管。在肝门蒂的主干被切开时,肝中静脉的大分支可能会被损伤,阻断前的超声检查有助于预防该风险。小心地切开靠近肝门蒂的分支可以在肝实质门蒂解剖时减少出血。

在肝实质横切时,笔者采用 Pringle 法间断阻断 5~10 分钟,然后打开肝脏流入道 3~5 分钟。依经验来看,这不会妨碍非肝硬化肝脏的切除效果,但在手术时会有少量出血[36]。

然而,如果肿瘤巨大靠近左或右肝门蒂主干,或对于合并肝纤维化/肝硬化性肝脏且肝功能储备较少的患者,需要对参与半肝血供的肝动脉和门静脉进行肝外切除和早期结扎。

2. 肝外/肝门流入道的控制

当肝脏疾病位置靠近肝门时,适合对肝门部结构进行切除和肝外控制。为了靠近肝门外主干结构,需要降低胆囊和肝门板的高度,且要探查到右或左肝动脉。此时各动脉被血管吊带控制,门静脉被切开且拿到肝外被血管吊带控制。为明确肝动脉解剖结构以进行充分的肝切除,需要分离动脉。进行多普勒超声检查以明确肝门外的解剖结构。因为流向门静脉分叉口常仅见于肝右或左动脉切开之后,此时各动脉被阻断了。一旦门静脉分叉口被安全识别,不管是运用血管吻合器还是血管钳和缝合技术等,要把左肝或右肝的各自分支分开来。对于操作困难的情况,要先对各自门静脉主干分支进行夹闭测试,而后对残肝进行多普勒超声检测。

十一、流出道控制的方法

如"肝脏的游离"部分所描述的,流出道控制可采用不同的方法。首先,在肝脏游离时,右和/或中和/或左肝静脉的控制可通过对各血管的周边进行仔细切开分离来实现。在把肝脏从下腔静脉处游离开来时,控制通向下腔静脉的小肝静脉。在肝实质横断时,尽可能多地控制这些小静脉对于预防血管撕裂大有裨益,尤其因为尾状叶充血很罕见且不常导致明显的术后并发症,因此,从尾状叶引流小静脉可以实现安全横断。

在血管阻断阶段,流入道分离到肝脏各部分之后,分离各肝静脉。运用血管吻合器分离肝静脉。在吻合器关闭之后且固定之前,需要仔细测量全身血压。在少数病例中,肝静脉的其中一支分离的血流通过下腔静脉回流到心脏。如果血压下降,移开血管钳并使血流复位,这样就没有静脉血流受阻。在其他肝静脉血流的监测中需要用到多普勒超声。如果计划切除后的残存肝脏没有静脉流出道的话,静脉血管就不应该被分离。这种情况不常见,但在术中有必要避免。

十二、肝实质离断技术

目前有各种不同的肝实质离断技术,但尚没有证实哪一种最佳[29,30,37,38]。谨慎离断术最近越来越受重视,但手指分离术和钳夹很少用到。对于解剖性肝切除,笔者在超声引导下,首先用超声刀分离1~2cm的肝实质。根据肝脏组织密度,超声离断可明确其分离程度。小血管通过电凝止血或任何双极电极血管封闭设备进行处理。

使用夹子、打结或血管钳等分离较大的肝蒂。在非解剖性切除时,如楔形切除,超声刀和/或电极血管封闭设备以及挤压钳一起使用可以提高效率但又不增加并发症发生率。表4-2 (Table 4-2)总结了肝实质离断设备的各种优点。

Table 4-2 Liver tissue transection devices

Authors	Technique	Resection Major	Resection Minor	Transfusion (n)	EBL (ml)	Pringle Maneuver (n)
Arnoletti & Brodsky,[41] 1999	Finger fracture with vascular occlusion	49	0	N/A	500	49
Arru et al,[42] 2007	Ultrasonic dissector and harmonic scalpel	69	31	N/A	500	58
Ayav et al,[43] 2008	Habib 4X	11	51	1	267	0
Lupo et al,[44] 2007 (randomized)	Crush clamp Linear RFA	10	19	13	N/A	N/A
		11	19	8	N/A	N/A
Cho et al,[45] 2009	Harmonic scalpel and water dissection	19	28	N/A	620	0
Wagman et al,[46] 2009	Habib 4X	31	45	11	427	20
Schmidbauer et al,[47] 2002	Ultracision	8	50	11	820	58
Takayama et al,[48] 2001 (randomized)	Ultrasonic dissector Crush clamp	24	42	N/A	515	48
		24	42	N/A	452	52

Abbreviations: EBL, estimated blood loss; N/A, not available; RFA, radiofrequency ablation.

Data from Wagman LD, Lee B, Castillo E, et al. Liver resection using a four-prong radiofrequency transection device. Am Surg 2009;75(10):991-4.

十三、具体步骤

1. 右半肝切除术

右半肝切除术中,一个关键步骤是右肝的完全游离。术中超声常用来明确主要右肝门蒂及其相关的肝中静脉的解剖结构。横断的边缘线经过胆囊窝和肝脏上部直至肝右和肝中静脉之间的平面。向下至胆囊窝的右侧,直到尾状叶和下腔静脉。研究者通常首先打开前部平面,然后离断右肝蒂。小心解剖肝蒂,如有可能且肿瘤学角度合理的话,选择性地暴露右前和右后蒂。此时,切记不可分离太远至左肝,尤其注意避免损伤左侧胆管系统。在分离肝蒂,明确左肝残存组织的流入道之前,进行夹闭试验很重要。如果可能的话,用血管钳分离肝蒂。另可选择使用 TA 吻合器夹闭、分离和缝合肝蒂。为了肝脏游离得更彻底,使用血管钳分离肝右静脉。

在进一步离断直至肝圆顶时,很有可能遇到肝中静脉。为避免该血管出血,离断过程必须足够仔细,且细小分支必须选择性地切开和处理。根据病灶的位置,离断可以沿着肝中静脉的右侧或左侧前行。但左侧离断可能会导致肝 4a/b 段的(部分)充血,因而需要通过左肝静脉进行引流。

一旦决定了做右半肝切除术,需要评估肝中静脉是否要保留,切开该血管并用血管钳分离。最后,在下腔静脉附近离断时需要特别注意,以免静脉残端的某一分支明显出血。

2. 扩大右肝切除术

随着右肝和肝门蒂至肝4段门静脉栓塞的广泛使用,扩大右肝切除术已变得更加安全、更加常用。需要再次强调的是,肝脏需要尽可能多地被游离开来,包括肝左外区。必须处理所有的肝静脉。离断的界线靠近肝镰状韧带的右边。根据肝中静脉的解剖结构和病灶的位置决定是否需要保留静脉。另外,在肝实质流入道的控制方面,肝实质离断手术需要同肝门部平行,直至胆囊窝并向下至尾状叶。当需要进行不连续尾状叶切除术时,必须在离断之前完全游离肝1段。另外,在尾状叶上方(在肝左外区的下方和沿着静脉韧带)进行肝切除术。但是,与右半肝切除术不同,扩大切除术首先打开肝脏前部平面时,需要通过结扎或运用吻合器处理一些深入肝4段的较大肝蒂。当离断向下进行到主要的肝门蒂时,需要特别注意避免损伤左侧肝门的结构。沿着门静脉分支至右侧,进行肝实质的离断,并按照右半肝切除术的描述去完成。在分离肝门之前,建议使用精确的多普勒超声辅助。在Klatskin肿瘤扩散到左侧肝门部的情况下,可能需要局部切除左胆管系统。这个过程常常会导致几个细小的胆管被阻断,这时就需要对胆管实施Roux en Y 胆管空肠吻合术。在肝膈顶部完成横切,需要谨慎解剖肝中静脉,以免损伤血管导致出血。由于残肝可能会移动,笔者主张重新用几个间断缝合来连接三角韧带。

3. 左半肝切除术

与右半肝切除术类似,左边切除的平面原则上位于肝脏5/8和4a/b段之间。这种手术并不少见且难度较低。除非尾状叶必须要切除之外,通常情况下是不需要移动右半肝的。中心静脉压需尽可能保持在低压状态。从肝5/8和4a/b段分割面的边缘画一条线作为横断面的切面,沿着胆囊窝延伸到肝脏左侧,沿着静脉韧带到尾状叶,直至下腔静脉左侧。在不连续性尾状叶切除术中,横断面取自主门静脉一直向下至腔静脉。在右肝切除术中,超声的作用是保证有血流流入右半肝。左侧主要肝门蒂在脐裂的底部分支,除非尾状叶被切除,否则离尾状叶流入道起点应较远。肝左静脉通常在向肝膈顶部横切的过程中,在肝实质内分支。

4. 中央肝切除术

对于肝脏的大段肿瘤,最佳方案为中央肝切除术。这种切除术在保证肿瘤清除率的情况下可以保持左右侧的肝功能。图4-1注明了手术方法和需要横切的主要结构。

手术过程通过游离大部分的右肝,以促进胆囊动脉和胆管的分离。随后,切开肝实质到右侧脐隙和肝门入口的横切Ⅳ处进行固定或缝合结扎(图4-2)。然后,从肝门内上方开始,切口向上到右主肝门蒂直达右前肝门蒂(Ⅴ,Ⅷ,图4-3),将门蒂环形包围并钳住。通过多普勒超声保证在肝门蒂切除之后仍有足够血流流至右肝门后方区域。右前部门蒂的分界应该很明显。肝门蒂分离后,应在5/8和6/7段之间的平面完成横断。当朝向段8的底部横切时,应小心操作以保护肝右静脉。分离肝中静脉以靠近下腔静脉,此时完成切除并考虑保存标本(图4-4)。

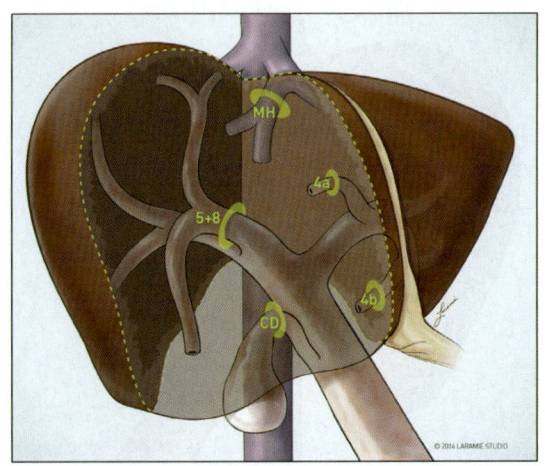

图 4-1 概观

CD:胆囊管;MH:肝中静脉

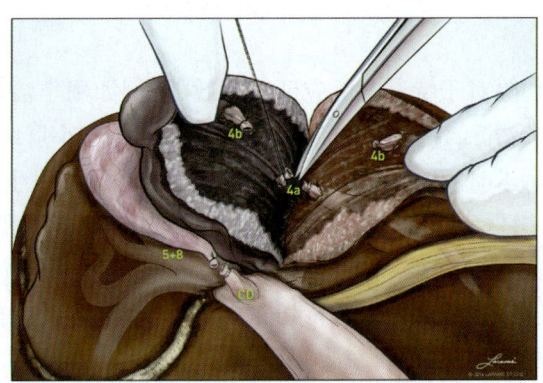

图 4-2 处理 4a 和 4b 处的肝门蒂

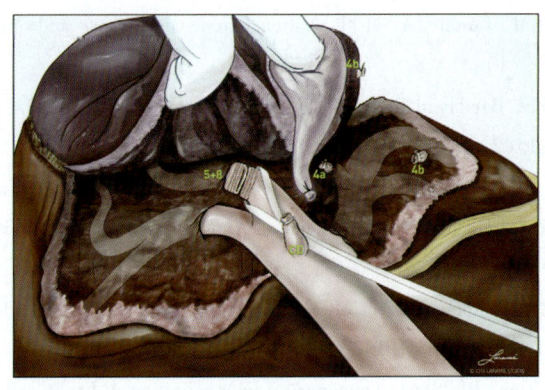

图 4-3 处理 5/7 段的肝门蒂和胆囊管

CD:胆囊管

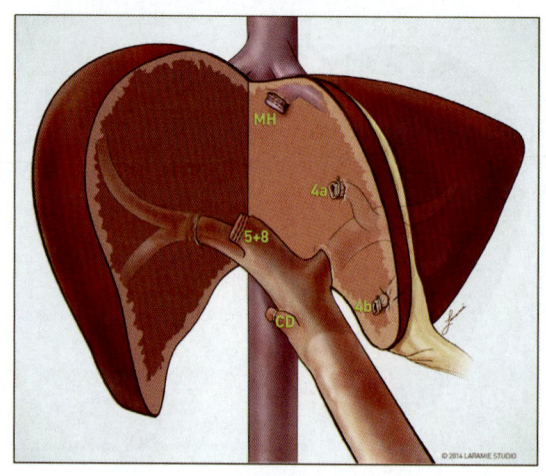

图 4-4 完成

CD:胆囊管;MH:肝中静脉

5. 肝段切除术

肝段切除或者楔形切除对于特定的适应证是有效的,例如用于治疗多发性双叶转移和分阶段肝切除术的理想单叶清除;治疗残肝疾病的复发;治疗潜在小肝综合征;当因为患者有其他合并症需要尽量缩短手术时间时;在众多类癌/神经内分泌肿瘤发生肝转移需要做减积手术时。虽然段切除术在组织保存方面存在优势,但却会增加失血量和增加胆道并发症的风险[39,40]。此外,因为这些切除部分经常与正常组织边缘相连,根据它们位置的不同,可能导致肝门重要结构意外损伤。在按照原计划进行切除术的情况下,这样的损伤使得无法再进行二次手术。另一方面,肝段切除往往可以在腹腔镜下进行,这样可显著缩短患者的住院时间。

参考文献

[1] Dimick JB, Wainess RM, Cowan JA, et al. National trends in the use and outcomes of hepatic resection. J Am Coll Surg 2004;199(1):31-8.

[2] Dokmak S, Fteriche FS, Borscheid R, et al. 2012 Liver resections in the 21st century: we are far from zero mortality. HPB 2013;15(2):908-15.

[3] Jarnagin WR, Gonen M, Fong Y, et al. Improvement in perioperative outcome after hepatic resection: analysis of 1,803 consecutive cases over the past decade. Ann Surg 2002;236(4):397-406 [discussion: 406-7].

[4] Karkar AM, Tang LH, Kashikar ND, et al. Management of hepatocellular adenoma: comparison of resection, embolization and observation. HPB (Oxford) 2013;15(3):235-43.

[5] Bieze M, Busch OR, Tanis PJ, et al. Outcomes of liver resection in hepatocellular adenoma and focal nodular hyperplasia. HPB (Oxford) 2014;16(2):140-9.

[6] de Jong MC, Pulitano C, Ribero D, et al. Rates and patterns of recurrence following curative intent surgery

[7] Scheele J, Stangl R, Altendorf-Hofmann A. Hepatic metastases from colorectal carcinoma: impact of surgical resection on the natural history. Br J Surg 1990; 77(11):1241-6.

[8] Tomlinson JS, Jarnagin WR, DeMatteo RP, et al. Actual 10-year survival after resection of colorectal liver metastases defines cure. J Clin Oncol 2007;25(29): 4575-80.

[9] Nordlinger B, Sorbye H, Glimelius B, et al. Perioperative chemotherapy with FOLFOX4 and surgery versus surgery alone for resectable liver metastases from colorectal cancer (EORTC Intergroup trial 40983): a randomised controlled trial. Lancet 2008;371(9617):1007-16.

[10] Nordlinger B, Sorbye H, Glimelius B, et al. Perioperative FOLFOX4 chemotherapy and surgery versus surgery alone for resectable liver metastases from colorectal cancer (EORTC 40983): long-term results of a randomised, controlled, phase 3 trial. Lancet Oncol 2013;14(12):1208-15.

[11] Frilling A, Modlin IM, Kidd M, et al. Recommendations for management of patients with neuroendocrine liver metastases. Lancet Oncol 2014;15(1):e8-21.

[12] Mayo SC, Herman JM, Cosgrove D, et al. Emerging approaches in the management of patients with neuroendocrine liver metastasis: role of liver-directed and systemic therapies. J Am Coll Surg 2013;216(1):123-34.

[13] Llovet JM, Fuster J, Bruix J, et al. The Barcelona approach: diagnosis, staging, and treatment of hepatocellular carcinoma. Liver Transpl 2004;10(2 Suppl 1): S115-20.

[14] Zhong JH, Ke Y, Gong WF, et al. Hepatic resection associated with good survival for selected patients with intermediate and advanced-stage hepatocellular carcinoma. Ann Surg 2014;260(2):329-40.

[15] Zaydfudim VM, Rosen CB, Nagorney DM. Hilar cholangiocarcinoma. Surg Oncol Clin N Am 2014;23(2): 247-63.

[16] Darwish Murad S, Kim WR, Harnois DM, et al. Efficacy of neoadjuvant chemoradiation, followed by liver transplantation, for perihilar cholangiocarcinoma at 12 US centers. Gastroenterology 2012;143(1):88-98. e3 [quiz: e14].

[17] Hoekstra LT, de Graaf W, Nibourg GA, et al. Physiological and biochemical basis of clinical liver function tests: a review. Ann Surg 2013;257(1):27-36.

[18] Ribero D, Amisano M, Bertuzzo F, et al. Measured versus estimated total liver volume to preoperatively assess the adequacy of the future liver remnant: which method should we use? Ann Surg 2013;258(5):801-6 [discussion: 806-7].

[19] Chun YS, Laurent A, Maru D, et al. Management of chemotherapy-associated hepatotoxicity in colorectal liver metastases. Lancet Oncol 2009;10(3):278-86.

[20] Huang SY, Aloia TA, Shindoh J, et al. Efficacy and safety of portal vein embolization for two-stage hepatectomy in patients with colorectal liver metastasis. J Vasc Interv Radiol 2014;25(4):608-17.

[21] Shindoh J, Tzeng CW, Aloia TA, et al. Safety and efficacy of portal vein embolization before planned major or extended hepatectomy: an institutional experience of 358 patients. J Gastrointest Surg 2014;18(1):45-51.

[22] Shindoh J, Vauthey JN, Zimmitti G, et al. Analysis of the efficacy of portal vein embolization for patients with extensive liver malignancy and very low future liver remnant volume, including a comparison with the as-

sociating liver partition with portal vein ligation for staged hepatectomy approach. J Am Coll Surg 2013;217(1):126-33 [discussion:133-4].

[23] Correa D, Schwartz L, Jarnagin WR, et al. Kinetics of liver volume changes in the first year after portal vein embolization. Arch Surg 2010;145(4):351-4 [discussion:354-5].

[24] Shindoh J, Truty MJ, Aloia TA, et al. Kinetic growth rate after portal vein embolization predicts posthepatectomy outcomes: toward zero liver-related mortality in patients with colorectal liver metastases and small future liver remnant. J Am Coll Surg 2013;216(2):201-9.

[25] Couinaud C. The liver: anatomical and surgical studies (in French). Paris: Masson; 1957.

[26] The Terminology Committee of the IHPBA. The Brisbane 2000 terminology of hepatic anatomy and resections. HPB 2000;2:333-9.

[27] Simillis C, Li T, Vaughan J, et al. Methods to decrease blood loss during liver resection: a network meta-analysis. Cochrane Database Syst Rev 2014;(4):CD010683.

[28] Pamecha V, Gurusamy KS, Sharma D, et al. Techniques for liver parenchymal transection: a meta-analysis of randomized controlled trials. HPB (Oxford) 2009;11(4):275-81.

[29] Rahbari NN, Elbers H, Koch M, et al. Randomized clinical trial of stapler versus clamp-crushing transection in elective liver resection. Br J Surg 2014;101(3):200-7.

[30] Raoof M, Aloia TA, Vauthey JN, et al. Morbidity and mortality in 1,174 patients undergoing hepatic parenchymal transection using a stapler device. Ann Surg Oncol 2014;21(3):995-1001.

[31] Rau HG, Duessel AP, Wurzbacher S. The use of water-jet dissection in open and laparoscopic liver resection. HPB (Oxford) 2008;10(4):275-80.

[32] Lochan R, Ansari I, Coates R, et al. Methods of haemostasis during liver resection-a UK national survey. Dig Surg 2013;30(4-6):375-82.

[33] Figueras J, Llado L, Ruiz D, et al. Complete versus selective portal triad clamping for minor liver resections: a prospective randomized trial. Ann Surg 2005;241(4):582-90.

[34] Hoekstra LT, van Trigt JD, Reiniers MJ, et al. Vascular occlusion or not during liver resection: the continuing story. Dig Surg 2012;29(1):35-42.

[35] Sugiyama Y, Ishizaki Y, Imamura H, et al. Effects of intermittent Pringle's manoeuvre on cirrhotic compared with normal liver. Br J Surg 2010;97(7):1062-9.

[36] Gur I, Diggs BS, Wagner JA, et al. Safety and outcomes following resection of colorectal liver metastases in the era of current perioperative chemotherapy. J Gastrointest Surg 2013;17(12):2133-42.

[37] Muratore A, Mellano A, Tarantino G, et al. Radiofrequency vessel-sealing system versus the clamp-crushing technique in liver transection: results of a prospective randomized study on 100 consecutive patients. HPB (Oxford) 2014;16:707-12.

[38] Savlid M, Strand AH, Jansson A, et al. Transection of the liver parenchyma with an ultrasound dissector or a stapler device: results of a randomized clinical study. World J Surg 2013;37(4):799-805.

[39] Lee SY. Central hepatectomy for centrally located malignant liver tumors: a systematic review. World J Hepatol 2014;6(5):347-57.

[40] Dokmak S, Agostini J, Jacquin A, et al. High risk of biliary fistula after isolated segment VIII liver resection. World J Surg 2012;36(11):2692-8.

[41] Arnoletti JP, Brodsky J. Reduction of transfusion requirements during major hepatic resection for metastatic

disease. Surgery 1999;125(2):166-71.

[42] Arru M, Pulitano C, Aldrighetti L, et al. A prospective evaluation of ultrasonic dissector plus harmonic scalpel in liver resection. The American surgeon 2007; 73(3):256-60.

[43] Ayav A, Jiao L, Dickinson R, et al. Liver resection with a new multiprobe bipolar radiofrequency device. Archives of surgery 2008;143(4):396-401; discussion 401.

[44] Lupo L, Gallerani A, Panzera P, et al. Randomized clinical trial of radiofrequencyassisted versus clamp-crushing liver resection. The British journal of surgery 2007;94(3):287-91.

[45] Cho JY, Han HS, Yoon YS, et al. Outcomes of laparoscopic liver resection for lesions located in the right side of the liver. Archives of surgery 2009;144(1):25-9.

[46] Wagman LD, Lee B, Castillo E, et al. Liver resection using a four-prong radiofrequency transection device. The American surgeon 2009;75(10):991-4.

[47] Schmidbauer S, Hallfeldt KK, Sitzmann G, et al. Experience with ultrasound scissors and blades (UltraCision) in open and laparoscopic liver resection. Annals of surgery 2002;235(1):27-30.

[48] Takayama T, Makuuchi M, Kubota K, et al. Randomized comparison of ultrasonic vs clamp transection of the liver. Archives of surgery 2001;136(8):922-8.

第五章　肝脏切除术并发症

Maria C. Russell, MD

【关键词】

肝切除；静脉血栓；胆漏；肝脏切除术后肝衰竭

要点

- 接受肝部分切除的患者越来越多，其中患有多种疾病的老年患者也越来越多。
- 有效的化疗以及门静脉栓塞等技术的出现，使日益复杂的肝切除率增加到了 75%。尽管从致死率角度来看手术已经变得更安全，但肝切除术并发症并未下降。
- 肝脏切除术后四大严重并发症：术后大出血、静脉血栓、胆漏、肝脏切除术后肝衰竭。

肝脏切除术仍然是原发性或继发性肝恶性肿瘤最有效的治疗手段。1996—2000 年，美国有超过 7000 例肝脏切除术，2000 年美国肝切除手术约是 1988 年的 2 倍[1]。由于原发性或继发性肝恶性肿瘤发病率的升高，肝脏切除术的数量也逐年上升。

由于手术技术的进步，肝脏切除术的死亡率由 20% 降至目前的 1%~5%，但术后并发症的发生率仍高达 20%~56%。根据患者情况、肝切除范围、疾病进展、医院以及医生的不同，发生率在这个范围内波动[2-8]。

大部分关于肝脏切除术后并发症的研究都出自单个研究机构。1977 年 Foster 和 Berman 通过回顾性综述总结出肝脏切除术后死亡率为 13%~20%，但后来，通过回顾 1991—2001 年在 Sloan Kettering 纪念医院接受肝脏切除术的 1800 例患者，Jarnagin 等反驳了前者总结出的

作者无其他声明。

Division of Surgical Oncology, Department of Surgery, Emory University Hospital, 550 Peachtree Street Northeast, 9th Floor MOT, Atlanta, GA 30308, USA

E-mail address: maria.c.russell@emory.edu

数据。在做这项回顾性研究的过程中,手术死亡率从4.0%降低至1.3%,手术并发症约45%。Benzoni等[9]调查了一家医疗中心的134例肝切除手术患者和153例肝转移灶切除术患者,估算出其死亡率为4.5%,并发症发生率为47.7%。在肝大部切除、扩大肝切除、Pringle法阻断>20分钟、输血量>600ml的患者中并发症发生率较高。而在HCC患者中,肝功能B级和C级、肝癌组织分化程度与并发症的发生率相关。Sadamori等[10]则发现,在行多次肝脏切除术或手术时间较长的肝细胞癌患者中,胆漏和手术区域感染发生率较高,分别为12.8%和8.6%。2007年,Virani等[11]利用NSQIP – PSS(National Surgical Quality Improvement Program – Patient Safety in Surgery)系统,评估了全美14家医院肝脏切除术后30天死亡率及并发症发生率,总并发症发生率为22.6%,败血症、切口感染、泌尿道感染、手术区域感染是最常见的并发症,其中5.2%的患者需再次手术处理并发症,发生术后并发症的患者死亡率仍然较高。因此,为降低术后死亡率,首先要找出肝脏切除术后并发症的高危患者。肝脏切除术后并发症发生率持续升高的原因是多方面的。总体来看,接受手术的患者平均年龄在上升,并伴随多种合并症,而肝切范围的扩大、次数的增多也使得手术越来越复杂。此外,在结直肠癌肝转移中,有效化疗方案可使不可切除的肝转移灶变为可切除,但化疗后数月肝脏出现脂肪变性或脂肪性肝炎可能性大。因为肝切术不断地被应用于此类患者,术后并发症发生率仍然很高。

肝脏切除术后的并发症与肝切除范围密切相关。肝脏切除术的范围从小的非解剖性楔形切除到75%肝3段切除。根据Couinaud定义,肝大部分切除是指3个或以上肝段的切除。大部分研究的结果显示切除范围和发生率相关。Zimmitti等[12]根据手术复杂程度分析术后并发症,发现除了胆漏,其他并发症的发生率与手术复杂程度无明显关系。Li等[13]比较了肝大部分切除、小肝切除术、肝消融术的并发症,严重并发症的发生率分别为35.1%、21.3%、9.3%($P<0.01$),总的并发症发生率为41.0%、26.9%、11.5%($P<0.01$)。与小肝切除术相比,肝大部分切除会导致感染(器官/腔或表层皮肤感染、肺炎、败血症、败血性休克)、肺部并发症(意外重插管、延长呼吸机支持)、肾脏并发症(进行性肾功能不全、急性肾衰竭)、血液系统并发症[72小时出血需输血,深静脉血栓(DVT)]发生率升高。

肝脏基础病与肝脏切除术后并发症也密切相关。约80%肝细胞癌的患者同时合并肝纤维化和肝硬化[14],因此残肝可能已受损害,也更易受损伤。是否切除或肝移植这些肝脏仍然存在争议[15-19]。有研究显示,在米兰标准内的患者行肝脏切除术总生存率(65.7% vs 43.8%,$P=0.005$)和无复发生存率(85.3% vs 22.7%,$P<0.001$)较高,尤其是慢性丙型肝炎的患者[19]。其他研究则显示,在有良好肝功能储备的单发肝细胞癌患者中,手术切除是首选治疗方法[20-22]。即便如此,相比无基础疾病的患者,肝硬化、肝纤维化、脂肪肝的患者行肝脏切除术后,发生并发症的可能性要高。

肝切除患者易发生的常见并发症有伤口感染、败血症、肺炎及其他并发症,但这些并发症并不是肝切除术中特有的。本章主要关注肝切除术特有并发症,包括肝脏切除术后出血、静脉血栓、胆漏和肝衰竭。

一、术后大出血

1977年,Foster和Berman[3]研究发现,肝大部分切除手术死亡率为20%,其中20%的死亡原因为大出血。随着影像学检查、手术技术和围术期管理方法的进步,需要输血的患者逐渐减少。考虑到输血可能引起不良反应,减少输血可以降低肝脏切除术后并发症的发生[23]。近年的文章显示,肝脏切除术后大出血发生率为0.6%~0.8%[5,24-27]。

目前对于术后出血的定义仍有争议。各机构对出血的定义范围从需要输浓缩红细胞(PRBCs)的数目到手术部位出血需要再次手术探查到出血引流量[11,28-33]。2011年,ISGLS(International Study Group of Liver Surgery)制定的指南中肝脏切除术后出血的定义为:血红蛋白较术后基线水平(术后即刻)降低3g/dl[24],或者术后血红蛋白降低以致需要输注红细胞,或者需要再次手术或介入栓塞来止血。其中定义术后出血A级为输注红细胞少于2单位,B级为大于2单位,C级为需要介入栓塞或再次手术止血(表5-1)。这一定义已在835例患者中得到验证,其中A、B、C级患者住院期间死亡率分别为0、17%和50%。直到现在,临床研究仍不能给出准确的定义。

表5-1 术后大出血

国际肝脏手术研究小组(ISGLS)对肝脏切除术后大出血的定义:
1. 设置术后基准线后,血红蛋白降低30g/L
2. 任何因血红蛋白降低引起的术后输血和/或用以止血的任何再次介入治疗(栓塞或再次手术)
3. 失血证据,如:通过引流管失血或影像证实活动性出血
A级:失血需输血最高至2单位浓缩红细胞(PRBCs)
B级:失血需输血>2单位浓缩红细胞,但无侵入性介入治疗
C级:失血需介入治疗或再次手术
排除:术中失血,术后需立即输血的患者

摘自 Rahbari NN, Garden OJ, Padbury R, et al. Post-hepatectomy haemorrhage: a definition and grading by the International Study Group of Liver Surgery (ISGLS). HPB (Oxford) 2011;13:531; with permission.

1. 致出血因素

确定导致术后出血的因素有一定难度。Lim等[27]的研究结果显示:肝硬化患者的出血更多,拔管后中心静脉压改变导致流出道系统改变。Yang等[34]比较了肝脏切除术后出血再次腹腔镜下止血的术后死亡率,发现晚期腹腔镜组(>6小时)的患者死亡率为25%,明显高于早期腹腔镜组(<6小时)患者的8.6%,$P=0.001$。住院期间死亡的独立危险因素包括:手术年份(1997—2004),肝硬化,无效止血,晚期再次腹腔镜手术,术后肝衰竭以及术后肾衰竭需要透析。

2. 处理方法

大部分术后大出血发生在术后48小时内,从肝脏表面或膈膜出血[35]。而引流管的有效性较低,因为凝血块极易堵塞引流管。建议术后出血后应密切监测血流动力学,如果有低血压或心动过速,应采取相应措施,及时纠正凝血功能异常或输血。再次腹腔镜手术的指征则包括:出血量大于 1L 或需要持续输血,血红蛋白降低 3~4g/dl,血流动力学不稳定需输血等[27,35]。

肝脏切除术后大出血的患者中 1%~8% 需要再次手术,而死亡率高达 17%~83%[24,36-38]。术后出血导致切除术后并发症发生率和死亡率明显升高。

二、肝脏切除术后静脉血栓形成/栓塞

腹部或盆腔肿瘤手术的患者术后极易形成静脉血栓栓塞(VTE)[39-41],其严重后果应得到充分重视。出现 VTE 者 8 年后死亡率为 12%~50%[42-43]。最近一篇以人群为基础的研究显示,深静脉血栓(DVE)和肺栓塞(PE)患者 30 天死亡率分别为 3% 和 31%,而对照组无静脉血栓栓塞患者的死亡率为 0.4%。虽然 VTE 患者第一年的死亡率最高,但 30 年总死亡危险比深静脉栓塞为 1.55%(95% CI 1.53~1.57),肺栓塞为 2.77%(95% CI 2.74~2.81),具有统计学意义[44]。

尽管此并发症有可能致死,但考虑到术后出血,肝脏切除术后肝功能损伤的风险,以及自体抗凝的可能[45-47],很多外科医生不愿意在肝脏切除术后使用抗凝药。近年的研究显示,肝脏切除术后肺栓塞的发生率约为 6%,而静脉血栓的发生率与其他腹部恶性肿瘤术后的发生率类似[45,48]。因此,药物预防规范可能改变。

由于缺乏标准的术后预防抗凝方法,很难对各方案的效果进行比较。虽然有些文献中提及了具体的药物方案,但大部分仍然是由外科医师自行决定,使得预防性药物的使用效果不明确。另外,很难确定术后患者的早期行走能力,以及后续使用加压装置的具体情况,使得各个研究之间的一致性更差。

1. 致栓塞因素

目前,尚无关于肝切除患者形成静脉血栓栓塞的前瞻性随机对照研究。多项回顾性研究以及一项前瞻性研究阐述了导致静脉血栓栓塞形成的因素包括:体重指数过高、手术时间长、肝大部分切除(表 5-2)[45,46,49-52]。其他因素包括:既往有静脉血栓栓塞的病史、术后并发症、住院时间长等。

值得注意的是,Nathan 等[49]关于"自体抗凝"的说法:即 INR 上升却使患者形成静脉血栓栓塞的风险增高,反驳了 Chitlur 等[53]认为 INR 不能完全代表患者凝血功能的观点。来自 M. D. Anderson 医院的 Tzeng 等[45]的研究结果也显示,INR 上升和肝切除的范围相关,但不是对抗静脉血栓栓塞形成的保护因素。

表 5-2 肝脏切除术后静脉血栓栓塞的危险因素

研究	比例	危险因素
Ejaz 等[52]（可变药物预防）	4.7% VTE 1.8% PE 3.3% DVT	VTE 病史 手术时间延长 住院时间延长
Nathan 等[49]（可变药物预防）	2.6% VTE 1.7% PE 1.1% DVT	高龄 BMI 过高 手术时间延长 主要并发症 术后 INR 偏高
Tzeng 等[45]（无预防数据）	2.9% VTE 1.3% PE 1.9% DVT	肝大部分切除 男性 术前 AST >27IU/L ASA 分级≥3 OR 时间 >222 分钟 术后器官间隙感染 住院时间≥7 天
Reddy 等[46]（可变药物预防）	3.6% VTE 2.8% PE 0.7% DVT	药物引起血栓
Melloul 等[50]（药物和机械预防）	6% PE	BMI >25kg/m^2 肝大部分切除 正常或小部分肝实质纤维化
Morris - Stiff 等[51]（预防不明确）	2.1% VTE 1.3% PE 0.7% DVT	DVT 或 PE 病史

缩写：ASA，美国麻醉医师协会；AST，天冬氨酸转氨酶；BMI，体重指数；DVT，深静脉血栓；INR，国际标准化比值；OR，手术室；PE，肺栓塞；VTE，静脉血栓栓塞

2. 处理方法

对于静脉血栓栓塞来说，预防是最好的方法。但是，目前此方法的循证医学证据大多是从普通外科的文献推测而来。Reddy 等[46]在文章中提出，让外科医生决定对患者的处理方法、处理时机以及使用何种药物预防 VTE，而机械性预防及尽早下床行走由患者掌握。Nathan 等[49]比较了药物预防 VTE 的效果，发现唯一有统计学差异的变量为有无药物预防，有药物预防比无药物预防的患者发生 VTE 的概率低(6.3% vs 2.2%，$P=0.03$)，而何时给药（即刻，早期，晚期/从不）无统计学差异。目前最佳的 VTE 预防方法也不能完全避免其发生，术后 24 小时内即采用预防手段的患者，有 70.4%最终也发生了静脉血栓栓塞。虽然药物预防可使手术

患者 VTE 发生率降低 75%，但事实是，即使使用了药物预防，还是会发生 VTE[54,55]。

药物预防 VTE 最大的隐患是可能发生术后出血，但目前文献对此结论不一。Tzeng 等[45]通过评估 NSQIP 数据发现，VTE 的发生率远远高于大出血的发生率，因此，他们建议在无出血风险的患者中使用药物预防术后 VTE。同样，Reddy 等[46]的结果显示，使用药物预防 VTE 的患者术后输血较少（16.7% vs 26.4%，$P=0.02$），总输血率与未使用预防手段的患者相似（35.0% vs 30.6%，$P=0.36$）。这两项研究结果说明，药物预防 VTE 不会增加出血风险。

虽然尚无严格的随机实验比较 VTE 预防手段在肝脏手术中的作用，但目前大多数研究认为，VTE 是个常见且潜在致死的并发症，并且预防 VTE 不会升高术后出血风险。因此，在更有效的方法出现之前，建议肝大部分切除的患者常规使用药物抗凝预防 VTE。

三、肝脏切除术后门静脉、肝动脉血栓形成

血管并发症，如门静脉或肝动脉血栓形成，是一类罕见的肝脏切除术后并发症，并且大多数仅存在于文献记载中。但随着扩大肝脏切除术和肝动脉、门静脉重建术的增多，导致门静脉、肝动脉血栓形成的因素越来越多，发生频率越来越高。

肝动脉血栓形成（HAT）是很少见的并发症，通常仅见于同时行肝动脉重建术的肝切除或移植术患者，而在肝动脉切除中很少见。Azoulay 等[56]报道，5 例行肝动脉重建的胆管癌患者，肝动脉均保持 100% 通畅。对于行肝移植术的患者，3%~9% 术后会形成肝动脉血栓，最终导致病情急剧进展以致移植器官功能不全[57]。肝动脉血栓的临床表现通常为急性肝功能衰竭、败血症、脓肿，或晚期的胆管炎、胆漏、肝功能不全[57,58]。

门静脉血栓形成亦主要发生于肝移植的患者，发生率为 2%~6%[59,60]。肝脏切除术后，门静脉血栓形成因缺乏特异性临床表现而导致经常被忽略；若血栓累及肠系膜上静脉，患者可有腹痛、肠梗阻或缺血，亦或恶心、呕吐、厌食、体重减轻、腹泻、腹水、腹胀[61,62]。若急性血栓形成未被发现，侧支循环形成后会引起门静脉海绵样变、门静脉高压，临床表现为食管胃底静脉曲张、脾亢以及大出血[63]。

1. 危险因素

最近，一项关于肝门区胆管癌血管切除术的 meta 分析综述显示，在行血管切除术的患者中，血管并发症发生率更高（OR 8.8，95% CI 3.5~22；$P<0.0001$），包括门静脉血栓形成、肝动脉血栓形成、狭窄、假性动脉瘤[64]。此外，血管切除的患者死亡率显著增高（OR 2.07，95% CI 1.21~3.57；$P=0.008$），行肝动脉切除术的患者死亡率更高（OR 4.48，95% CI，1.97~10.16；$P=0.0003$）。肝移植术相关文献显示，导致肝动脉并发症的因素包括：动脉直径较小、供体年龄大（>60 岁）、出血时间延长、输血、手术时间长、胆漏、胆管炎等[57,65,66]。其他研究显示，活供体移植受体发生肝动脉并发症时，解剖外吻合术是唯一与之独立相关的多变量因素。

超声是移植患者术后常规检查项目，肝动脉血栓一般都可以通过多普勒超声检查发现。当然，CT 检查也可以发现。由于肝动脉切除不是肝脏切除术中的常规手段，因此很难明确这些患者的相关危险因素。

和肝动脉血栓一样,门静脉血栓也可通过超声、MRI、CT等方法发现。彩超在诊断门静脉血栓、门静脉海绵样变方面有效,甚至优于CT检查,但此方法对操作者的要求较高。磁共振血管造影可提供血流和解剖结构的动态影像,但性价比较低。门静脉造影可同时用于确诊和治疗,但属于侵入性检查,易引起相关并发症。

2. 处理方法

肝动脉血栓处理方法取决于其严重程度。若程度较轻,肝功能正常,可以行保守治疗,如肝素、容量管理;若要血流重建,也可考虑介入治疗手段,如血管成形术;或者急诊行外科取栓术[67]。

2010年,Thomas和Ahmad[68]在文章中表示,门静脉血栓的处理方法很多。肝素加华法林抗凝可减少血栓形成风险,促进静脉再通[63,69],而且越早使用,血管再通的可能性越大[70,71]。肝移植术相关指南提示其他治疗方法包括溶栓、血管成形术、支架植入[72,73],早期溶栓效果卓越,甚至可能优于全身抗凝[68]。最后,开腹血栓切除术也可以用于重建门静脉系统血流[61],但通常用于由门静脉-肠系膜静脉血栓引起的肠缺血。它的优点在于可以立即处理血栓,同时手术修复可能引起血栓形成的吻合口,最大缺点是手术规模较大。

四、胆漏

胆漏是肝脏切除术后相当严重的并发症,发生率为2.6%~33.0%[74-77]。Zimmitti等[12]调查了M. D. Anderson肿瘤中心行肝切除的患者,结果显示,术后并发症发生率为9.8%,其中胆漏发生率为4.8%。虽然这么多年来,术中失血量和输血率一直在下降,但胆漏的发生率却从早年的3.7%上升至近年来的5.9%。尽管切除术的死亡率和其他并发症的发生率都下降了,但是胆道系统的并发症仍然是一个重要的问题。

胆漏的定义有许多种:腹部伤口或引流管中引流出胆汁,引流管或再次手术中探查到胆漏,或者胆道造影发现胆汁外泄[76]。国际肝脏手术研究小组(ISGLS)将胆漏定义为:引流液中胆红素水平高于血浆水平3倍,或术后3天上升3倍,或需要放射或手术介入治疗胆汁积聚、胆汁性腹膜炎[78]。

胆漏会导致住院时间明显延长,并且需要额外的影像学检查或介入治疗。严重的胆漏会引起腹腔内脓肿,死亡率为40%~50%[79,81];胆漏患者平均住院时间延长8~12天,$P<0.001$。

1. 危险因素

许多研究对胆漏危险因素进行了探讨。Lo等[76]发现,高龄、手术前白细胞增高、肝左叶切除、手术时间较长为致胆漏的危险因素。Nagano等认为,高龄、切口面积大、高危手术为致胆漏因素[82,83]。除此之外,Benzoni等[9]还发现,Pringle法阻断超过20分钟、输血量大于600ml、胸膜渗漏、扩大肝切除是肝脏切除术后致胆漏的因素。而高龄在不同的研究结果中,不能确定是否为致病因素[76,84]。详见表5-3。

表 5-3 胆漏因素

研究者	胆漏发生率(%)		重要因素
Lo 等[76]	8.1	年龄 非 HCC 平均血红蛋白 EBL 血小板 非肝硬化肝脏 Logistic 回归： 　高龄 　术前白细胞增多	肝功能 Child 分级为 B 和 C 级 肝脏大部分切除 肝尾叶切除 T 管引流 伴随胆肠吻合术 平均手术时间 左肝切除 延长手术时间
Sadamori 等[10] (全部肝细胞癌)	12.9	三段切除 重复肝脏切除 MVA OR 时间 >300 分钟	OR 时间 >300 分钟 输血
Zimmitti 等[12]	4.8	术前黄疸 门静脉栓塞 胆管肿瘤 重复肝脏切除 两段肝切除 扩大切除 肝尾叶切除 整块膈膜切除 MVA 重复肝脏切除 胆管切除 术中输血	胆管切除/重建 肝脏相关流程手术时间 >180 分钟 EBL >1000ml 肿瘤直径 >30mm 肝门淋巴结清扫 术中输血 整块膈膜切除 扩大切除
Benzoni 等[9]	6	肝脏大部分切除 左肝切除 三段切除 两段肝切除术/左肝叶切除	段/楔形切除 Pringle 法 >20 分钟 输血 >600ml 囊肿 肝功能不全 胸腔积液

续表

研究者	胆漏发生率(%)	重要因素	
adamori 等[83]	12.8	重复肝脏切除 OR 时间 >300 分钟 预计输血量 >2000ml MVA 重复肝切除 手术时间 >300 分钟	输血 肝实质横切时间
Nagano 等[82]	5.4	年龄 切面面积 高风险手术	
Okumura 等[85]	6.5	肝脏纤维化或肝硬化 OR 时间 >5 小时 肝脏大部分切除 MVA 手术时间 肝 4 段切除	包括肝脏 4 段或 5 段的肝脏切除术

EBL:预计失血量;HCC:肝细胞癌;MVA:多因素分析;OR,手术室

对于肝细胞癌的患者,致胆漏因素包括肝硬化、肝大部分切除、手术时间等,胆漏发生率与非肝细胞癌患者之间无统计学差异(表 5 - 4)[85]。Sadamori 等[10]的研究结果显示,重复肝脏切除术的单变量因素:手术时间 >300 分钟,失血 >2L,输血,断肝时间等是肝细胞癌患者胆漏的危险致病因素。虽然很多文献都分析了致胆漏的危险因素,但由于胆漏的定义和各个实验设计的不同,使得各个研究之间很难相互对比。

表 5 - 4 不同病理学的胆漏情况

研究者	病理	胆漏数量(百分比)
Tanaka 等[103] 2002	HCC(316)	23(7.3%)
	CCC(9)	3(33.3%)
	转移性癌症(33)	0(0%)
	其他(5)	0(0%)
Nagano 等[82] 2003	HCC(126)	9(7.1%)
	转移性癌症(187)	17(5.4%)
Sadamori 等[10] 2013	HCC(359)	46(12.8%)

缩写:CCC,胆管癌;HCC,肝细胞癌

2. 处理方法

针对各大并发症,预防是最好的处理方法。有很多文献提供了预防或术中发现、修补胆漏的策略[86-92],但没有哪一种术式可以彻底避免胆漏。钳夹法、缝合器缝合、超声吸引刀(CUSA)、射频切割闭合器、超声刀、血管缝合系统都有可能导致胆漏。一项 meta 分析显示,和钳夹法、超声吸引刀、射频切割闭合器相比,使用血管缝合系统胆漏发生率较低,但仍需要随机对照研究来验证[93]。同样,有人建议使用其他方法,如纤维蛋白胶水、大网膜包裹法,但缺乏大型随机或多中心实验研究,专家也未在其有效性方面达成共识[94-97]。

预防术后胆漏的备选策略为术中即刻探查并修补胆漏。有许多研究分析了术中探查胆漏的方法,但各有优缺点。M. D. Anderson 肿瘤中心的 Zimmitti 等[98]最近提出"air leak test"法在术中检测胆漏,使用该方法的患者术后胆漏发生率较低(1.9% vs 10.8%,$P = 0.008$)。染色剂吲哚菁绿、亚甲蓝也可用于术中胆漏的探查,但这些染色剂同时也会浸染周围的软组织,使探查难度加大[74,99]。注射生理盐水检查也可用于胆漏的探查,但 Ljichi 等[100]的随机对照研究未发现该方法可降低术后胆漏发生(6% vs 4%,$P = 0.99$)。Li 等[101]最近设计了一个"白色实验",即往导管内注入脂肪乳浊液来探查有无胆漏,实验组和对照组术后胆漏发生率分别为 5.3% 和 22.9%,$P < 0.01$,但这只是小样本单中心实验。Kaibori 等[102]在术中使用吲哚菁绿荧光胆道造影来探查有无胆漏,实验组和对照组术后胆漏发生率分别为 10% 和 0,$P = 0.019$。尽管这些研究结果十分乐观,但大多为小样本或单中心的回顾性研究,将来仍需要大样本多中心研究来证实。

很多患者的胆漏可以自愈。2002 年,Tanaka 等[103]的研究显示,363 例行肝脏切除术的患者,7.2%(26/338)术后出现胆漏,其中 69%(18/26)的患者未经治疗自愈了。2003 年,Nagano 等[82]的结果也显示了类似的结果,大多数患者仅靠引流就可自愈,术后胆漏平均自愈时间为 37.8 天。Vigano 等[104]的结果示,593 例有胆漏的患者,其中 76.5% 可以自愈,多变量因素分析发现,保守治疗失败的唯一因素为引流量大于 100ml/d。

对于没有预留有效引流管的患者,可用介入治疗放置引流管,治疗腹腔积液、预防并治疗败血症。对于持续性胆漏患者,内窥镜逆行胰胆管造影(ERPCs)和经皮肝胆管造影(PTCs)常用来提高胆道引流效果,目的是减少胆囊创口流出液。但是,常常因为未在术后及早进行胆道扩张而无法使用经皮肝胆管造影术。最近发现,在胆道减压和治疗胆漏方面,内窥镜逆行胰胆管造影非常有效,但不适用于胆道分流术后[105,106]。较小的胆漏可以使用纤维蛋白胶水修补。有的研究人员建议,每天胆漏量少于 50ml 可使用该方法修补,但具体的量尚未确定[74,103]。这种方法仍存在一定争议。

胆漏需要再次手术的患者死亡率极高。肝脏在首次手术后已创伤累累,很难有足够的肝功能储备耐受第二次大手术。而且,胆漏也常出现在术后炎症应答最严重时,很有可能发生吻合口粘连。有研究结果显示,再次手术的患者死亡率为 37.5%[76,107]。Lo 等[76]的结果则是:5 例需要再次手术修补胆漏的患者中仅 1 例生存。

五、肝脏切除术后肝衰竭

肝衰竭是肝脏切除术后最严重的并发症。虽然临时支持体系正在发展,然而目前,除了给予支持性密切监护外,对于肝衰竭这一致死性并发症暂无他法。肝脏切除术后肝衰竭(RHLF)的发生率为4%~19%,在不同人群和肝切除范围内有所不同[108-112]。近年随着术前评估、术中手术技术及术后支持治疗的进步,肝切除术后肝衰竭的发生率已经低于10%[78,113]。肝衰竭是肝脏切除术后主要的死亡原因,有的研究中死亡率为18%~75%[114-116],而另一些研究中死亡率为60%~100%[117-119]。

超过50项研究对肝脏切除术后肝衰竭给出不同的定义。有人根据实验室检查指标,如胆红素、INR,另外有些人则是根据临床表现,如肝性脑病、腹水的出现,还有人则是结合实验室检查和临床表现给出定义[6,78,120-122]。不同时期肝衰竭的定义也是不同的,比如,"50-50标准"采用术后5天胆红素和INR来预测肝脏切除术后死亡率[123]。Hyder等[4]则采用综合算法来预测肝脏切除术后肝衰竭。Mullen等[6]定义术后胆红素峰浓度大于7mg/dl为肝衰竭。2011年,ISGLS定义肝脏切除术后肝衰竭为肝脏合成、分泌、解毒能力受损,手术5天以后INR值和胆红素同时升高,并根据程度不同分为A、B、C级[78]。Erta等[124]定义,术后3天胆红素高于3mg/dl是早期肝功能不全特异且敏感的指标。这些不同的肝衰竭定义,使得很难在不同研究之间进行横向比较。

1. 危险因素

确定肝脏切除术后肝衰竭的危险因素很重要,可以避免这些患者在接受手术后发生致死性的严重并发症。危险因素包括患者及基础肝脏疾病、术中术后患者管理两大方面(表5-5)。

表5-5 肝脏切除术后肝衰竭危险因素

类别	危险因素
患者相关	年龄
	男性
	合并症
	先前存在的(基础)肝脏疾病
	脂肪肝
	肝脏纤维化
	肝硬化
	化疗导致的肝损伤
手术/术后	手术时间延长
	过度失血
	残肝过小
	缺血/再灌注
	感染

(1)患者及疾病因素

年龄和性别可能是肝脏切除术后肝衰竭的危险因素,但各研究结果却不一致。有的研究结果显示,经过选择的高龄患者不易发生肝脏切除术后肝衰竭,但有些研究显示,年龄大于65岁的患者术后更易出现肝功能不全,尤其在行扩大肝切除术的时候[123,125-132]。从肝再生能力这一点来看,Fernandes等[132]的结果显示,不同年龄患者肝脏再生能力无差别。就性别因素而言,男性易发生肝脏切除术后肝衰竭,有研究认为,男性肝衰竭发生率加倍[6,133]。

由于新辅助化疗的作用,越来越多患者在化疗后接受肝脏切除术[134]。结直肠癌常用的化疗药物包括5氟尿嘧啶、奥沙利铂、伊立替康,另外还有贝伐单抗、西妥昔单抗等靶向治疗。虽然化疗及靶向治疗可使不可切除的结直肠癌肝转移变为可切除,但使用化疗或靶向治疗后可能引起脂肪变性、脂肪性肝炎、肝窦瘀血等[135-141]。

2006年,Karoul等[142]发表文章,探讨术前化疗对肝大部分切除的影响。结果显示,术后并发症的发生率与术前化疗周期明显相关,对照组中无肝脏切除术后肝衰竭,化疗组11%的患者出现明显的肝衰竭,$P=0.046$。实验组中位化疗周期为15,其中90%患者中50%的肝细胞出现脂肪变性。Shindoh等[143]研究了无化疗组、短程化疗(<12周)、长程化疗(>12周)的患者,其术后肝功能不全发生率分别为0%、5.1%、16.3%,$P=0.04$。因此,他们建议,在化疗时间长于12周的患者中残肝(future liver remnant,FLR)的量至少应为30%,从而减少术后肝功能不全的发生率。

除了化疗引起的毒性,肝硬化是另一个致肝衰竭的重要因素,尤其在肝细胞癌患者中。这些患者肝功能储备、再生能力都较差,使得手术本身风险就较高,因此需要更多的残肝来避免肝脏切除术后肝衰竭。肝硬化患者肝脏切除术后肝衰竭发生率为2%~19%[144-151]。Chlid-Pugh评分或终末期肝脏疾病模型(Model for End-Stage Liver Disease)虽然可以评估肝硬化的程度,但也可能低估患者耐受手术的能力。因此在此类患者中,至少是在亚洲患者中,有必要进行术前肝功能储备测试,如吲哚菁绿清除率[139,152]。肝硬化患者至少需要40%残肝[153-155]。对于一些肝脏储备能力特别差,如吲哚菁绿清除率为10%~20%的患者,有人建议残肝至少为50%,以减少术后肝衰竭的发生[153,156]。

(2)术中、术后危险因素

手术中及术后也存在致肝衰竭危险因素,其中,术后肝功能不全与残肝、肝血流阻断时间、手术时间、失血量有关。

对于正常肝组织,20%~25%的残肝就可避免术后肝功能不全,但对于术前接受过化疗或本身合并肝硬化、脂肪肝、肝脏纤维化的患者,残肝至少应达到40%[154,157]。门静脉栓塞等手段可用于确保有足够的残肝。外科医生在术前应认真考虑残肝量[133,158]。

肝脏耐受Pringle法缺血/再灌注周期的能力可能会有限,术后肝功能储备也会减少,因此有人提出间断或持续夹闭可以提高患者的耐受力。Clavien等[159]提出,若在肝脏血流断流30分钟前进行缺血预处理,即10分钟缺血、10分钟再灌注,可以降低术后肝衰竭发生率,特别是年轻患者及阻断时间较长、合并脂肪肝的患者。有研究显示,间断性夹闭可提高术后肝功能,但另一些研究则认为持续性夹闭失血较少、术中断肝时间较短[159-161]。而对肝硬化患者需谨慎考虑血流阻断方式。如确有必要阻断血流,选择性断流可保证在门静脉阻塞期间,残肝可通过肝动脉为肝脏供血[162]。

失血量和输血与肝功能不全呈直接正相关[5,23,75]。虽然不同文献中具体数值不同,但失血量达 1000~1250 ml 的患者术后并发症发生率明显升高。失血量增加可能引起低血压、心动过速、需要输血等[163]。失血还与凝血功能障碍有关,也意味着需要输血,存在感染隐患[23]。血液成分中的免疫调节因子也可能引起疾病复发[23,164]。以上各个因素都会在术后影响肝脏再生。

肝大部分切除术后感染率可高达50%,术后肝衰竭的患者80%以上合并细菌感染。感染可引起或加速由败血症引起的肝衰竭。而肝衰竭又会增加免疫抑制引起的感染或者败血症[116]。此外,肝衰竭也可能引起继发于免疫防御反应和败血症的感染[165]。负责肝脏再生、先天免疫系统的 Kupffer 细胞,受肝切除和细菌内毒素的双重影响,后者在肝脏和门脉血流易位的情况下,有可能增多。这些都会给肝脏带来进一步的负担,导致肝功能不全。

2. 治疗

肝衰竭最佳治疗方法是预防,主要的预防手段有:围手术期加强监控伴随疾病,仔细考量术前化疗周期次数,术后保留足够的残肝,尽量减少手术时间和失血量,术后严密监测肝功能、凝血指标和电解质水平等。患者一旦出现肝衰竭,治疗手段很有限。

一旦患者出现肝衰竭的征象,要马上对其严密监测,首先要保障患者的心肺肾功能[166],而新鲜冰冻血浆、维生素 K、白蛋白、利尿剂等都可用于支撑肝功能,必要时应透析或插管用呼吸机维持。

目前有两种主要的肝脏支持系统:分子吸收循环系统和普罗米修斯系统,前者是一种白蛋白透析机器,实际效果有待确认,而后者的解毒能力更佳[167,168]。未来需要更精细的研究对它们的疗效进行验证。肝衰竭患者有时也可考虑肝移植,但鉴于大部分肝脏切除术患者基础疾病为恶性肿瘤,肝移植的适应证较窄。

六、总结

美国肝脏切除术的数量及难度都在逐年增加,肝脏切除术后死亡率明显下降,但并发症的发生率仍保持稳定,甚至有文献称有上升趋势。虽然各研究分别比较了并发症的发生,但仍不确定术前、术中有哪些因素可影响患者预后。

应十分注意并发症的危害。2008年美国财政在医疗保健上的支出为 2.3 万亿美元,比 2007 年增加了 4.4%[169]。术后并发症的发生率是评价医疗质量的标准[170-172]。瑞士的一项研究显示,肝脏手术后30天死亡率为3.1%,总的并发症发生率为56%,29%的患者至少出现一种并发症[173]。无并发症的手术平均费用为 13 625 美元,有并发症时则为 69 369 美元。显而易见的是,并发症类型、数目越多,花费越多。无并发症和有并发症的平均住院时间分别为 7.3 ± 4.5 天和 15.0 ± 12.2 天,$P < 0.001$。而且发生并发症的患者30天内再次手术的可能性较大。

最近，Lucas 等[174]利用美国外科医师学会（NSQIP）的结果，分析了肝、胆、胰、脾术后并发症发生时间及再入院率。总的并发症发生率为20.9%，但并发症发生的时间各不相同。泌尿道感染、呼吸道并发症、手术出血、心血管并发症发生较早，而伤口、深部组织器官裂开等并发症发生则较晚。出现较早的并发症导致的再次住院率较低，而出现较晚的并发症则更容易导致再次入院治疗，两者再次住院校正后比率分别为3.13%和8.45%。随着再住院人数的上升，对门诊患者进行充分随访、管理也更加重要。

越来越多高龄、身患多种疾病、合并肝炎肝硬化的患者接受外科肝脏切除术，虽然术后死亡率在不断下降，但并发症发生率不断升高。对各种并发症没有统一的定义，接受治疗的患者基础病、肝脏切除手术类型不一致，导致很难将各研究进行比较。ISGLS 已为几种高发并发症设置定义，这样，定义并发症的实际发生情况也更加简单。接下来，关键是要确定导致术后并发症或死亡的术前危险因素，为高风险手术选择合适的患者。

参考文献

[1] Dimick JB, Wainess RM, Cowan JA, et al. National trends in the use and outcomes of hepatic resection. J Am Coll Surg 2004;199:31－8.

[2] Asiyanbola B, Chang D, Gleisner AL, et al. Operative mortality after hepatic resection: are literature－based rates broadly applicable? J Gastrointest Surg 2008;12:842－51.

[3] Foster JH, Berman MM. Solid liver tumors. Major Probl Clin Surg 1977;22:1－342.

[4] Hyder O, Pulitano C, Firoozmand A, et al. A risk model to predict 90－day mortality among patients undergoing hepatic resection. J Am Coll Surg 2013;216:1049－56.

[5] Jarnagin WR, Gonen M, Fong Y, et al. Improvement in perioperative outcome after hepatic resection: analysis of 1,803 consecutive cases over the past decade. Ann Surg 2002;236:397－406 [discussion: 406－7].

[6] Mullen JT, Ribero D, Reddy SK, et al. Hepatic insufficiency and mortality in 1,059 noncirrhotic patients undergoing major hepatectomy. J Am Coll Surg 2007;204:854－62 [discussion: 862－4].

[7] McKay A, Sutherland FR, Bathe OF, et al. Morbidity and mortality following multivisceral resections in complex hepatic and pancreatic surgery. J Gastrointest Surg 2008;12:86－90.

[8] Mathur AK, Ghaferi AA, Osborne NH, et al. Body mass index and adverse perioperative outcomes following hepatic resection. J Gastrointest Surg 2010;14:1285－91.

[9] Benzoni E, Cojutti A, Lorenzin D, et al. Liver resective surgery: a multivariate analysis of postoperative outcome and complication. Langenbecks Arch Surg 2007;392:45－54.

[10] Sadamori H, Yagi T, Shinoura S, et al. Risk factors for major morbidity after liver resection for hepatocellular carcinoma. Br J Surg 2013;100:122－9.

[11] Virani S, Michaelson JS, Hutter MM, et al. Morbidity and mortality after liver resection: results of the patient safety in surgery study. J Am Coll Surg 2007;204:1284－92.

[12] Zimmitti G, Roses RE, Andreou A, et al. Greater complexity of liver surgery is not associated with an increased incidence of liver－related complications except for bile leak: an experience with 2,628 consecutive resections. J Gastrointest Surg 2013;17:57－64 [discussion: 64－5].

[13] Li GZ, Speicher PJ, Lidsky ME, et al. Hepatic resection for hepatocellular carcinoma: do contemporary morbidity and mortality rates demand a transition to ablation as first - line treatment? J Am Coll Surg 2014; 218:827 - 34.

[14] Okuda K. Hepatocellular carcinoma. J Hepatol 2000;32:225 - 37.

[15] Adam R, Azoulay D, Castaing D, et al. Liver resection as a bridge to transplantation for hepatocellular carcinoma on cirrhosis: a reasonable strategy? Ann Surg 2003;238:508 - 18 [discussion: 518 - 9].

[16] Bigourdan JM, Jaeck D, Meyer N, et al. Small hepatocellular carcinoma in Child A cirrhotic patients: hepatic resection versus transplantation. Liver Transpl 2003; 9:513 - 20.

[17] Cha CH, Ruo L, Fong Y, et al. Resection of hepatocellular carcinoma in patients otherwise eligible for transplantation. Ann Surg 2003;238:315 - 21 [discussion: 321 - 3].

[18] Margarit C, Escartin A, Castells L, et al. Resection for hepatocellular carcinoma is a good option in Child - Turcotte - Pugh class A patients with cirrhosis who are eligible for liver transplantation. Liver Transpl 2005;11:1242 - 51.

[19] Squires MH 3rd, Hanish SI, Fisher SB, et al. Transplant versus resection for the management of hepatocellular carcinoma meeting Milan Criteria in the MELD exception era at a single institution in a UNOS region with short wait times. J Surg Oncol 2014;109:533 - 41.

[20] Bismuth H, Majno PE. Hepatobiliary surgery. J Hepatol 2000;32:208 - 24.

[21] Arii S, Yamaoka Y, Futagawa S, et al. Results of surgical and nonsurgical treatment for small - sized hepatocellular carcinomas: a retrospective and nationwide survey in Japan. The Liver Cancer Study Group of Japan. Hepatology 2000;32:1224 - 9.

[22] Bruix J, Sherman M, Llovet JM, et al. Clinical management of hepatocellular carcinoma. Conclusions of the Barcelona - 2000 EASL conference. European Association for the Study of the Liver. J Hepatol 2001; 35:421 - 30.

[23] Kooby DA, Stockman J, Ben - Porat L, et al. Influence of transfusions on perioperative and long - term outcome in patients following hepatic resection for colorectal metastases. Ann Surg 2003;237:860 - 9 [discussion: 869 - 70].

[24] Rahbari NN, Garden OJ, Padbury R, et al. Post - hepatectomy haemorrhage: a definition and grading by the International Study Group of Liver Surgery (ISGLS). HPB (Oxford) 2011;13:528 - 35.

[25] Belghiti J, Hiramatsu K, Benoist S, et al. Seven hundred forty - seven hepatectomies in the 1990s: an update to evaluate the actual risk of liver resection. J Am Coll Surg 2000;191:38 - 46.

[26] Schroeder RA, Marroquin CE, Bute BP, et al. Predictive indices of morbidity and mortality after liver resection. Ann Surg 2006;243:373 - 9.

[27] Lim C, Dokmak S, Farges O, et al. Reoperation for post - hepatectomy hemorrhage: increased risk of mortality. Langenbecks Arch Surg 2014;399:735 - 40.

[28] Fujii M, Shimada M, Satoru I, et al. A standardized safe hepatectomy: selective Glissonean transection using endolinear stapling devices. Hepatogastroenterology 2007;54:906 - 9.

[29] Fujii Y, Shimada H, Endo I, et al. Management of massive arterial hemorrhage after pancreatobiliary surgery: does embolotherapy contribute to successful outcome? J Gastrointest Surg 2007;11:432 - 8.

[30] Ogata S, Belghiti J, Farges O, et al. Sequential arterial and portal vein embolizations before right hepatectomy in patients with cirrhosis and hepatocellular carcinoma. Br J Surg 2006;93:1091 - 8.

[31] Cho JY, Suh KS, Kwon CH, et al. Mild hepatic steatosis is not a major risk factor for hepatectomy and regenerative power is not impaired. Surgery 2006;139:508-15.

[32] Azoulay D, Lucidi V, Andreani P, et al. Ischemic preconditioning for major liver resection under vascular exclusion of the liver preserving the caval flow: a randomized prospective study. J Am Coll Surg 2006;202:203-11.

[33] Vauthey JN, Pawlik TM, Abdalla EK, et al. Is extended hepatectomy for hepatobiliary malignancy justified? Ann Surg 2004;239:722-30 [discussion:730-2].

[34] Yang T, Li L, Zhong Q, et al. Risk factors of hospital mortality after re-laparotomy for post-hepatectomy hemorrhage. World J Surg 2013;37:2394-401.

[35] Jin S, Fu Q, Wuyun G, et al. Management of post-hepatectomy complications. World J Gastroenterol 2013;19:7983-91.

[36] Tsao JI, Loftus JP, Nagorney DM, et al. Trends in morbidity and mortality of hepatic resection for malignancy. A matched comparative analysis. Ann Surg 1994;220:199-205.

[37] Finch MD, Crosbie JL, Currie E, et al. An 8-year experience of hepatic resection: indications and outcome. Br J Surg 1998;85:315-9.

[38] Sitzmann JV, Greene PS. Perioperative predictors of morbidity following hepatic resection for neoplasm. A multivariate analysis of a single surgeon experience with 105 patients. Ann Surg 1994;219:13-7.

[39] Catheline JM, Capelluto E, Gaillard JL, et al. Thromboembolism prophylaxis and incidence of thromboembolic complications after laparoscopic surgery. Int J Surg Investig 2000;2:41-7.

[40] Agnelli G, Bolis G, Capussotti L, et al. A clinical outcome-based prospective study on venous thromboembolism after cancer surgery: the @RISTOS project. Ann Surg 2006;243:89-95.

[41] Alcalay A, Wun T, Khatri V, et al. Venous thromboembolism in patients with colorectal cancer: incidence and effect on survival. J Clin Oncol 2006;24:1112-8.

[42] Flinterman LE, van Hylckama Vlieg A, Cannegieter SC, et al. Long-term survival in a large cohort of patients with venous thrombosis: incidence and predictors. PLoS Med 2012;9:e1001155.

[43] Ng AC, Chung T, Yong AS, et al. Long-term cardiovascular and noncardiovascular mortality of 1023 patients with confirmed acute pulmonary embolism. Circ Cardiovasc Qual Outcomes 2011;4:122-8.

[44] Sogaard KK, Schmidt M, Pedersen L, et al. 30-year mortality following venous thromboembolism: a population-based cohort study. Circulation 2014;130:829-36.

[45] Tzeng CW, Katz MH, Fleming JB, et al. Risk of venous thromboembolism outweighs post-hepatectomy bleeding complications: analysis of 5651 National Surgical Quality Improvement Program patients. HPB (Oxford) 2012;14:506-13.

[46] Reddy SK, Turley RS, Barbas AS, et al. Post-operative pharmacologic thromboprophylaxis after major hepatectomy: does peripheral venous thromboembolism prevention outweigh bleeding risks? J Gastrointest Surg 2011;15:1602-10.

[47] Kakkar AK, Levine M, Pinedo HM, et al. Venous thrombosis in cancer patients: insights from the FRONTLINE survey. Oncologist 2003;8:381-8.

[48] De Martino RR, Goodney PP, Spangler EL, et al. Variation in thromboembolic complications among patients undergoing commonly performed cancer operations. J Vasc Surg 2012;55:1035-40. e4.

[49] Nathan H, Weiss MJ, Soff GA, et al. Pharmacologic prophylaxis, postoperative INR, and risk of venous

thromboembolism after hepatectomy. J Gastrointest Surg 2014;18:295-302 [discussion:302-3].

[50] Melloul E, Dondero F, Vilgrain V, et al. Pulmonary embolism after elective liver resection: a prospective analysis of risk factors. J Hepatol 2012;57:1268-75.

[51] Morris-Stiff G, White A, Gomez D, et al. Thrombotic complications following liver resection for colorectal metastases are preventable. HPB (Oxford) 2008;10:311-4.

[52] Ejaz A, Spolverato G, Kim Y, et al. Defining incidence and risk factors of venous thromboembolism after hepatectomy. J Gastrointest Surg 2014;18:1116-24.

[53] Chitlur M. Challenges in the laboratory analyses of bleeding disorders. Thromb Res 2012;130:1-6.

[54] Collins R, Scrimgeour A, Yusuf S, et al. Reduction in fatal pulmonary embolism and venous thrombosis by perioperative administration of subcutaneous heparin. Overview of results of randomized trials in general, orthopedic, and urologic surgery. N Engl J Med 1988;318:1162-73.

[55] Mismetti P, Laporte S, Darmon JY, et al. Meta-analysis of low molecular weight heparin in the prevention of venous thromboembolism in general surgery. Br J Surg 2001;88:913-30.

[56] Azoulay D, Pascal G, Salloum C, et al. Vascular reconstruction combined with liver resection for malignant tumours. Br J Surg 2013;100:1764-75.

[57] Silva MA, Jambulingam PS, Gunson BK, et al. Hepatic artery thrombosis following orthotopic liver transplantation: a 10-year experience from a single centre in the United Kingdom. Liver Transpl 2006;12:146-51.

[58] Bhattacharjya S, Gunson BK, Mirza DF, et al. Delayed hepatic artery thrombosis in adult orthotopic liver transplantation—a 12-year experience. Transplantation 2001;71:1592-6.

[59] Woo DH, Laberge JM, Gordon RL, et al. Management of portal venous complications after liver transplantation. Tech Vasc Interv Radiol 2007;10:233-9.

[60] Wozney P, Zajko AB, Bron KM, et al. Vascular complications after liver transplantation: a 5-year experience. AJR Am J Roentgenol 1986;147:657-63.

[61] Cohen J, Edelman RR, Chopra S. Portal vein thrombosis: a review. Am J Med 1992;92:173-82.

[62] Witte CL, Brewer ML, Witte MH, et al. Protean manifestations of pylethrombosis. A review of thirty-four patients. Ann Surg 1985;202:191-202.

[63] Sheen CL, Lamparelli H, Milne A, et al. Clinical features, diagnosis and outcome of acute portal vein thrombosis. QJM 2000;93:531-4.

[64] Abbas S, Sandroussi C. Systematic review and meta-analysis of the role of vascular resection in the treatment of hilar cholangiocarcinoma. HPB (Oxford) 2013;15:492-503.

[65] Varotti G, Grazi GL, Vetrone G, et al. Causes of early acute graft failure after liver transplantation: analysis of a 17-year single-centre experience. Clin Transplant 2005;19:492-500.

[66] Langnas AN, Marujo W, Stratta RJ, et al. Vascular complications after orthotopic liver transplantation. Am J Surg 1991;161:76-82 [discussion:82-3].

[67] Iida T, Kaido T, Yagi S, et al. Hepatic arterial complications in adult living donor liver transplant recipients: a single-center experience of 673 cases. Clin Transplant 2014;28:1025-30.

[68] Thomas RM, Ahmad SA. Management of acute post-operative portal venous thrombosis. J Gastrointest Surg 2010;14:570-7.

[69] Condat B, Pessione F, Hillaire S, et al. Current outcome of portal vein thrombosis in adults: risk and ben-

efit of anticoagulant therapy. Gastroenterology 2001;120:490 – 7.

[70] Turnes J, Garcia – Pagan JC, Gonzalez M, et al. Portal hypertension – related complications after acute portal vein thrombosis: impact of early anticoagulation. Clin Gastroenterol Hepatol 2008;6:1412 – 7.

[71] Plessier A, Darwish – Murad S, Hernandez – Guerra M, et al. Acute portal vein thrombosis unrelated to cirrhosis: a prospective multicenter follow – up study. Hepatology 2010;51:210 – 8.

[72] Sobhonslidsuk A, Reddy KR. Portal vein thrombosis: a concise review. Am J Gastroenterol 2002;97:535 – 41.

[73] Bhattacharjya T, Olliff SP, Bhattacharjya S, et al. Percutaneous portal vein thrombolysis and endovascular stent for management of posttransplant portal venous conduit thrombosis. Transplantation 2000;69:2195 – 8.

[74] Yamashita Y, Hamatsu T, Rikimaru T, et al. Bile leakage after hepatic resection. Ann Surg 2001;233:45 – 50.

[75] Imamura H, Seyama Y, Kokudo N, et al. One thousand fifty – six hepatectomies without mortality in 8 years. Arch Surg 2003;138:1198 – 206 [discussion:1206].

[76] Lo CM, Fan ST, Liu CL, et al. Biliary complications after hepatic resection: risk factors, management, and outcome. Arch Surg 1998;133:156 – 61.

[77] Capussotti L, Ferrero A, Vigano L, et al. Bile leakage and liver resection: Where is the risk? Arch Surg 2006;141:690 – 4 [discussion: 695].

[78] Rahbari NN, Garden OJ, Padbury R, et al. Posthepatectomy liver failure: a definition and grading by the International Study Group of Liver Surgery (ISGLS). Surgery 2011;149:713 – 24.

[79] Kohno H, Nagasue N, Chang YC, et al. Comparison of topical hemostatic agents in elective hepatic resection: a clinical prospective randomized trial. World J Surg 1992;16:966 – 9 [discussion: 970].

[80] Bismuth H, Chiche L, Castaing D. Surgical treatment of hepatocellular carcinomas in noncirrhotic liver: experience with 68 liver resections. World J Surg 1995;19:35 – 41.

[81] Lai EC, Fan ST, Lo CM, et al. Hepatic resection for hepatocellular carcinoma. An audit of 343 patients. Ann Surg 1995;221:291 – 8.

[82] Nagano Y, Togo S, Tanaka K, et al. Risk factors and management of bile leakage after hepatic resection. World J Surg 2003;27:695 – 8.

[83] Sadamori H, Yagi T, Matsuda H, et al. Risk factors for major morbidity after hepatectomy for hepatocellular carcinoma in 293 recent cases. J Hepatobiliary Pancreat Sci 2010;17:709 – 18.

[84] Yamanaka N, Okamoto E, Kuwata K, et al. A multiple regression equation for prediction of posthepatectomy liver failure. Ann Surg 1984;200:658 – 63.

[85] Okumura K, Sugimachi K, Kinjo N, et al. Risk factors of bile leakage after hepatectomy for hepatocellular carcinoma. Hepatogastroenterology 2013;60:1717 – 9.

[86] Kim J, Ahmad SA, Lowy AM, et al. Increased biliary fistulas after liver resection with the harmonic scalpel. Am Surg 2003;69:815 – 9.

[87] Weber JC, Navarra G, Jiao LR, et al. New technique for liver resection using heat coagulative necrosis. Ann Surg 2002;236:560 – 3.

[88] Poon RT, Fan ST, Wong J. Liver resection using a saline – linked radiofrequency dissecting sealer for transection of the liver. J Am Coll Surg 2005;200:308 – 13.

[89] Delis SG, Bakoyiannis A, Karakaxas D, et al. Hepatic parenchyma resection using stapling devices: peri-operative and long-term outcome. HPB (Oxford) 2009;11:38-44.

[90] Castaldo ET, Earl TM, Chari RS, et al. A clinical comparative analysis of crush/clamp, stapler, and dissecting sealer hepatic transection methods. HPB (Oxford) 2008;10:321-6.

[91] Romano F, Garancini M, Caprotti R, et al. Hepatic resection using a bipolar vessel sealing device: technical and histological analysis. HPB (Oxford) 2007;9:339-44.

[92] Geller DA, Tsung A, Maheshwari V, et al. Hepatic resection in 170 patients using saline-cooled radiofrequency coagulation. HPB (Oxford) 2005;7:208-13.

[93] Alexiou VG, Tsitsias T, Mavros MN, et al. Technology-assisted versus clamp-crush liver resection: a systematic review and meta-analysis. Surg Innov 2013;20:414-28.

[94] Kobayashi S, Nagano H, Marubashi S, et al. Fibrin sealant withPGAfelt for prevention of bile leakage after liver resection. Hepatogastroenterology 2012;59:2564-8.

[95] Sanjay P, Watt DG, Wigmore SJ. Systematic review and meta-analysis of haemostatic and biliostatic efficacy of fibrin sealants in elective liver surgery. J Gastrointest Surg 2013;17:829-36.

[96] Nanashima A, Tobinaga S, Abo T, et al. Usefulness of omental wrapping to prevent biliary leakage and delayed gastric emptying in left hepatectomy. Hepatogastroenterology 2012;59:847-50.

[97] de Boer MT, Boonstra EA, Lisman T, et al. Role of fibrin sealants in liver surgery. Dig Surg 2012;29:54-61.

[98] Zimmitti G, Vauthey JN, Shindoh J, et al. Systematic use of an intraoperative air leak test at the time of major liver resection reduces the rate of postoperative biliary complications. J Am Coll Surg 2013;217:1028-37.

[99] Lam CM, Lo CM, Liu CL, et al. Biliary complications during liver resection. World J Surg 2001;25:1273-6.

[100] Ijichi M, Takayama T, Toyoda H, et al. Randomized trial of the usefulness of a bile leakage test during hepatic resection. Arch Surg 2000;135:1395-400.

[101] Li J, Malago M, Sotiropoulos GC, et al. Intraoperative application of "white test" to reduce postoperative bile leak after major liver resection: results of a prospective cohort study in 137 patients. Langenbecks Arch Surg 2009;394:1019-24.

[102] Kaibori M, Ishizaki M, Matsui K, et al. Intraoperative indocyanine green fluorescent imaging for prevention of bile leakage after hepatic resection. Surgery 2011;150:91-8.

[103] Tanaka S, Hirohashi K, Tanaka H, et al. Incidence and management of bile leakage after hepatic resection for malignant hepatic tumors. J Am Coll Surg 2002;195:484-9.

[104] Vigano L, Ferrero A, Sgotto E, et al. Bile leak after hepatectomy: predictive factors of spontaneous healing. Am J Surg 2008;196:195-200.

[105] Sherman S, Shaked A, Cryer HM, et al. Endoscopic management of biliary fistulas complicating liver transplantation and other hepatobiliary operations. Ann Surg 1993;218:167-75.

[106] Cheung KL, Lai EC. Endoscopic stenting for malignant biliary obstruction. Arch Surg 1995;130:204-7.

[107] Pace RF, Blenkharn JI, Edwards WJ, et al. Intra-abdominal sepsis after hepatic resection. Ann Surg 1989;209:302-6.

[108] Capussotti L, Muratore A, Amisano M, et al. Liver resection for hepatocellular carcinoma on cirrhosis: analysis of mortality, morbidity and survival – a European single center experience. Eur J Surg Oncol 2005;31:986 – 93.

[109] Chok KS, Ng KK, Poon RT, et al. Impact of postoperative complications on longterm outcome of curative resection for hepatocellular carcinoma. Br J Surg 2009;96:81 – 7.

[110] Kawano Y, Sasaki A, Kai S, et al. Short – and long – term outcomes after hepatic resection for hepatocellular carcinoma with concomitant esophageal varices in patients with cirrhosis. Ann Surg Oncol 2008; 15:1670 – 6.

[111] Mizuguchi T, Nagayama M, Meguro M, et al. Prognostic impact of surgical complications and preoperative serum hepatocyte growth factor in hepatocellular carcinoma patients after initial hepatectomy. J Gastrointest Surg 2009;13:325 – 33.

[112] Okamura Y, Takeda S, Fujii T, et al. Prognostic significance of postoperative complications after hepatectomy for hepatocellular carcinoma. J Surg Oncol 2011;104:814 – 21.

[113] Paugam – Burtz C, Janny S, Delefosse D, et al. Prospective validation of the "fiftyfifty" criteria as an early and accurate predictor of death after liver resection in intensive care unit patients. Ann Surg 2009; 249:124 – 8.

[114] Detroz B, Sugarbaker PH, Knol JA, et al. Causes of death in patients undergoing liver surgery. Cancer Treat Res 1994;69:241 – 57.

[115] Simmonds PC, Primrose JN, Colquitt JL, et al. Surgical resection of hepatic metastases from colorectal cancer: a systematic review of published studies. Br J Cancer 2006;94:982 – 99.

[116] Garcea G, Maddern GJ. Liver failure after major hepatic resection. J Hepatobiliary Pancreat Surg 2009; 16:145 – 55.

[117] McCall J, Koea J, Gunn K, et al. Liver resections in Auckland 1998 – 2001: mortality, morbidity and blood product use. N Z Med J 2001;114:516 – 9.

[118] Sun HC, Qin LX, Wang L, et al. Risk factors for postoperative complications after liver resection. Hepatobiliary Pancreat Dis Int 2005;4:370 – 4.

[119] Schindl MJ, Redhead DN, Fearon KC, et al. The value of residual liver volume as a predictor of hepatic dysfunction and infection after major liver resection. Gut 2005;54:289 – 96.

[120] Pawlik TM, Olino K, Gleisner AL, et al. Preoperative chemotherapy for colorectal liver metastases: impact on hepatic histology and postoperative outcome. J Gastrointest Surg 2007;11:860 – 8.

[121] Zorzi D, Chun YS, Madoff DC, et al. Chemotherapy with bevacizumab does not affect liver regeneration after portal vein embolization in the treatment of colorectal liver metastases. Ann Surg Oncol 2008;15: 2765 – 72.

[122] Adam R, Aloia T, Levi F, et al. Hepatic resection after rescue cetuximab treatment for colorectal liver metastases previously refractory to conventional systemic therapy. J Clin Oncol 2007;25:4593 – 602.

[123] Balzan S, Belghiti J, Farges O, et al. The "50 – 50 criteria" on postoperative day 5: an accurate predictor of liver failure and death after hepatectomy. Ann Surg 2005;242:824 – 8 [discussion: 828 – 9].

[124] Etra JW, Squires MH 3rd, Fisher SB, et al. Early identification of patients at increased risk for hepatic insufficiency, complications and mortality after major hepatectomy. HPB (Oxford) 2014;16:875 – 83.

[125] Menon KV, Al – Mukhtar A, Aldouri A, et al. Outcomes after major hepatectomy in elderly patients. J

Am Coll Surg 2006;203:677 - 83.

[126] Aldrighetti L, Arru M, Caterini R, et al. Impact of advanced age on the outcome of liver resection. World J Surg 2003;27:1149 - 54.

[127] Ferrero A, Vigano L, Polastri R, et al. Hepatectomy as treatment of choice for hepatocellular carcinoma in elderly cirrhotic patients. World J Surg 2005;29: 1101 - 5.

[128] Hanazaki K, Kajikawa S, Shimozawa N, et al. Hepatic resection for hepatocellular carcinoma in the elderly. J Am Coll Surg 2001;192:38 - 46.

[129] Mastoraki A, Tsakali A, Papanikolaou IS, et al. Outcome following major hepatic resection in the elderly patients. Clin Res Hepatol Gastroenterol 2014;38:462 - 6.

[130] Alfieri S, Carriero C, Caprino P, et al. Avoiding early postoperative complications in liver surgery. A multivariate analysis of 254 patients consecutively observed. Dig Liver Dis 2001;33:341 - 6.

[131] Koperna T, Kisser M, Schulz F. Hepatic resection in the elderly. World J Surg 1998;22:406 - 12.

[132] Fernandes AI, Tralhao JG, Abrantes A, et al. Functional hepatocellular regeneration in elderly patients undergoing hepatectomy. Liver Int 2013. [Epub ahead of print].

[133] Shoup M, Gonen M, D'Angelica M, et al. Volumetric analysis predicts hepatic dysfunction in patients undergoing major liver resection. J Gastrointest Surg 2003;7:325 - 30.

[134] Brouquet A, Nordlinger B. Neoadjuvant therapy of colorectal liver metastases: lessons learned from clinical trials. J Surg Oncol 2010;102:932 - 6.

[135] Fowler WC, Eisenberg BL, Hoffman JP. Hepatic resection following systemic chemotherapy for metastatic colorectal carcinoma. J Surg Oncol 1992;51:122 - 5.

[136] Bismuth H, Adam R, Levi F, et al. Resection of nonresectable liver metastases from colorectal cancer after neoadjuvant chemotherapy. Ann Surg 1996;224: 509 - 20 [discussion: 520 - 2].

[137] Shankar A, Leonard P, Renaut AJ, et al. Neo - adjuvant therapy improves resectability rates for colorectal liver metastases. Ann R Coll Surg Engl 2001;83:85 - 8.

[138] King PD, Perry MC. Hepatotoxicity of chemotherapy. Oncologist 2001;6:162 - 76.

[139] Makuuchi M, Kokudo N, Arii S, et al. Development of evidence - based clinical guidelines for the diagnosis and treatment of hepatocellular carcinoma in Japan. Hepatol Res 2008;38:37 - 51.

[140] Rubbia - Brandt L, Lauwers GY, Wang H, et al. Sinusoidal obstruction syndrome and nodular regenerative hyperplasia are frequent oxaliplatin - associated liver lesions and partially prevented by bevacizumab in patients with hepatic colorectal metastasis. Histopathology 2010;56:430 - 9.

[141] Soubrane O, Brouquet A, Zalinski S, et al. Predicting high grade lesions of sinusoidal obstruction syndrome related to oxaliplatin - based chemotherapy for colorectal liver metastases: correlation with post - hepatectomy outcome. Ann Surg 2010;251:454 - 60.

[142] Karoui M, Penna C, Amin - Hashem M, et al. Influence of preoperative chemotherapy on the risk of major hepatectomy for colorectal liver metastatses. Ann Surg 2006;243(1):1 - 7.

[143] Shindoh J, Tzeng CW, Aloia TA, et al. Optimal future liver remnant in patients treated with extensive preoperative chemotherapy for colorectal liver metastases. Ann Surg Oncol 2013;20(8):2493 - 500.

[144] Fong Y, Sun RL, Jarnagin W, et al. An analysis of 412 cases of hepatocellular carcinoma at a Western center. Ann Surg 1999;229:790 - 9 [discussion: 799 - 800].

[145] Midorikawa Y, Kubota K, Takayama T, et al. A comparative study of postoperative complications after

hepatectomy in patients with and without chronic liver disease. Surgery 1999;126:484 - 91.

[146] Poon RT, Fan ST, Lo CM, et al. Extended hepatic resection for hepatocellular carcinoma in patients with cirrhosis: is it justified? Ann Surg 2002;236:602 - 11.

[147] Hsu KY, Chau GY, Lui WY, et al. Predicting morbidity and mortality after hepatic resection in patients with hepatocellular carcinoma: the role of Model for End - Stage Liver Disease score. World J Surg 2009;33:2412 - 9.

[148] Choi GH, Park JY, Hwang HK, et al. Predictive factors for long - term survival in patients with clinically significant portal hypertension following resection of hepatocellular carcinoma. Liver Int 2011;31:485 - 93.

[149] Ruzzenente A, Valdegamberi A, Campagnaro T, et al. Hepatocellular carcinoma in cirrhotic patients with portal hypertension: is liver resection always contraindicated? World J Gastroenterol 2011;17:5083 - 8.

[150] Cucchetti A, Ercolani G, Vivarelli M, et al. Is portal hypertension a contraindication to hepatic resection? Ann Surg 2009;250:922 - 8.

[151] Capussotti L, Ferrero A, Vigano L, et al. Portal hypertension: contraindication to liver surgery? World J Surg 2006;30:992 - 9.

[152] Scheingraber S, Richter S, Igna D, et al. Indocyanine green disappearance rate is themost usefulmarker for liver resection. Hepatogastroenterology 2008;55:1394 - 9.

[153] Kubota K, Makuuchi M, Kusaka K, et al. Measurement of liver volume and hepatic functional reserve as a guide to decision - making in resectional surgery for hepatic tumors. Hepatology 1997;26:1176 - 81.

[154] Shirabe K, Shimada M, Gion T, et al. Postoperative liver failure after major hepatic resection for hepatocellular carcinoma in the modern era with special reference to remnant liver volume. J Am Coll Surg 1999;188:304 - 9.

[155] Zorzi D, Laurent A, Pawlik TM, et al. Chemotherapy - associated hepatotoxicity and surgery for colorectal liver metastases. Br J Surg 2007;94:274 - 86.

[156] Makuuchi M, Kosuge T, Takayama T, et al. Surgery for small liver cancers. Semin Surg Oncol 1993;9:298 - 304.

[157] de Santibanes E, Alvarez FA, Ardiles V. How to avoid postoperative liver failure: a novel method. World J Surg 2012;36:125 - 8.

[158] Vauthey JN, Chaoui A, Do KA, et al. Standardized measurement of the future liver remnant prior to extended liver resection: methodology and clinical associations. Surgery 2000;127:512 - 9.

[159] Clavien PA, Selzner M, Rudiger HA, et al. A prospective randomized study in 100 consecutive patients undergoing major liver resection with versus without ischemic preconditioning. Ann Surg 2003;238:843 - 50 [discussion: 851 - 2].

[160] Serafin A, Rosello - Catafau J, Prats N, et al. Ischemic preconditioning increases the tolerance of fatty liver to hepatic ischemia - reperfusion injury in the rat. Am J Pathol 2002;161:587 - 601.

[161] Petrowsky H, McCormack L, Trujillo M, et al. A prospective, randomized, controlled trial comparing intermittent portal triad clamping versus ischemic preconditioning with continuous clamping for major liver resection. Ann Surg 2006;244:921 - 8 [discussion: 928 - 30].

[162] Jin S, Dai CL. Hepatic blood inflow occlusion without hemihepatic artery control in treatment of hepatocellular carcinoma. World J Gastroenterol 2010;16: 5895 - 900.

[163] van den Broek MA, Olde Damink SW, Dejong CH, et al. Liver failure after partial hepatic resection: definition, pathophysiology, risk factors and treatment. Liver Int 2008;28:767-80.

[164] Jensen LS, Andersen AJ, Christiansen PM, et al. Postoperative infection and natural killer cell function following blood transfusion in patients undergoing elective colorectal surgery. Br J Surg 1992;79:513-6.

[165] Lipka JM, Zibari GB, Dies DF, et al. Spontaneous bacterial peritonitis in liver failure. Am Surg 1998; 64:1155-7.

[166] Schreckenbach T, Liese J, Bechstein WO, et al. Posthepatectomy liver failure. Dig Surg 2012;29:79-85.

[167] van de Kerkhove MP, de Jong KP, Rijken AM, et al. MARS treatment in posthepatectomy liver failure. Liver Int 2003;23(Suppl 3):44-51.

[168] Chiu A, Chan LM, Fan ST. Molecular adsorbent recirculating system treatment for patients with liver failure: the Hong Kong experience. Liver Int 2006;26:695-702.

[169] Sisko A, Truffer C, Smith S, et al. Health spending projections through 2018: recession effects add uncertainty to the outlook. Health Aff (Millwood) 2009;28:w346-57.

[170] Birkmeyer JD, Dimick JB, Birkmeyer NJ. Measuring the quality of surgical care: structure, process, or outcomes? J Am Coll Surg 2004;198:626-32.

[171] Barkun JS, Aronson JK, Feldman LS, et al. Evaluation and stages of surgical innovations. Lancet 2009; 374:1089-96.

[172] Ergina PL, Cook JA, Blazeby JM, et al. Challenges in evaluating surgical innovation. Lancet 2009;374: 1097-104.

[173] Vonlanthen R, Slankamenac K, Breitenstein S, et al. The impact of complications on costs of major surgical procedures: a cost analysis of 1200 patients. Ann Surg 2011;254:907-13.

[174] Lucas DJ, Sweeney JF, Pawlik TM. The timing of complications impacts risk of readmission after hepatopancreatobiliary surgery. Surgery 2014;155:945-53.

第六章 肝细胞癌、胆管细胞癌和结直肠癌肝转移的消融治疗

Paul D. Hansen, MD*, Maria A. Cassera, bsc, Ronald F. Wolf, MD

【关键词】

肝脏；消融；射频；微波；冷冻疗法；肝细胞癌；结直肠癌肝转移

要点

- 选择消融技术治疗时，术者应根据实际情况，综合考虑各种不同的消融方法，不局限于单一的消融方法。
- 无论良性、恶性、原发性或转移性肿瘤，均可选取合适的消融疗法。
- 一般而言，消融治疗更常用于少量或较小的肿瘤，同时，对于不适合或者不愿接受手术切除的患者，消融治疗也是很好的选择。
- 消融技术可以分为化学消融和物理消融（热、冷冻消融）。每种消融方法都可通过经皮穿刺、经腹腔镜或手术开腹等途径进行。

一、简介

对于肝细胞癌、胆管细胞癌、结直肠癌肝转移以及其他肝内肿瘤，手术切除一直被认为是治愈性治疗的金标准。然而，由于肿瘤大小、位置、体积、多灶性、肝功能不全等因素，只有5%～15%的患者适合进行手术治疗[1]。消融技术已成为除肝脏切除术以外另一种安全有效

的治疗方法。近年来,一系列随机、对照临床实验结果显示[2,3],对于某些特定病例,消融治疗可以达到和手术治疗相同的效果。

近几十年来,一系列消融治疗技术得以陆续开展,而且可以根据不同患者情况选取相应的消融方法。目前,消融技术主要分为两大类:化学消融和物理消融。最近,不可逆电穿孔(IRE)也成为电诱导细胞破坏的一种代替形式。在这一章中,我们主要论述几种肝肿瘤消融技术、患者选择标准、目前的消融方案和整体疗效等内容。

二、消融技术

肿瘤消融并不是一个新的概念。几个世纪之前,就已经出现了粗略的关于组织或肿瘤消融的报道。随着对肿瘤、现代影像学技术和消融技术研究的深入,我们目前可以更好地评估肿瘤组织的情况,并准确地定位肿瘤,从而安全进行消融治疗。尽管与消融治疗相关的更深入的研究还在进行,目前已经可以证明,对于特定病例,消融技术可以治愈肿瘤,并保证最小并发症发生率。

目前,肿瘤消融常使用的方式为化学消融或物理消融。对每种方法的具体介绍将在后文进行详述。总体而言,非切除性治疗方式有多方面优势。近20年来,尽管肝脏切除术在安全性上有明显的改善,而且可以使用微创技术完成手术,但消融治疗的并发症发生率仍远小于手术切除。除此之外,因为消融治疗可以对单个肿瘤进行定位治疗,周围的肝实质不会受到很大影响,所以特别适合那些病灶弥散、肝功能受损,以及需要长期进行重复性介入治疗的患者。

1. 化学消融

最常用的化学消融法是酒精注入,也有一些医院使用5%乙酸作为替代品[4]。向肿瘤组织内缓慢注入纯度95%的酒精可以导致局部肿瘤凝固性坏死,肿瘤血管形成血栓以及组织缺血。

化学消融的优点是操作简单,手术治疗费用较低。其使用的药物价格都较低廉,如果病灶易于定位,则可以在门诊超声引导下进行。相对于热消融,化学消融另一个很重要的优势是精确定位,明显减少对周围组织、胆管及血管结构的损伤。

化学消融的局限性在于其治疗效果依赖于化学药物在肿瘤内的扩散程度。尽管肝细胞癌和神经内分泌性肿瘤相对较软,而且有包膜包裹,治疗药物弥散较好。但对于致密的肿瘤,如转移性的腺癌,常常质地较硬而且纤维化程度较高,往往化学药物在瘤内不能均匀扩散。

由于复发率相对较高,化学消融通常只用于不适合切除或热消融治疗(比如肿瘤贴近胆管等情况),且肿瘤小于2cm的患者。

2. 冷冻消融

冷冻消融术利用超冷消融针,连接液氮、液氩循环系统进行消融。温度低于-170℃时,细胞内冰晶形成,细胞壁被破坏,微血管血栓形成,进而细胞坏死。

冷冻消融的优势在于,可见消融冰球的边缘,进而明确消融的范围。冰球的边缘是一个回波反射器,使用超声即可观察到。

冷冻消融也有明显局限性。消融针头的直径为5~10mm,单根消融针产生的最大冰球直径为5cm。为了扩大消融范围,常常会使用多根消融针。在解冻循环中,消融更易使组织结冰,就像在温水中放入冰块一样。这种冷冻方式可导致血管受损,明显出血。在拔出针头的过程中,管腔内大出血的情况比较常见,需向管腔中注入栓塞剂进行栓塞止血。基于上述特点,冷冻消融的穿刺路径局限性较大。冷冻消融特有的治疗后全身反应包括血小板严重降低、凝血功能障碍、肌红蛋白尿、急性肾功能损伤、电解质紊乱以及心律不齐等[5-11]。这些潜在的问题导致冷冻消融的患者需要额外监护,以及术后住院时间延长(图6-1)。

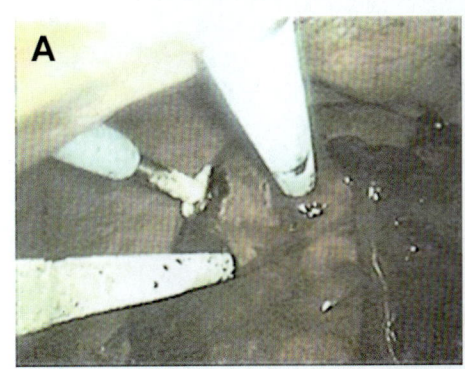
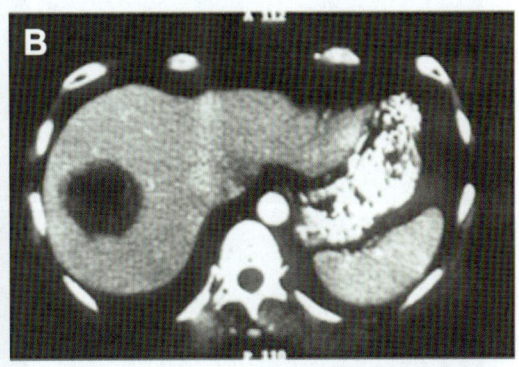

图6-1

A. 三根冷冻消融针在肝内产生了5cm的冰球;B. CT扫描显示,接受治疗10天后,肿瘤坏死区域

3. 热消融

很多消融技术是使组织升温至50℃以上,在这个温度下,蛋白质开始凝固,细胞壁被破坏,微血管血栓形成;在高于60℃时,细胞立即坏死。可以安全准确地导致靶病灶100%坏死,又不损伤周围组织的技术,即为消融技术。最常用的热消融技术是射频消融(RFA)和微波消融(MWA)。

热消融技术也存在一定的局限性。热消融的效果取决于是否在治疗区域达到合适的治疗温度。尽管目前临床上可以使用温度监测,测定消融区域多个点的温度,也有人仅在单一消融点测量温度,或经验性的设定消融时间,或通过阻抗测量。在对贴近中央胆管的肿瘤进行消融时,消融针可能在灭活靶病灶的同时引起脓肿或胆道狭窄。此外,邻近的器官,如十二指肠和结肠,也容易在消融过程中受损。术者应避免在离上述结构1~2cm范围内进行消融,或在消融过程中将以上组织剥离开来。

(1) 射频消融

射频消融是最常用的热消融治疗方式。射频消融使用高频交流电改变肿瘤和周围组织的电场离子运转方向,离子搅拌产生摩擦能量和热量,通过热传导分散开。单个靶病灶的消融时间取决于病灶大小及位置,通常在10~30分钟。直径2cm的肿瘤平均消融时间为20分钟。射频消融的优点是易操作,可通过经皮穿刺、经腹腔镜或手术开腹等途径进行。单个消融针的最大消融范围为6~7cm。这种治疗方式适用于单针大病灶消融。和微波消融相比较，射频消融升温较慢，且大血管较少受到损伤(图6-2)[12]。

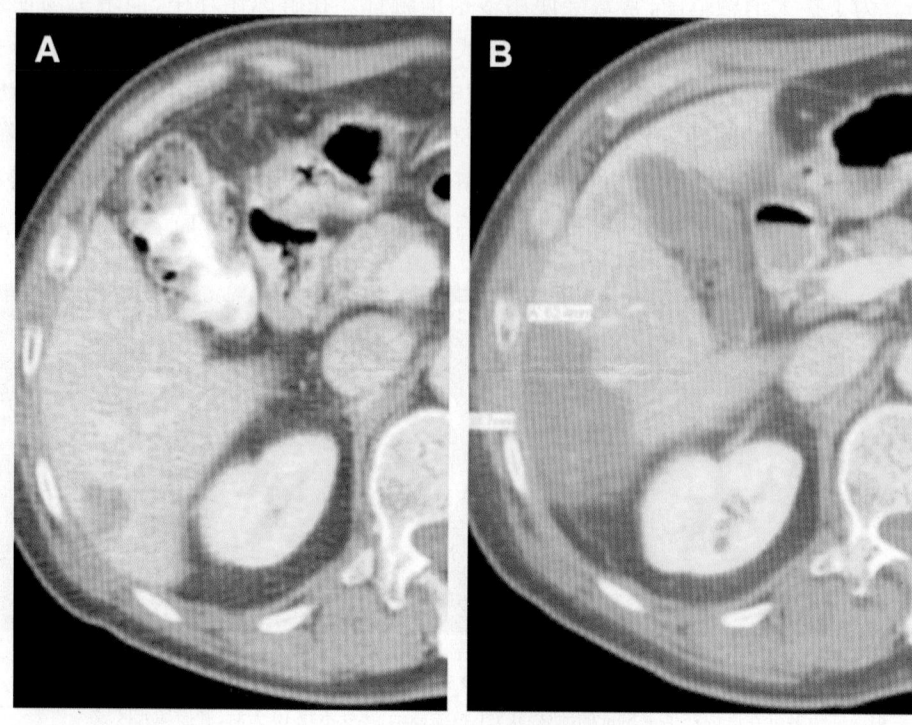

图6-2 射频消融治疗结直肠癌肝转移
A. 治疗前；B. 治疗后

(2) 微波消融

微波消融依据介质磁滞现象产热。由于磁场的作用，组织在加热时被破坏，通常磁场频率为900~2500MHz。组织中的极性分子不断与振荡电场对齐，增加动能，引起组织温度升高，含有较多水分的肿瘤组织适用于此种治疗方法。

微波能有效地使多种类型的组织间产生热传导，甚至低电导率、高阻抗或导热系数低的组织都可以使用微波治疗。微波可以穿透其他热消融涂敷器附近的炭化组织，而不受电流传导和炭化的影响。

微波治疗的优势是消融速度快(5~20分钟，直径2cm的肿瘤平均消融时间12分钟)以及治疗邻近血管的肿瘤时无热损失(这是血液流动冷辐射效应的结果)。微波消融的主要缺陷在于单针消融范围受限。单针微波消融的最大治疗范围为4.6cm。因此，只用单针消融时，边界1cm的肿瘤，其最大消融范围只有2.6cm。所以，大范围的消融需要单针多重使用或多根消融。两者都可能存在治疗失败或覆盖范围不够等问题(图6-3)。

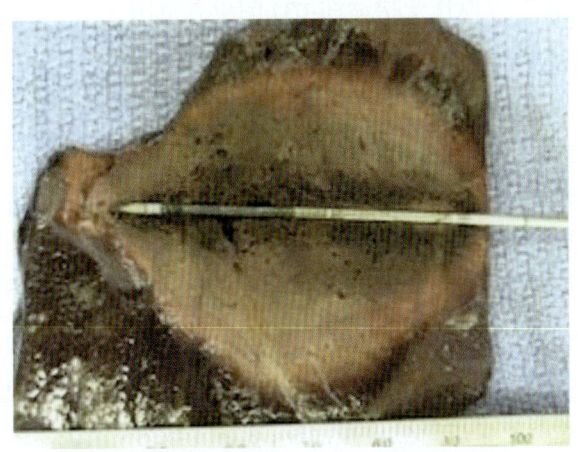

图 6-3　离体肝组织微波消融

4. 不可逆电穿孔

不可逆电穿孔是一种新的非热传导的消融技术，使用脉冲直流电致细胞死亡。它利用跨细胞膜的电位梯度和高压直流电，改变细胞中的跨膜电位和破坏脂质双分子层，使之产生小孔洞，细胞外离子内流增加。当施加的电压足够高，这些孔隙便永久形成[13]。这些离子由三磷酸腺苷（ATP）附属离子泵清除，致使细胞内 ATP 耗竭，进而细胞死亡，24 小时后组织达到最大凋亡率[14]。目前认为细胞凋亡是由于在细胞膜上形成固定孔导致的，故细胞外基质、血管和胆管的胶原结构仍会保持完整。

不同于热消融技术，不可逆电穿孔不会产生热沉效应，即不会因为血液流动带走部分热量而导致治疗效果变差。此方法能安全地靠近重要结构而不造成伤害，因其运行机制是非热能的。不过近来一些文献报道，不可逆电穿孔可能也会产热[14]。

三、患者选择

1. 肿瘤类型

除了肝外胆管肿瘤，基本上所有肝内原发性和继发性肿瘤患者都是消融治疗的适应人群。肿瘤消融的适应证很多，其治疗的指南和手术切除类似。尽管消融治疗的并发症和创伤影响要少于手术切除，但其临床适应证并不会因此扩大。

一般情况下，对于肝脏良性肿瘤，只有出现症状或增大时，才建议对其进行消融治疗。很少建议对局灶结节性增生和血管瘤进行切除或消融治疗。但腺瘤有潜在恶性和出血倾向，当腺瘤有切除适应证时，消融治疗可作为一种选择。在消融良性病变时，对于消融边缘正常组织的要求不是很严格，因此，较大的肿瘤可达到根治性治疗的效果。

肝脏恶性肿瘤消融治疗的适应证大致和手术切除相同。其优点是，减少手术创伤、降低死亡率、保护正常肝组织、扩大可以接受根治性治疗的患者范围。

(1) 肝细胞癌

肝细胞癌的治疗有其独特之处。首先，大多数肝细胞癌患者都有肝硬化，其较少的肝功能储备决定了大多数此类患者不能进行治愈性治疗。消融治疗能不伤及肝实质，继而对肝功能影响较小。其次，肝细胞癌是具有包膜、质软的肿瘤，因此化学消融药物易于在其中分散开来，从而达到较好的治疗效果。最后，肝细胞癌往往是多灶性肿瘤，可能有多个分散的原发灶、肝内转移灶及非原发性卫星灶，这导致不管使用哪种消融方法治疗成功率均不高。

(2) 结直肠癌肝转移

结直肠癌肝转移也适合进行消融治疗。胃肠道腺瘤质地较硬，不适合化学消融。但有越来越多的文献报道，对此类患者进行热消融治疗，取得了较好的临床效果。对于不适合手术切除及病灶弥散或双叶病变的患者，可推荐使用消融治疗。

(3) 神经内分泌肿瘤

神经内分泌肿瘤也是消融治疗的适应证。一般来讲，肝脏的神经内分泌肿瘤往往是继发性多于原发性，一些有激素活性并且引起症状。典型神经内分泌肿瘤生长较慢，但保持持续生长，一旦转移到肝脏很难治愈，需要在此类患者疾病进展过程中多次进行干预治疗。因为此类肿瘤质地较软，所以毗邻中央胆管结构的病灶可使用化学消融进行治疗。

(4) 其他

关于消融治疗其他肿瘤的文献报道也有很多，如肝内胆管细胞癌、非结直肠的胃肠道恶性肿瘤、乳腺癌、头颈部肿瘤、胸部肿瘤及肉瘤等。需仔细考虑消融治疗这些肿瘤的临床适应证。如果有切除适应证，那么消融往往也是可选择的治疗方式。

2. 一般情况

肝肿瘤消融治疗的一个优点是可通过几种包括经皮穿刺和手术开腹等方式进行。因此，对于一个特定的患者，我们不仅要考虑肿瘤消融的可行性，而且还要考虑患者的耐受能力。

经皮穿刺被公认是创伤性最小的方式。腹腔镜和开腹手术都需要全身麻醉。腹腔镜途径通常需要开2个10mm大小的孔，尽管这种创伤大于经皮穿刺，但在实际操作中很少引起损伤。开放性的方式需要手术开腹，因此选择这种方式的患者须能承受大幅度的侵入治疗。化学消融术可以在镇静下进行，而因为疼痛，热消融患者几乎全部需要深度镇静或全身麻醉。

3. 消融的局限性

尽管消融治疗已经在临床上广泛应用，但仍存在明显的局限性。所有的消融治疗都对肿瘤的大小有要求，对于较大的肿瘤疗效一般。大量文献报道，消融治疗小于3cm的肿瘤疗效较好；3~5cm的肿瘤疗效一般；而大于5cm的肿瘤疗效相对较差。因此，临床上一些医生使用多种消融方式治疗单个大肿瘤，但实际上未能取得理想的疗效。

同样，肿瘤个数也是一个相对禁忌证。尽管对肿瘤个数并没有明确的上限规定，但通常认为肿瘤个数越多，原位和局部治疗效果就越差。对于多发性肿瘤，消融治疗面临的一个问题是肿瘤的可视度,这是由于消融治疗不能进行深层次成像导致的。术中及术后评估多发性肿瘤消融情况也是目前面临的一个问题。肿瘤体积越大,治疗的风险也越高。此外,尽管没有明确的规定,但大多数医生在操作时不会消融超过肝脏体积的30%。对于较大的肿瘤,往往将手术切除与消融结合起来进行治疗。而大量的酒精注射可能会导致急性低血压和治疗后毒性反应。

如前所述,消融中央胆管附近(右、左肝管和肝总管)1~2cm的组织有较高的风险。因为热损伤不能识别,不同于大血管,胆管不能通过血液的流动散热。一些医生使用降温技术,如在消融时使用冰盐水进行冲洗,试图解决这一问题[15]。加热的程度很难准确评估和控制,而更多的临床医生避免在这一区域进行热消融,而是使用化学消融或手术切除的方法(图6-4)。

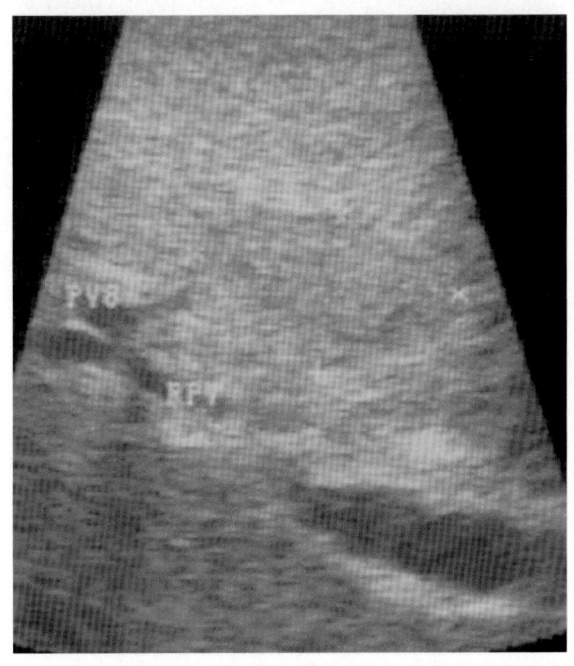

图6-4 贴近右侧门脉的神经内分泌肿瘤。热消融会损伤右肝管,因此这个病例使用酒精注射进行治疗

四、消融的途径

1. 经皮穿刺/经腹腔镜、开腹手术

每种方法都有各自的优缺点。经皮穿刺消融在治疗小的肝脏肿瘤时具有安全、侵入性小、费用较低等优点。无论是化学消融还是热消融,仅需要一定程度的镇静,不需要花费较高、风险较大的全身麻醉。

经皮穿刺治疗失败率较高,其原因有很多。经皮穿刺未经腹腔镜和肝内超声进行术前评估,因此常常因为术中有未发现的肿瘤或肝外病变而导致治疗效果较差。另一问题是肿瘤的定位,相对于腹腔镜或开腹后使用超声,腹壁或胸壁会影响经皮超声,导致成像质量下降。

由于缺乏对比剂,CT 或 MRI 引导下的消融治疗也有局限性。尽管在诊断时由于使用了对比剂,CT 和 MRI 可以很准确地呈现出肿瘤的形态,但是在进行消融时不会使用对比剂,因此进针位置往往不那么准确,进而影响治疗效果。

无论使用超声、CT 还是 MRI,膈下的肿瘤很难通过经皮穿刺的方式进行治疗。此外,肝脏表面肿瘤邻近的器官在进行热消融时有可能受到损害。而这些情况下,使用经腹腔镜或开腹方式消融是相对较好的选择,这样既可以接近肝膈顶,又能保护肝脏周围器官(图 6-5)。

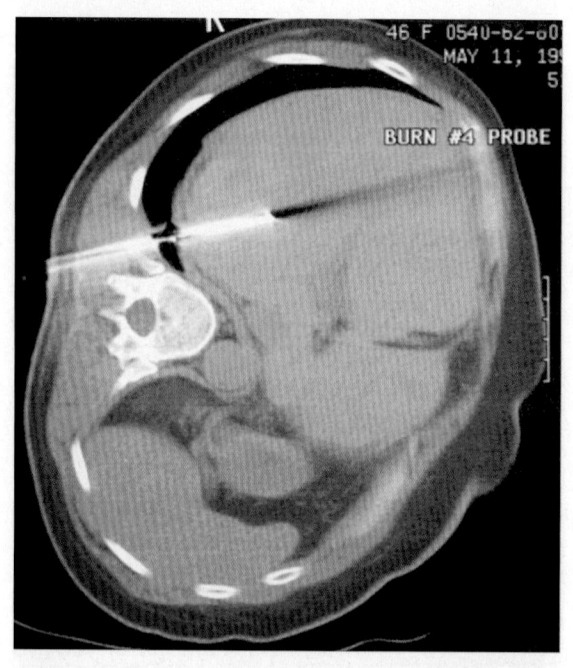

图 6-5　CT 引导下射频消融探头的位置位于肝膈顶。在穿刺时,对比剂已经廓清。最后针头的位置是通过与其他已知解剖标志的三角关系来确定的

经腹腔镜途径的消融治疗需要在腹部开两个孔,一个孔(5~10mm)伸入镜头,另一个孔(10mm)伸入超声,其并发症发生率与经皮穿刺途径大致相同。但经腹腔镜途径消融常常需要对患者进行全身麻醉,有时还需要在肝脏进行粘连松解术以便针头到达病灶。对于存在肝硬化的患者,手术创口可能导致术后肝功能失代偿以及腹水渗漏等并发症。

开放性的治疗方式会对患者造成更大的创伤及心理压力,影响恢复过程。尽管肝脏的所有部分都可以通过腹腔镜进行治疗,但开放性的方式可以为后续治疗提供便利,如大型肝脏切除术。如果医师没有腹腔镜器材或操作不熟练,开放性的方式就是非常好的选择。

2. 定位技术——超声肿瘤定位

基本的技术包括使用超声定位肿瘤。在向肿瘤靠近时,消融设备与超声图像的长轴保持平行,便于医生从上到下调整角度和深度。通过左、右、上、下移动超声探头,医生可以逐渐将消融针对准目标肿瘤。

通过开腹途径进行消融时,消融的针头往往位于超声探头的末端,最合适的进针角度是45°。如果角度太陡,很难看到消融针的针头。使用腹腔镜时,选择皮肤和肝脏表面的进针点则更具挑战性,因为医生需要评估腹壁的厚度、到肝脏的距离以及肝内进针的深度(图6-6)。

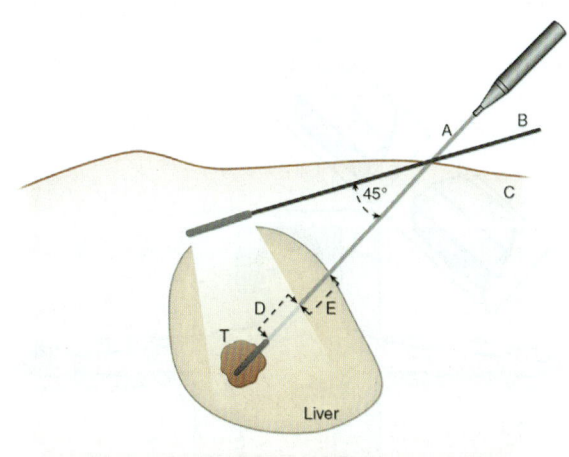

图6-6 在超声引导下的消融。超声探头和消融针头穿过腹壁。超声探头和消融针头保持45°,可以在腹壁进针点调整消融针头的角度。超声探头提供了一个纵向的视野,操作者在肝实质的视野之外进针时必须特别注意

A. 消融针;B. 超声探头;C. 腹壁;D. 超声可视范围;E. 超声可视范围之外;T. 肿瘤

五、围术期准备

1. 术前评估

一般评估项目包括常规病史、体格检查、实验室检查以及CT或MRI横断面成像。

2. 患者体位

(1)经皮穿刺

患者仰卧位,无菌消毒手术区。一般需要深度镇静或全身麻醉,因为热消融会引起剧烈的疼痛。一般要在影像学设备引导下进行消融,这样可以确保穿刺路径是安全的,而且避免损伤邻近器官。进行化学消融时,观察低回声反应确保酒精在肿瘤里均匀分布。使用热消融时,针头位于肿瘤里面并进行精确定位,确保靶病灶以及1cm边界内的正常肝组织都得到消融治

疗。

(2) 经腹腔镜途径

患者仰卧位,进行全身麻醉,无菌消毒手术区。术者在患者左侧,腹腔镜和超声在患者右肩侧。这样术者就可以兼顾超声屏幕和靶病灶。在腹直肌外侧肝脏边缘开一个 10mm 的孔,脐部再开一个孔用来伸入镜头 (5~10 mm)。全麻诱导后,将套管置入腹腔,并进行腹腔镜操作。如果没有明显不能切除的肝外病灶,就可以使用术中超声诊断肝内病灶,并指导治疗。在超声引导下,射频消融针头穿刺入肿瘤,肿瘤及 1cm 边界内的正常肝组织也应得到消融治疗(图 6-7)。

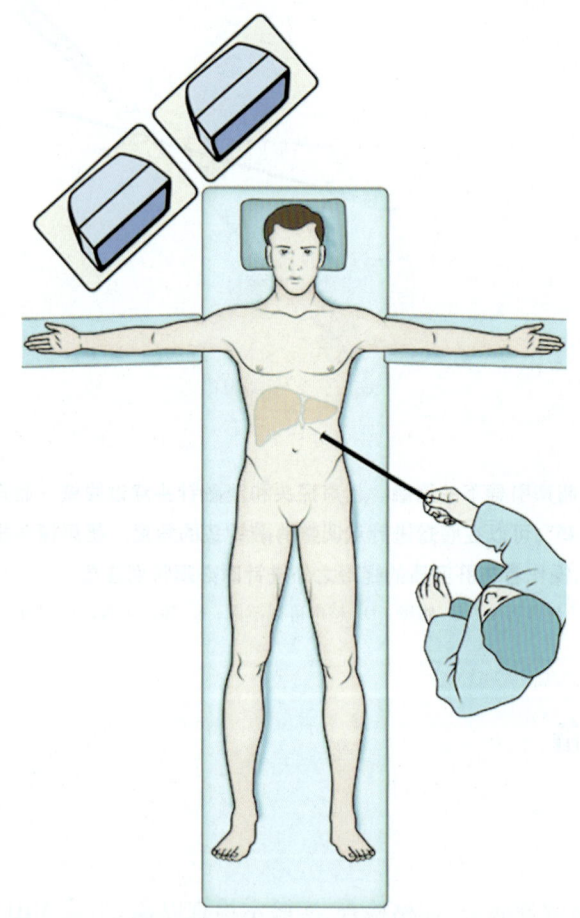

图 6-7 肝脏消融患者体位

超声(左侧显示器);腹腔镜视野(右侧显示器)

(3) 开腹手术路径

一般来说,选择右肋下或腹中线切口,术者站在患者的左侧,方便射频消融的操作。超声显示器在患者右肩侧,这样便于术者兼顾靶病灶和显示器。切开后,使用超声探查腹部,如果发现其他的肿瘤,选择合适的术式进行切除。使用直接接触的超声定位,将消融针插入病灶进行消融。开放性的射频消融一般更适合右后叶的消融,尤其是 S_7、S_8 段,因为消融角度可灵活多变,经验丰富的术者可以对整个 S_8 进行消融。

(4)化学消融

消融时酒精的用量取决于影像学显示的肿瘤大小[16,17]。注射的酒精量大致要和靶病灶的体积保持一致。对于球形肿瘤,可以利用公式($4/3 \times \pi \times r^3$)计算体积。95%酒精往往用量较小,而使用生理盐水稀释的50%酒精的用量较大。若注射酒精量大于50ml,操作时需要格外小心,因为有可能会引起一过性低血压和毒性反应。

注射酒精时要从肿瘤深处开始,这是由于注射时会产生高回声区域,掩盖更深层结构的信号。一般使用标准的15.2cm,20G或22G腰椎消融针,或特制的多侧孔的穿刺针进行操作。注射时针尖可以在肿瘤内移动,保证均匀注射、覆盖病灶。

3. 术后观察

(1)经皮穿刺和经腹腔镜热消融

一般来讲,CT引导下消融治疗的患者需要观察24小时后才能出院,而部分情况良好的患者可以手术当天出院。

在腹腔镜射频消融术后,患者需要在医院过夜观察,术后第二天出院,也有患者当天出院。出院之前,必须保证患者可以走动,能口服液体,可以控制疼痛并愿意在出现问题时及时返院。建议肝功能较差或存在静脉高压的患者术后留院观察。

(2)开放性热消融

通常情况下,开放性射频消融患者的住院时间取决于疼痛控制情况以及开腹后反应,同时也应该及时评估其术后肝功能。

4. 并发症及处理

消融术后并发症并不常见(发生率为1%~5%)。尽管由于组织结构破坏,大范围的消融可能导致暂时性的发热,这种情况通常可以承受且消失较快。大多数患者会出现右上腹和右侧腹疼痛,这种情况可能持续1~2周。也有可能出现肝脓肿,不过主要出现在进行过胆道手术的患者。出血和胆漏的情况并不多见。罕见却更严重的并发症是肠道损伤或胆汁胸膜瘘(图6-8)。

大面积的消融以及术前肝硬化肝功能较差的患者可能发生肝衰竭。因此,根据肿瘤大小以及肝功能损伤情况,肝硬化患者术后需留院观察一段时间。

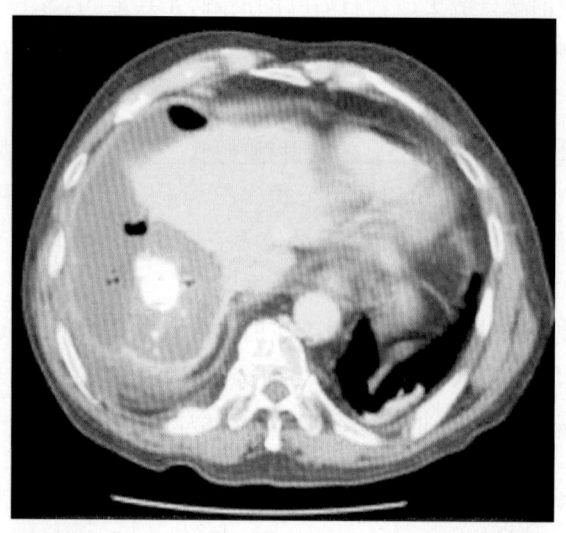

图6-8 虽然有些热消融靶点术后会产生气体,但如果气泡很大则可能是脓肿形成的标志。患者可能会出现感染的迹象,甚至发生脓毒症。对此,治疗方法是使用抗生素和经皮穿刺引流。一般很少使用清创手术

5. 长期随访

术后10~14天要行增强对比、多期扫描的影像学检查评估消融情况。消融后的组织无血流灌注。靶病灶和周围1cm的肝组织应该是无血流灌注区域。肿瘤内或附近1cm内仍有血流灌注,表示消融不彻底。如果有残余病灶,应此时进行治疗。否则,虽然消融区域体积缩小,但肿瘤也很难消失。

六、疗效

1. 肝细胞癌

目前,手术切除和肝移植被认为是肝细胞癌的治愈性治疗方式,据文献报道,肝细胞癌患者5年生存率分别为36%~70%[18]和60%~70%。然而,由于肿瘤负荷、肝功能储备、伴随疾病等因素,只有10%~20%的患者可以接受手术切除治疗。原位消融技术,如经皮穿刺酒精注射及热消融尤其适用于此类患者。由于每种治疗方法的适应人群存在差异性,前瞻性随机对照研究很难开展。

(1)肝细胞癌的射频消融

射频消融是最常用的热消融技术。据文献报道,主要并发症发生率为0~10%,治疗失败率为1.7%~29.4%[19-31]。治疗的成功率与肿瘤大小及治疗方式有关。与经皮穿刺方式相比,手术切除对小于3cm肿瘤的治疗成功率更高。

据文献报道,经皮穿刺方式及经腹腔镜方式治疗的 1 年、3 年及 5 年生存率分别为 79%～100%、42%～91% 及 20%～72.8%。表 6-1 列出了切除和移植在生存率和并发症发生率降低方面的对比。

表 6-1 肝细胞癌射频消融疗效

作者	时间	n	方式	1 年生存率(%)	3 年生存率(%)	5 年生存率(%)	并发症(%)	原位治疗失败(%)
Cillo 等[20]	2013	103	Lap	79	49	40	—	—
Wong 等[30]	2013	76	Lap/开放性	87.3	61	48.6	4.7（所有诊断）	24.7
Shiina 等[29]	2005	118	Perc	—	—	74 (4 年)	—	1.7
Guglielmi 等[21]	2008	109	Perc	—	42	20	10	—
Wong 等[30]	2013	100	Perc	92.8	68.7	47.2	4.7（所有诊断）	29.4
Chen 等[19]	2006	71	Perc	95.8	71.4	64	4.2	4.2
Hong 等[22]	2005	55	Perc	100	72.7	—	—	—
Lu 等[27]	2006	51	Perc	93.5	87.1	—	7.8	—
Wong 等[31]	2013	36	Perc	97.1	91	72.8	0	—

缩写:Lap:腹腔镜;n:患者数量;Perc:经皮穿刺

(2)肝细胞癌经皮酒精注射消融

文献报道的主要并发症发生率为 0～2.2%[4,16,23,24,29,32-40]。原位治疗失败率在 0～34.5%,多数和肿瘤大小相关。一些研究表明,小于 2～3cm 的肿瘤、小于 3cm 的肿瘤、大于 3cm 的肿瘤,肿瘤完全缓解率分别为 90%～100%、70%～80% 以及 50%～60%[41-43]。因此,对于 5cm 以上的肿瘤,不推荐使用无水酒精注入术。

文献报道,肝细胞癌经皮酒精注射消融术 1 年、3 年及 5 年生存率分别为 88%～97%、62%～81.6% 及 39%～60.3%[4,16,23,24,29,32,40]。

一些随机临床试验显示,对于小肝细胞癌,射频消融治疗效果要优于酒精注射,因此,热消融更受青睐(表 6-2)[29,37,44,45]。

表6-2 无水酒精注射治疗肝细胞癌疗效

作者	时间	n	1年生存率(%)	3年生存率(%)	5年生存率(%)	并发症(%)	原位治疗失败(%)
Ebara 等[34]	2005	270	—	81.6	60.3	2.2	10
Shiina 等[29]	2005	114	—	63	—	—	0
Pompili 等[39]	2001	111	97	62	41	0	—
Fartoux 等[35]	2005	102	—	70	—	0	24
Brunello 等[33]	2008	69	—	57	—	—	—
Sung 等[40]	2006	64	—	71	39	0	—
Lin 等[37]	2005	62	88	81	—	0	34.5

缩略词:n:患者数量

(3)肝细胞癌的冷冻消融

冷冻消融已用于治疗小肝细胞癌,然而目前唯一的文献数据来源于非随机小样本的试验及一些回顾性综述。此外,冷冻消融治疗肝细胞癌的效果很难评估,因为几乎所有的报道都将仅进行冷冻消融的患者与又进行了切除的患者、多发疾病的患者结合起来进行分析。冷冻消融治疗肝细胞癌的并发症发生率为0~59%,原位治疗失败率为13.6%~27.3%,1年生存率为63.9%~66%(表6-3)[46-51]。

表6-3 冷冻消融治疗肝细胞癌疗效

作者	时间	n	1年生存率(%)	3年生存率(%)	5年生存率(%)	并发症(%)	原位治疗失败(%)
Zhou & Tang[51]	1998	78	63.9	40.3	26.9	0	—
Pearson 等[48]	1999	54(所有诊断,7例肝细胞癌)	—	—	—	40.7	13.6
Haddad 等[47]	1998	31	59	22	—	59	—
Adam 等[46]	2002	31	66	—	—	29	27.3
Wren 等[5]	1997	12	64	—	—	8.3	—

n:患者数量

(4)肝细胞癌的微波消融

微波消融对于小肝癌(small series)有显著的治疗效果。术后并发症发生率为0~15.9%,原位治疗失败率为2.9%~11.8%。其1年、3年及5年生存率分别为38%~92.5%、19%~50.5%及36.8%~70%(表6-4)[52-57]。

表6-4　微波消融治疗肝细胞癌疗效

作者	时间	n	1年生存率(%)	3年生存率(%)	5年生存率(%)	并发症(%)	原位治疗失败(%)
Groeschl 等[54]	2014	139	38	19	—	15.9 开放性,9.3 Lap,11.1 Perc	6
Dong 等[53]	2003	82	92.5	75.3(2年)	—	—	—
Swan 等[57]	2013	54	72.3	58.8(2年)	—	28.9	2.9
Lu 等[55]	2005	49	81.6	50.5	36.8(4年)	8.2	11.8
Dong 等[52]	1998	41	—	—	—	—	11
Seki 等[56]	1999	23	—	—	70	0	8

缩写:Lap:腹腔镜;n:患者数量;Perc:经皮穿刺

(5)不可逆电穿孔治疗肝细胞癌

近来,不可逆电穿孔开始用于不可切除的肝细胞癌,因相关研究较少,其长期疗效还没有明确的定论。在治疗小肝癌方面,并发症发生率为0~10%,还没有原位复发的报道。据报道,1年生存率为50%~100%[58-60]。Cheung 等[59]的研究显示,不可逆电穿孔是治疗肝细胞癌的一种安全可行手段,对于小于3cm的肿瘤有93%的成功率;对于大于3cm的肿瘤,成功率降至72%。在随访的18个月内,没有患者复发或死亡(表6-5)。

表6-5　不可逆电穿孔治疗肝细胞癌疗效

作者	时间	n	1年生存率(%)	3年生存率(%)	5年生存率(%)	并发症(%)	原位治疗失败(%)
Cannon 等[58]	2013	14	50	—	—	10(所有诊断)	0
Philips 等[60]	2013	13	—	—	—	8.5(所有诊断)	0
Cheung 等[59]	2013	11	100	—	—	0	0

n:患者数量

2. 结直肠癌肝转移

(1)射频消融治疗结直肠癌肝转移

主要并发症发生率为0~10.6%,治疗失败率为2.6%~37%[2,61-74]。使用经皮穿刺方式,1年、3年及5年生存率分别为79%~98%、38%~69%及19%~25.5%。使用腹腔镜和开腹方式,1年、3年及5年生存率分别为87%~93.5%、20.2%~57%及18.4%~33.1%[2,61-74]。

根据Mulier 等[75]的一项大型meta分析研究单因素分析结果提示,肿瘤较大、包膜下肿瘤位置、靠近大血管、血管闭塞以及1cm的边界是影响肿瘤复发的高危因素。多因素分析结果提示,对于小于3cm的肿瘤,外科手段(开腹或腹腔镜)和经皮穿刺的疗效不同,经皮穿刺消融的复发率更高。

因为存在选择偏见,很难在行射频消融的患者身上直接比较射频消融和手术切除的效果。然而,Hammill 等[2]最近的一项研究结果表明,对于接受射频消融的患者,可认为其在技术上可接受切除治疗,5 年生存率为 48%,疗效和肝脏切除术大致相同。但是由于确定治疗失败时间(消融点肿瘤复发)和总生存时间这一难题,使得射频消融的疗效难以知晓。除此之外,将以治愈为目标的消融术和因不可行手术切除而实施的消融术比较,使得生存结果的分析更加复杂(表 6 - 6)。

表 6 - 6 射频消融治疗结直肠癌肝转移疗效

作者	时间	n	射频消融方式	1 年生存率(%)	3 年生存率(%)	5 年生存率(%)	并发症(%)	原位治疗失败(%)
Veltri 等[3]	2008	122	Perc	79	38	22	1.1	26.3
Sorensen 等[72]	2007	102	Perc	87	46	—	6.9	—
Solbiati 等[70]	2012	99	Perc	98	69.3	25	2	6.9
Park 等[68]	2008	30	Perc	—	—	19	—	23
White 等[74]	2007	22	Perc	—	28	—	—	36
Hur 等[65]	2009	25	Perc/Lap	—	60	25.5	0	28
Siperstein 等[69]	2007	234	Lap	—	20.2	18.4	—	—
Kennedy 等[67]	2013	130	Lap	93.5	50.1	28.8	1.5	9.2 (3.6% <3 cm 肿瘤)
Hammill 等[2]	2011	113	Lap	87	52	33.1	1.8	2.6
Berber 等[64]	2008	68	Lap	—	35	30	2.9	—
Aloia 等[63]	2006	30	开放性	—	57	27	—	37
Abitabile 等[62]	2007	47	开放性/Perc	88	57	21	10.6	—

Lap:腹腔镜;n:患者数量;Perc:经皮穿刺

(2)结直肠癌肝转移的微波治疗

结直肠癌肝转移的患者行微波消融术后,并发症发生率为 0～19%,原位复发率为6%～14%。据文献报道,1 年、3 年和 5 年生存率分别为 45%～91.4%、46.4%～57% 以及 14%～32%[54,76-80]。

Shibata 等[79]进行了一项将微波消融与肝脏切除术对比的随机试验。实验显示,微波消融组的 1 年、3 年和 5 年生存率分别为 71%、57% 以及 14%,平均生存时间为 25 个月,平均原位复发率为 4.2%～14%,与手术切除组相比无统计学差异。这些结果提示,在治疗结直肠癌肝转移方面,微波消融和手术切除的疗效相当,但仍需更大样本临床试验支持这一结论(表 6 - 7)。

表6-7 微波消融治疗结直肠癌肝转移疗效

作者	时间	n	1年生存率(%)	3年生存率(%)	5年生存率(%)	并发症(%)	原位治疗失败(%)
Tanaka 等[80]	2006	16（微波+切除）	80	51	17	19	—
Groeschl 等[54]	2014	198	45	17	—	—	6（所有诊断）
Ogata 等[8]	2008	32	—	—	32	—	—
Liang 等[77]	2003	21	91.4	46.4	—	0	14
Shibata 等[79]	2000	14	71	57	14	14.3	—

n：患者数量

3. 神经内分泌肿瘤

一些小型研究结果表明，肝脏神经内分泌肿瘤射频消融后，并发症发生率为1%~10%，复发率为3.8%~22%，5年生存率为80%[81-87]。

因为神经内分泌肿瘤常伴随其他疾病，或是射频消融常常结合肝脏切除术，因此，射频消融治疗神经内分泌肿瘤的效果评估较为困难。接受射频消融同时又接受肝脏切除术的患者5年生存率为48%~80%（表6-8）[88-90]。

表6-8 神经内分泌肿瘤的消融治疗疗效

作者	时间	数量	方式	1年生存率(%)	3年生存率(%)	5年生存率(%)	并发症(%)	原位治疗失败(%)
Berber & Siperstein[83]	2007	74	Lap	—	—	—	5	—
Karabulut 等[84]	2011	69	Lap	—	—	—	10	22
Berber & Siperstein[82]	2008	63	Lap	—	—	48	—	—
Mazzaglia 等[85]	2007	63	Lap	98	—	57	—	6.3
Taner 等[87]	2013	94	肝切除+开放性消融	100	93.6	80	1	3.8

Lap：腹腔镜；n：患者数量；Perc：经皮穿刺

参考文献

[1] Weng M, Zhang Y, Zhou D, et al. Radiofrequency ablation versus resection for colorectal cancer liver metastases: a meta-analysis. PLoS One 2012;7(9):21.

[2] Hammill CW, Billingsley KG, Cassera MA, et al. Outcome after laparoscopic radiofrequency ablation of technically resectable colorectal liver metastases. Ann Surg Oncol 2011;18(7):1947-54.

[3] Livraghi T, Meloni F, Di Stasi M, et al. Sustained complete response and complications rates after radio-

frequency ablation of very early hepatocellular carcinoma in cirrhosis: is resection still the treatment of choice? Hepatology 2008;47(1):82-9.

[4] Huo TI, Huang YH, Wu JC, et al. Comparison of percutaneous acetic acid injection and percutaneous ethanol injection for hepatocellular carcinoma in cirrhotic patients: a prospective study. Scand J Gastroenterol 2003;38(7):770-8.

[5] McKinnon JG, Temple WJ, Wiseman DA, et al. Cryosurgery for malignant tumours of the liver. Can J Surg 1996;39(5):401-6.

[6] Morris DL, Ross WB. Australian experience of cryoablation of liver tumors: metastases. Surg Oncol Clin N Am 1996;5(2):391-7.

[7] Onik G, Rubinsky B, Zemel R, et al. Ultrasound - guided hepatic cryosurgery in the treatment of metastatic colon carcinoma. Preliminary results. Cancer 1991;67(4):901-7.

[8] Onik GM, Atkinson D, Zemel R, et al. Cryosurgery of liver cancer. Semin Surg Oncol 1993;9(4):309-17.

[9] Ravikumar TS, Kane R, Cady B, et al. A 5 - year study of cryosurgery in the treatment of liver tumors. Arch Surg 1991;126(12):1520-3 [discussion: 1523-4].

[10] Ross WB, Horton M, Bertolino P, et al. Cryotherapy of liver tumours – a practical guide. HPB Surg 1995;8(3):167-73.

[11] Weaver ML, Atkinson D, Zemel R. Hepatic cryosurgery in treating colorectal metastases. Cancer 1995;76(2):210-4.

[12] Hansen PD, Rogers S, Corless CL, et al. Radiofrequency ablation lesions in a pig liver model. J Surg Res 1999;87(1):114-21.

[13] Rubinsky B. Irreversible electroporation in medicine. Technol Cancer Res Treat 2007;6(4):255-60.

[14] Silk MT, Wimmer T, Lee KS, et al. Percutaneous ablation of peribiliary tumors with irreversible electroporation. J Vasc Interv Radiol 2014;25(1):112-8.

[15] Stippel DL, Bangard C, Kasper HU, et al. Experimental bile duct protection by intraductal cooling during radiofrequency ablation. Br J Surg 2005;92(7):849-55.

[16] Livraghi T, Giorgio A, Marin G, et al. Hepatocellular carcinoma and cirrhosis in 746 patients: long - term results of percutaneous ethanol injection. Radiology 1995;197(1):101-8.

[17] Shiina S, Tagawa K, Unuma T, et al. Percutaneous ethanol injection therapy for hepatocellular carcinoma. A histopathologic study. Cancer 1991;68(7):1524-30.

[18] Tiong L, Maddern GJ. Systematic review and meta - analysis of survival and disease recurrence after radiofrequency ablation for hepatocellular carcinoma. Br J Surg 2011;98(9):1210-24.

[19] Chen MS, Li JQ, Zheng Y, et al. A prospective randomized trial comparing percutaneous local ablative therapy and partial hepatectomy for small hepatocellular carcinoma. Ann Surg 2006;243(3):321-8.

[20] Cillo U, Vitale A, Dupuis D, et al. Laparoscopic ablation of hepatocellular carcinoma in cirrhotic patients unsuitable for liver resection or percutaneous treatment: a cohort study. PLoS One 2013;8(2):21.

[21] Guglielmi A, Ruzzenente A, Valdegamberi A, et al. Radiofrequency ablation versus surgical resection for the treatment of hepatocellular carcinoma in cirrhosis. J Gastrointest Surg 2008;12(1):192-8.

[22] Hong SN, Lee SY, Choi MS, et al. Comparing the outcomes of radiofrequency ablation and surgery in patients with a single small hepatocellular carcinoma and well - preserved hepatic function. J Clin Gastroen-

terol 2005;39(3):247-52.

[23] Lencioni RA, Allgaier HP, Cioni D, et al. Small hepatocellular carcinoma in cirrhosis: randomized comparison of radio-frequency thermal ablation versus percutaneous ethanol injection. Radiology 2003;228(1):235-40.

[24] Lin SM, Lin CJ, Lin CC, et al. Radiofrequency ablation improves prognosis compared with ethanol injection for hepatocellular carcinoma < or 54 cm. Gastroenterology 2004;127(6):1714-23.

[25] Livraghi T, Goldberg SN, Lazzaroni S, et al. Small hepatocellular carcinoma: treatment with radio-frequency ablation versus ethanol injection. Radiology 1999; 210(3):655-61.

[26] Llovet JM, Vilana R, Bru C, et al. Increased risk of tumor seeding after percutaneous radiofrequency ablation for single hepatocellular carcinoma. Hepatology 2001;33(5):1124-9.

[27] Lu MD, Kuang M, Liang LJ, et al. Surgical resection versus percutaneous thermal ablation for early-stage hepatocellular carcinoma: a randomized clinical trial. Zhonghua Yi Xue Za Zhi 2006;86(12):801-5 [in Chinese].

[28] Rossi S, Di Stasi M, Buscarini E, et al. Percutaneous RF interstitial thermal ablation in the treatment of hepatic cancer. AJR Am J Roentgenol 1996;167(3): 759-68.

[29] Shiina S, Teratani T, Obi S, et al. A randomized controlled trial of radiofrequency ablation with ethanol injection for small hepatocellular carcinoma. Gastroenterology 2005;129(1):122-30.

[30] Wong J, Lee KF, Yu SC, et al. Percutaneous radiofrequency ablation versus surgical radiofrequency ablation for malignant liver tumours: the long-term results. HPB (Oxford) 2013;15(8):595-601.

[31] Wong KM, Yeh ML, Chuang SC, et al. Survival comparison between surgical resection and percutaneous radiofrequency ablation for patients in Barcelona Clinic Liver Cancer early stage hepatocellular carcinoma. Indian J Gastroenterol 2013;32(4):253-7.

[32] Arii S, Yamaoka Y, Futagawa S, et al. Results of surgical and nonsurgical treatment for small-sized hepatocellular carcinomas: a retrospective and nationwide survey in Japan. The Liver Cancer Study Group of Japan. Hepatology 2000;32(6):1224-9.

[33] Brunello F, Veltri A, Carucci P, et al. Radiofrequency ablation versus ethanol injection for early hepatocellular carcinoma: a randomized controlled trial. Scand J Gastroenterol 2008;43(6):727-35. http://dx.doi.org/10.1080/00365520701885481.

[34] Ebara M, Okabe S, Kita K, et al. Percutaneous ethanol injection for small hepatocellular carcinoma: therapeutic efficacy based on 20-year observation. J Hepatol 2005;43(3):458-64.

[35] Fartoux L, Arrive L, Andreani T, et al. Treatment of small hepatocellular carcinoma with acetic acid percutaneous injection. Gastroenterol Clin Biol 2005;29(12): 1213-9.

[36] Hasegawa S, Yamasaki N, Hiwaki T, et al. Factors that predict intrahepatic recurrence of hepatocellular carcinoma in 81 patients initially treated by percutaneous ethanol injection. Cancer 1999;86(9):1682-90.

[37] Lin SM, Lin CJ, Lin CC, et al. Randomised controlled trial comparing percutaneous radiofrequency thermal ablation, percutaneous ethanol injection, and percutaneous acetic acid injection to treat hepatocellular carcinoma of 3 cm or less. Gut 2005;54(8):1151-6.

[38] Livraghi T, Benedini V, Lazzaroni S, et al. Long term results of single session percutaneous ethanol injection in patients with large hepatocellular carcinoma. Cancer 1998;83(1):48-57.

[39] Pompili M, Rapaccini GL, Covino M, et al. Prognostic factors for survival in patients with compensated

cirrhosis and small hepatocellular carcinoma after percutaneous ethanol injection therapy. Cancer 2001;92(1):126-35.

[40] Sung YM, Choi D, Lim HK, et al. Long-term results of percutaneous ethanol injection for the treatment of hepatocellular carcinoma in Korea. Korean J Radiol 2006; 7(3):187-92.

[41] El-Serag HB, Marrero JA, Rudolph L, et al. Diagnosis and treatment of hepatocellular carcinoma. Gastroenterology 2008;134(6):1752-63. http://dx.doi.org/10.1053/j.gastro.2008.02.090.

[42] Lencioni R, Llovet JM. Percutaneous ethanol injection for hepatocellular carcinoma: alive or dead? J Hepatol 2005;43(3):377-80.

[43] Livraghi T, Bolondi L, Lazzaroni S, et al. Percutaneous ethanol injection in the treatment of hepatocellular carcinoma in cirrhosis. A study on 207 patients. Cancer 1992;69(4):925-9.

[44] Bouza C, Lopez-Cuadrado T, Alcazar R, et al. Meta-analysis of percutaneous radiofrequency ablation versus ethanol injection in hepatocellular carcinoma. BMC Gastroenterol 2009;9:31. http://dx.doi.org/10.1186/1471-230X-9-31.

[45] Orlando A, Leandro G, Olivo M, et al. Radiofrequency thermal ablation vs. percutaneous ethanol injection for small hepatocellular carcinoma in cirrhosis: meta-analysis of randomized controlled trials. Am J Gastroenterol 2009;104(2):514-24. http://dx.doi.org/10.1038/ajg.2008.80.

[46] Adam R, Hagopian EJ, Linhares M, et al. A comparison of percutaneous cryosurgery and percutaneous radiofrequency for unresectable hepatic malignancies. Arch Surg 2002;137(12):1332-9 [discussion: 1340].

[47] Haddad FF, Chapman WC, Wright JK, et al. Clinical experience with cryosurgery for advanced hepatobiliary tumors. J Surg Res 1998;75(2):103-8.

[48] Pearson AS, Izzo F, Fleming RY, et al. Intraoperative radiofrequency ablation or cryoablation for hepatic malignancies. Am J Surg 1999;178(6):592-9.

[49] Tait IS, Yong SM, Cuschieri SA. Laparoscopic in situ ablation of liver cancer with cryotherapy and radiofrequency ablation. Br J Surg 2002;89(12):1613-9.

[50] Wren SM, Coburn MM, Tan M, et al. Is cryosurgical ablation appropriate for treating hepatocellular cancer? Arch Surg 1997;132(6):599-603 [discussion: 603-4].

[51] Zhou XD, Tang ZY. Cryotherapy for primary liver cancer. Semin Surg Oncol 1998; 14(2):171-4.

[52] Dong BW, Liang P, Yu XL, et al. Sonographically guided microwave coagulation treatment of liver cancer: an experimental and clinical study. AJR Am J Roentgenol 1998;171(2):449-54.

[53] Dong BW, Zhang J, Liang P, et al. Sequential pathological and immunologic analysis of percutaneous microwave coagulation therapy of hepatocellular carcinoma. Int J Hyperthermia 2003;19(2):119-33.

[54] Groeschl RT, Pilgrim CH, Hanna EM, et al. Microwave ablation for hepatic malignancies: a multiinstitutional analysis. Ann Surg 2014;259(6):1195-200.

[55] Lu MD, Xu HX, Xie XY, et al. Percutaneous microwave and radiofrequency ablation for hepatocellular carcinoma: a retrospective comparative study. J Gastroenterol 2005;40(11):1054-60.

[56] Seki T, Wakabayashi M, Nakagawa T, et al. Percutaneous microwave coagulation therapy for patients with small hepatocellular carcinoma: comparison with percutaneous ethanol injection therapy. Cancer 1999;85(8):1694-702.

[57] Swan RZ, Sindram D, Martinie JB, et al. Operative microwave ablation for hepatocellular carcinoma:

complications, recurrence, and long-term outcomes. J Gastrointest Surg 2013;17(4):719-29.

[58] Cannon R, Ellis S, Hayes D, et al. Safety and early efficacy of irreversible electroporation for hepatic tumors in proximity to vital structures. J Surg Oncol 2013; 107(5):544-9.

[59] Cheung W, Kavnoudias H, Roberts S, et al. Irreversible electroporation for unresectable hepatocellular carcinoma: initial experience and review of safety and outcomes. Technol Cancer Res Treat 2013;12(3): 233-41. http://dx.doi.org/10.7785/tcrt.2012.500317.

[60] Philips P, Hays D, Martin RC. Irreversible electroporation ablation (IRE) of unresectable soft tissue tumors: learning curve evaluation in the first 150 patients treated. PLoS One 2013;8(11):e76260.

[61] Abdalla EK, Vauthey JN, Ellis LM, et al. Recurrence and outcomes following hepatic resection, radiofrequency ablation, and combined resection/ablation for colorectal liver metastases. Ann Surg 2004;239(6): 818-25 [discussion:825-7].

[62] Abitabile P, Hartl U, Lange J, et al. Radiofrequency ablation permits an effective treatment for colorectal liver metastasis. Eur J Surg Oncol 2007;33(1): 67-71.

[63] Aloia TA, Vauthey JN, Loyer EM, et al. Solitary colorectal liver metastasis: resection determines outcome. Arch Surg 2006;141(5):460-6 [discussion: 466-7].

[64] Berber E, Tsinberg M, Tellioglu G, et al. Resection versus laparoscopic radiofrequency thermal ablation of solitary colorectal liver metastasis. J Gastrointest Surg 2008;12(11):1967-72. http://dx.doi.org/10.1007/s11605-008-0622-8.

[65] Hur H, Ko YT, Min BS, et al. Comparative study of resection and radiofrequency ablation in the treatment of solitary colorectal liver metastases. Am J Surg 2009; 197(6):728-36. http://dx.doi.org/10.1016/j.amjsurg.2008.04.013.

[66] Iannitti DA, Dupuy DE, Mayo-Smith WW, et al. Hepatic radiofrequency ablation. Arch Surg 2002;137(4):422-6 [discussion: 427].

[67] Kennedy TJ, Cassera MA, Khajanchee YS, et al. Laparoscopic radiofrequency ablation for the management of colorectal liver metastases: 10-year experience. J Surg Oncol 2013;107(4):324-8.

[68] Park IJ, Kim HC, Yu CS, et al. Radiofrequency ablation for metachronous liver metastasis from colorectal cancer after curative surgery. Ann Surg Oncol 2008;15(1):227-32.

[69] Siperstein AE, Berber E, Ballem N, et al. Survival after radiofrequency ablation of colorectal liver metastases: 10-year experience. Ann Surg 2007;246(4):559-65[discussion: 565-7].

[70] Solbiati L, Ahmed M, Cova L, et al. Small liver colorectal metastases treated with percutaneous radiofrequency ablation: local response rate and long-term survival with up to 10-year follow-up. Radiology 2012;265(3):958-68.

[71] Solbiati L, Livraghi T, Goldberg SN, et al. Percutaneous radio-frequency ablation of hepatic metastases from colorectal cancer: long-term results in 117 patients. Radiology 2001;221(1):159-66.

[72] Sorensen SM, Mortensen FV, Nielsen DT. Radiofrequency ablation of colorectal liver metastases: long-term survival. Acta Radiol 2007;48(3):253-8.

[73] Veltri A, Sacchetto P, Tosetti I, et al. Radiofrequency ablation of colorectal liver metastases: small size favorably predicts technique effectiveness and survival. Cardiovasc Intervent Radiol 2008;31(5):948-56. http://dx.doi.org/10.1007/s00270-008-9362-0.

[74] White RR, Avital I, Sofocleous CT, et al. Rates and patterns of recurrence for percutaneous radiofrequen-

cy ablation and open wedge resection for solitary colorectal liver metastasis. J Gastrointest Surg 2007;11(3):256-63.

[75] Mulier S, Ni Y, Jamart J, et al. Local recurrence after hepatic radiofrequency coagulation: multivariate meta-analysis and review of contributing factors. Ann Surg 2005;242(2):158-71.

[76] Bhardwaj N, Strickland AD, Ahmad F, et al. Microwave ablation for unresectable hepatic tumours: clinical results using a novel microwave probe and generator. Eur J Surg Oncol 2010;36(3):264-8.

[77] Liang P, Dong B, Yu X, et al. Prognostic factors for percutaneous microwave coagulation therapy of hepatic metastases. AJR Am J Roentgenol 2003;181(5):1319-25.

[78] Ogata Y, Uchida S, Hisaka T, et al. Intraoperative thermal ablation therapy for small colorectal metastases to the liver. Hepatogastroenterology 2008;55(82-83):550-6.

[79] Shibata T, Niinobu T, Ogata N, et al. Microwave coagulation therapy for multiple hepatic metastases from colorectal carcinoma. Cancer 2000;89(2):276-84.

[80] Tanaka K, Shimada H, Nagano Y, et al. Outcome after hepatic resection versus combined resection and microwave ablation for multiple bilobar colorectal metastases to the liver. Surgery 2006;139(2):263-73.

[81] Berber E, Flesher N, Siperstein AE. Laparoscopic radiofrequency ablation of neuroendocrine liver metastases. World J Surg 2002;26(8):985-90.

[82] Berber E, Siperstein A. Local recurrence after laparoscopic radiofrequency ablation of liver tumors: an analysis of 1032 tumors. Ann Surg Oncol 2008;15(10):2757-64. http://dx.doi.org/10.1245/s10434-008-0043-7.

[83] Berber E, Siperstein AE. Perioperative outcome after laparoscopic radiofrequency ablation of liver tumors: an analysis of 521 cases. Surg Endosc 2007;21(4):613-8.

[84] Karabulut K, Akyildiz HY, Lance C, et al. Multimodality treatment of neuroendocrine liver metastases. Surgery 2011;150(2):316-25.

[85] Mazzaglia PJ, Berber E, Milas M, et al. Laparoscopic radiofrequency ablation of neuroendocrine liver metastases: a 10-year experience evaluating predictors of survival. Surgery 2007;142(1):10-9.

[86] Siperstein A, Garland A, Engle K, et al. Local recurrence after laparoscopic radiofrequency thermal ablation of hepatic tumors. Ann Surg Oncol 2000;7(2):106-13.

[87] Taner T, Atwell TD, Zhang L, et al. Adjunctive radiofrequency ablation of metastatic neuroendocrine cancer to the liver complements surgical resection. HPB (Oxford) 2013;15(3):190-5.

[88] Landry CS, McMasters KM, Scoggins CR, et al. Proposed staging system for gastrointestinal carcinoid tumors. Am Surg 2008;74(5):418-22.

[89] Musunuru S, Chen H, Rajpal S, et al. Metastatic neuroendocrine hepatic tumors: resection improves survival. Arch Surg 2006;141(10):1000-4[discussion:1005].

[90] Touzios JG, Kiely JM, Pitt SC, et al. Neuroendocrine hepatic metastases: does aggressive management improve survival? Ann Surg 2005;241(5):776-83[discussion:783-5].

第七章　肝恶性肿瘤的肝动脉灌注化疗方案

Julie N. Leal, MD, FRCSC, T. Peter Kingham, MD*

【关键词】

局部治疗；肝脏定向治疗；原发性肝癌；肝转移

要点

- 原发性和转移性肝脏肿瘤供血的主要血管是肝动脉。
- 经肝动脉将化疗药物直接灌注病灶内，可选择性地使细胞毒素类药物作用于肿瘤细胞，而相对减少对正常肝细胞的损害。
- 通过手术插入肝动脉导管和植入式化疗泵被认为是最佳药物输送方式，且在技术上是可行的。相关数据显示，其并发症发生率在可接受范围内。
- 大量证据表明，肝动脉灌注（hepatic artery infusion，HAI）化疗在辅助治疗无法手术切除的结直肠癌肝转移（colorectal cancer liver metastasis，CRLM）和可手术切除的结直肠癌肝转移中，均有重要的作用。
- 目前，运用肝动脉灌注化疗来治疗原发性肝癌和无法手术切除的结直肠癌肝转移的临床试验较少，这种治疗方案仍需要进一步的临床研究。

一、简介

肝脏是全身唯一一个既接受动脉系统血供，又接受肝肠循环血供的器官。正常的肝脏组织大部分血供来自门静脉,而肝脏肿瘤细胞的绝大部分血供却来自肝动脉(hepatic artery, HA)[1]。在过去的数十年中,研究者为了利用肝脏双重血供这一特点,尝试了多种治疗方案,对肝脏肿瘤进行局部治疗。在20世纪60年代早期,Sullivan等[2]率先报道了运用持续性肝动脉灌注化疗治疗肝恶性肿瘤。尽管样本量较小而且包含了各种类型的肿瘤,但这项开创性的研究初步揭示,肝动脉灌注化疗是可行的,并且肿瘤对化疗药物的反应程度是可量化的。不过,由于缺乏标准的化疗方案和肿瘤反应率的量化方法,肝动脉灌注化疗的应用十分有限。此外,由于置入导管、延长的灌注时间和笨重的外部输液泵引发较高的并发症,进一步的临床应用受到阻碍[3]。尽管早期研究有各种不足,但是为了安全有效地行肝动脉灌注化疗,以下3个基本要素被认为是必需的:①为了能持续灌注化疗,必须置入耐用的动脉导管;②选择合适的化疗药物;③为了能够持续、可靠和便捷地使用化疗药物,必须建立一个有效的药物转运系统[4]。

肝动脉灌注化疗的主要目的是选择性地将高浓度化疗药物送至肿瘤细胞,并尽可能地减少药物对正常肝细胞组织的损害。为了达到此目的,用于肝动脉灌注化疗的药物必须具备可量化的抗肿瘤活性和最佳药代动力学特征,即:①应首先被肝脏摄取;②在血浆中的半衰期较短;③具备较陡剂量-反应曲线的一级药物代谢动力学特点[5]。目前为止,一些可用于治疗原发性肝癌和肝转移瘤药物的药代动力学特点已在肝动脉灌注化疗中得到评估[6-11]。表7-1显示的是几种肝动脉灌注化疗术中常用药物的药代动力学特点。相对于其他几种化疗药物,氟尿嘧啶脱氧核苷(FUDR)应用最为广泛。应用于肝动脉灌注化疗术的FUDR在肝脏中的聚集浓度是其他器官的100~400倍,同时,其在肝脏肿瘤细胞中的浓度是正常肝细胞的15倍。超过92%的FUDR会首先被肝脏摄取,减少了其他器官的暴露剂量,并且FUDR在人体内的清除速度较快[4,12]。

表7-1 经肝动脉化疗药物的药代动力学

药物	肝脏摄取量(%)	血浆半衰期(分钟)	灌注暴露增长倍数	保留全身暴露相对静脉注射(%)
5-氟尿嘧啶(5-FU)	22~45	10	5~10	60~70
氟脲苷(FUDR)	69~92	<10	100~400	<5
丝裂霉素C(MMC)	22	<10	6~8	80~90
顺铂(CDDP)	—	20~30	4~7	100
多柔比星	45~50	60	2	40~50

HA:肝动脉;IV:静脉内。

[引自:Ensminger WD, Gyves JW. Clinical pharmacology of hepatic arterial chemotherapy. Semin Oncol 1983;10(2):176-82.]

成功进行肝动脉灌注化疗的关键在于正确使用药物并放置耐用的肝动脉导管,以保障药物灌注长期安全有效。目前,肝动脉导管主要是通过开腹手术置入的[13]。为了减少开腹手术相关的并发症,也会使用经皮穿刺方法。最近,Arru等[14]开展了一项经腋下皮肤穿刺(PCT)

置入肝动脉导管和手术开腹(LPT)置入肝动脉导管的对比研究。结果表明,在 LPT 组,平均住院时间更长、使用的止痛药剂量更大。然而,由于导管引起并发症而导致治疗延期或停止,在 PCT 组为43%,而在 LPT 组仅为7%($P=0.005$)。这项研究显示,在 PCT 组,可接受的化疗周期数远少于 LPT 组(4.3 vs 6.5,$P=0.038$)。这说明,尽管在手术过程中并发症的发生率较高,通过 LPT 放置肝动脉导管使机体更加耐受,可保证较长时间的药物灌注。近期,已有文献报道了将微创技术应用于肝动脉化疗栓塞术[15,16]。在一项单中心临床研究中,27 例患者通过腹腔镜手术置入肝动脉导管,导管置入成功率为100%,平均手术时间为45~55 分钟,有11%的患者产生了导管相关并发症[17]。在规范的医疗中心,应用腹腔镜手术置入肝动脉导管是可行的,而且并发症发生率也在可接受范围内。近来,已经有文献报道了将机器人应用于肝动脉导管置入术中[18]。

早期的肝动脉化疗输药系统包括:肝动脉导管口系统和与外部输液泵相连的经皮导管系统。这些器材不仅笨重而且引起的并发症发生率较高。这些不利因素使得肝动脉灌注化疗术发展缓慢。1979 年,首个可长时间持续灌注化疗的可置入输液泵系统开始在临床应用[19]。随后,针对此系统的评估也显示出置入的有效性和安全性,而设备引起的并发症发生率也在可接受范围内[20]。Heinrich 等[21]选择180 例患者,将可置入输液泵和肝动脉口系统进行比对。在肝动脉口组中,因发生严重并发症而停止治疗的比例为47%,而在可置入泵组中,此比例为30%。置入泵组中,无并发症生存期为12.2 个月,而肝动脉口组 z 仅为7.3 个月($P=0.002$)。后续研究发现,肝动脉口组中需要干预治疗的人数比置入泵组多了3 倍($P=0.003$)[22]。此外,最近一项含超过3000 例患者的系统研究显示,肝动脉口组并发症发生率超过30%,而置入泵组并发症的发生率仅为16%[23]。这项回顾性研究中有关化疗周期数的报道较少,但可以知道,置入泵组中平均可接受化疗周期数为12,而肝动脉口组仅为8。这说明,在肝动脉灌注化疗中,可置入泵在耐用性及可靠性方面优于肝动脉口。

为了研究的全面性,通过门静脉(Portalvein,PVI)进行肝内病灶直接灌注化疗的疗效也已被评估。通过门静脉的属支(回结肠静脉、结肠静脉、肠系膜下静脉、胃网膜静脉)可以较容易地置入门静脉导管,进行局部药物灌注。一项在1987 年前完成的关于门静脉灌注化疗的 meta 分析显示(包含了10 个临床研究和超过4000 例患者),绝对生存获益率为4.7%[24]。然而,最近一些运用5-FU 作为门静脉灌注药物的回顾性研究并不支持这一观点[25-28]。所有此类研究均提示,在无复发生存期(Recurrence-free survival,RFS)或总生存期(Overall survival,OS)方面,门静脉灌注化疗无明显生存获益。因此,通过门静脉进行肝内直接灌注化疗效果不明显,很少在临床使用。

二、技术方面

1. 输液泵

全置入式输液泵的特点有:可长时间、可靠、持续地对门诊患者行药物灌注治疗;现已经生产了几种型号;有些依靠化学电源,有些则用电池供电。目前应用最广泛的持续性输液泵是一种钛合金圆盘,它的直径约7cm,容量在20~50ml(图7-1)。它的两个腔由一支焊接波纹管分开。输液腔内有作用于肿瘤的药物,而外部的功能腔内有液体和蒸气混合物,用来提供化学能源。这个输液泵设计的非常巧妙,在药物填充进灌注腔的过程中,可以对化学能源进行充电,并且唯一使药物持续流入病灶的能量来源来自周期性的再灌注。

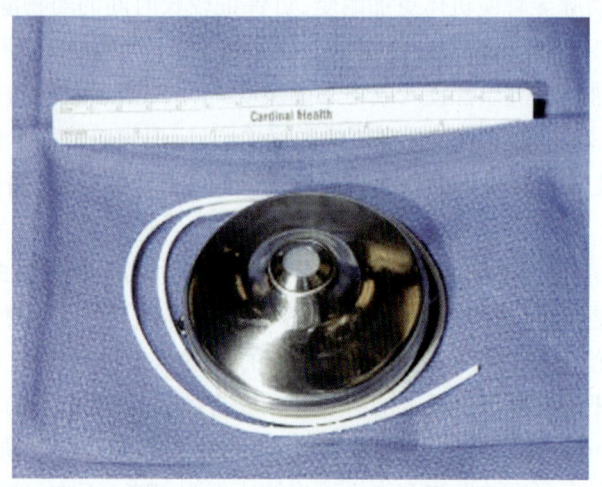

图7-1　Codman 3000 植入灌注泵

(可植入式持续灌注泵。Codman 公司,Johnson & Johnson 公司,Raynham, MA.)

2. 患者

所有考虑接受肝动脉灌注化疗术的患者必须接受影像学检查、内窥镜检查或肝外疾病(Extrahepatic disease,EHD)的筛查[29]。表7-2中显示的是相对不适合行肝动脉灌注化疗的患者和肿瘤类型。通常来说,无明显肝外疾病、PS 评分较低和肝功能储备良好的患者更适合接受肝动脉灌注化疗[30]。对于适合手术的患者,为了更好地了解肝动脉情况,必须评估其腹腔干和肠系膜上动脉[31]。血管造影一直都是评估肝动脉的金标准。然而最近,速度快、质量高的 CT 扫描将无创伤血管造影引领到新的水平。使用最新 CT 血管造影技术可以快速获得图像,并且可以通过三维重建发现肝动脉畸形,甚至可以取代传统的血管成像,从而避免了动脉穿刺并发症[32]。目前,CT 血管造影已成为许多医疗中心术前肝动脉评估首选的检查方法。

表7-2　持续性肝动脉灌注化疗相对禁忌证

患者因素	肿瘤/解剖因素
PS 较高(Karnofsky <60%)	肝外疾病
肝功能不全(总胆红素≥1.5 mg/dl)	弥散性肝转移灶(肝肿瘤浸润>70%)
	门静脉栓塞

3. 手术过程

术前必须详细评估肝动脉的解剖结构。表7-1列出了化疗泵置入的技术要点。手术通常采取腹正中切口,但若需同时行肝脏切除术,则要在肋下切口或曲棍球棒形切口。进入腹腔后,首先要排除肝外疾病。如果将输液泵放置在不可切除的病灶内,应在开腹探查前预先采用腹腔镜检查排除肝外疾病[33]。一旦排除肝外疾病,需行胆囊切除术,避免化学性胆囊炎。在行肝脏切除术的患者中,可在肝门区探查到肝总动脉和胃十二指肠动脉(图7-2)。当确定肝总动脉位置后,从近端1cm处分离胃十二指肠动脉。将远端的肝总动脉、胃十二指肠动脉和肝固有动脉游离,结扎胃右动脉。将所有肝总动脉、胃十二指肠动脉和肝固有动脉的侧支结扎,以免肝外灌注。将输液泵袋放置在合适的位置,通常是在左腹部。横切口要达到8cm,以防灌注泵接触到肋骨的边缘和髂前上棘。灌注泵袋要放置在前腹壁较浅的部位,以便在体表用针穿过腹壁。只有当灌注泵袋放置完成,且胃十二指肠动脉已准备好插管后,才能将灌注泵

表7-1　肝动脉化疗泵植入的主要技术要点

技术要点:
导管放置应允许统一的肝脏双叶灌注
结扎导管远端和肝脏近端的所有侧支,以避免肝外灌注
将导管端放置在胃十二指肠动脉和肝总动脉的连接处,以避免栓塞
识别并结扎任何副/替代肝动脉

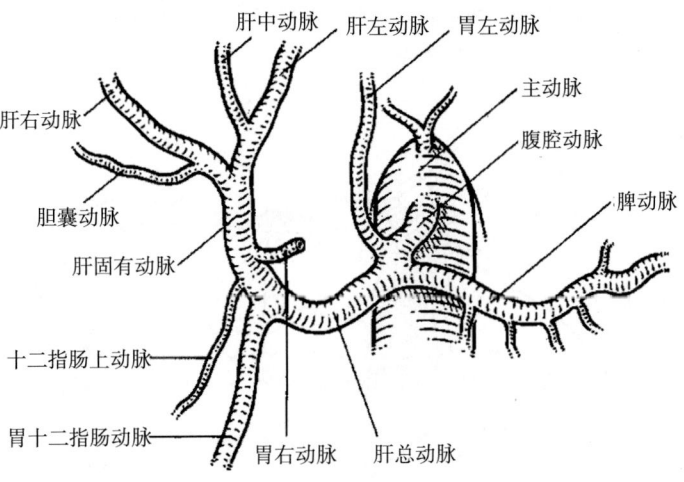

图7-2　正常肝动脉解剖图

[引自 Chamberlain RS. Essential functional hepatic and biliary anatomy for the surgeon. In: Abdeldayem H, editor. Hepatic surgery. 2013. (Figure 5). Available at: http://www.intechopen.com/books/hepatic-surgery. Accessed September 5, 2014; with permission.]

放入手术区。在泵内注入肝素生理盐水冲洗导管,在灌注泵袋的中央筋膜穿一个孔,并将导管送入腹腔。然后将连接好导管的输液泵缝入泵袋中(图7-3)。将胃十二指肠动脉的远端用不可吸收的缝线结扎,以控制远处、近处的胃十二指肠血管,并将血管缝合器放置在肝总动脉和肝固有动脉上,或在肝总动脉与胃十二指肠动脉连接处,将胃十二指肠动脉夹闭,以控制游离的胃十二指肠动脉。后一种方法需将导管放置在合适的位置,以防导管无意滑落至肝总动脉。确认已处理血管后,对胃十二指肠动脉行动脉切开术,将导管的远端送至肝总动脉和胃十二指肠动脉的连接处(图7-4)。将导管放置在肝总动脉可能会导致湍流或血栓,而将导管放置在胃十二指肠动脉,会直接使血管暴露在细胞毒性药物中。导管若未放置至合适的位置,会导致血管壁硬化、血栓或者假性动脉瘤。正如图7-4B所示,将导管缝在2~3个不可吸收的结上。

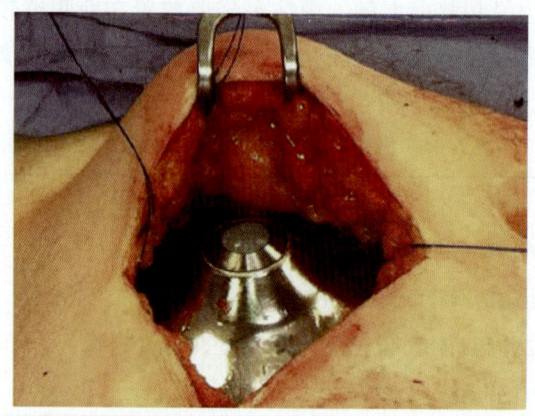

图7-3 完全置入式肝动脉灌注泵,在下腹壁前面皮下输液泵袋内

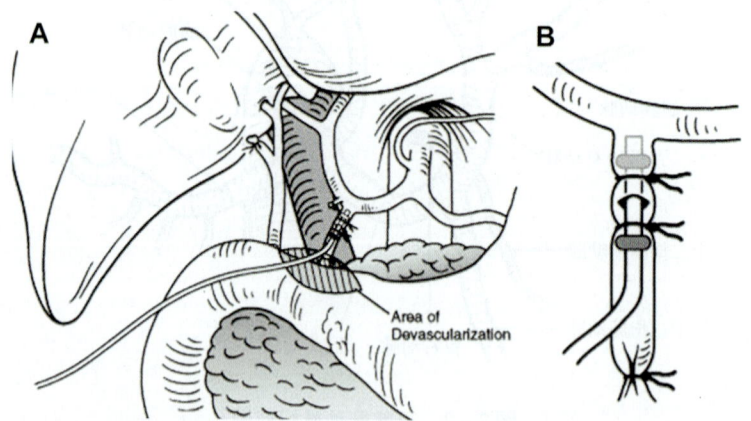

图7-4 A. 导管置入胃十二指肠动脉(GDA)。胃右动脉毗邻胃十二指肠动脉,并结扎。B. 胃十二指肠灌注导管置入和安全保障技术。[改自 Skitzki JJ, Chang AE. Hepatic artery chemotherapy for colorectal liver metastases: technical considerations and review of clinical trials. Surg Oncol 2002; 11 (3): 126; with permission.]

当导管进入胃十二指肠动脉后,需要评估导管放置位置和肝脏灌注情况。将亚甲蓝(使用可见光源)或荧光素(使用伍德灯和黑光)通过输液泵注入肝脏,通过染料分布情况可以评估染料的外渗及意外的肝外灌注情况(图7-5)。若发现异常的肝脏灌注或者肝外灌注,则需行血管造影,以明确有无副肝动脉或其他侧支血管。一旦发现此类血管,必须准确定位并将其结扎。当导管放置完成后,通过冲洗确保灌注通畅,然后缝合切口,手术完成。

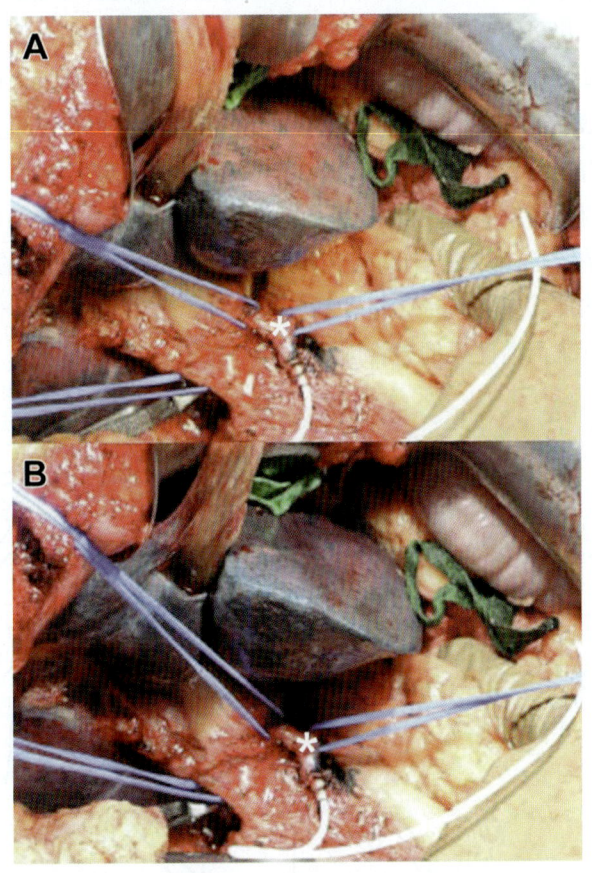

图7-5 亚甲蓝注入后动脉导管置入和肝脏灌注
A. 注入后早期;B. 注入后晚期,双叶灌注充分,无肝外灌注。
*表示胃十二指肠动脉导管固定在合适位置

三、处理不同解剖形态的肝动脉

一系列尸检表明,只有50%~60%的人肝动脉解剖形态正常。在Michels[34]的解剖学著作中,他定义了10种不同类型的异常肝脏血管。大体可归纳为异常肝右动脉或异常肝左动脉,进一步细分为副肝动脉(相对于正常的分支)或者替代肝动脉(取代了正常的肝动脉)。一项针对超过1900例患者的回顾性研究发现,发自肠系膜动脉的副肝右动脉或替代肝右动脉是最为常见的变异(14.9%)。其次是发自副胃左动脉的副肝左动脉或替代肝左动脉

$(11.3\%)^{[30]}$。

　　肝动脉解剖学变异一般不会影响肝动脉灌注化疗泵的置入。以前使用的双腔灌注泵可以同时对胃十二指肠动脉和异常的血管进行插管,这样,可对整个肝脏进行稳定灌注$^{[35]}$,但已经停产了。通常来说,处理畸变血管的最佳方法是结扎异常血管,并将灌注泵导管置入胃十二指肠动脉中(图7-6A,7-6B)。结扎的安全性已被一项研究证实:在接受肝叶动脉结扎术5天后,所有参与研究患者的两个肝叶仍可灌注$^{[36]}$。另一项针对544例患者的研究也证实,这种方法可避免插入胃十二指肠动脉以外的血管。这项研究也发现,接受肝动脉灌注泵置入的患者,其并发症发生率及置入失败率也会增加$^{[37]}$。胃十二指肠动脉起始端的变异也偶有发生,包括由肝总动脉直接发出,由肝左动脉、肝右动脉和胃十二指肠动脉共同构成的三根分叉血管。如图7-6C所示,这种情况下,处理方法同替代左/右肝动脉的副动脉一样,即结扎较小的叶动脉,并对胃十二指肠动脉插管。更加罕见的情况是,血管虽未畸变,但管径较小,需要使用专门的微导管进行插管。对于胃十二指肠动脉无法插管或者胃十二指肠动脉缺失而肝动脉被完全替代者,则需考虑自体血管移植或采用人造血管来为灌注泵的导管创造空间$^{[38]}$。

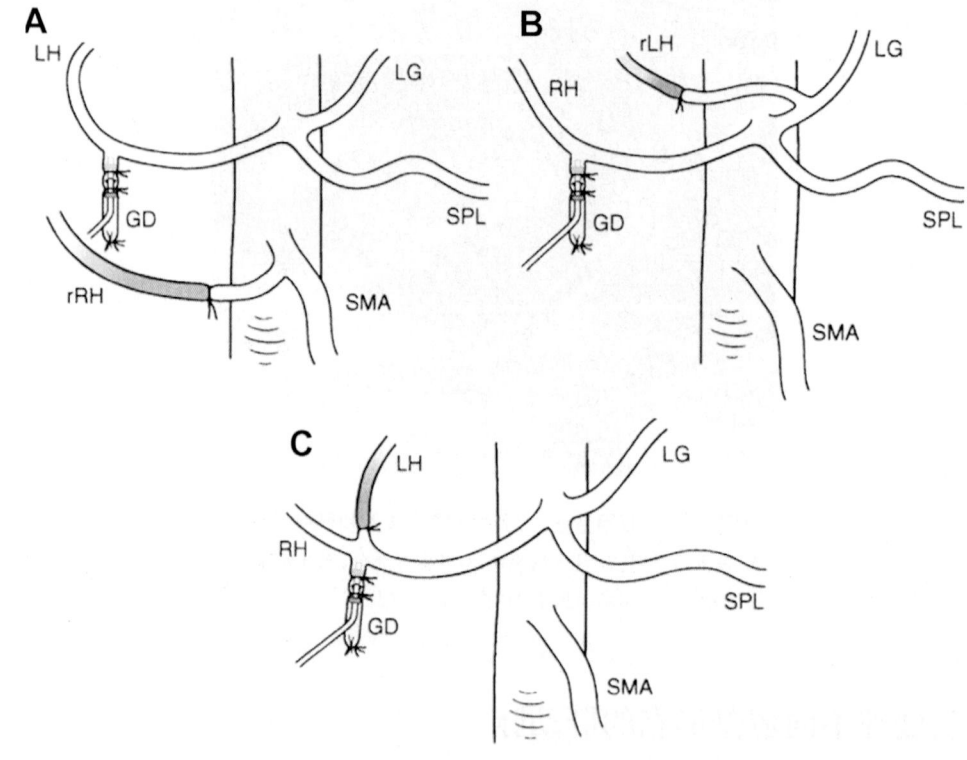

图7-6　A. 替代肝右动脉从肠系膜上动脉分离,结扎并将导管置入从肝左动脉分离的胃十二指肠动脉;B. 替代肝左动脉从左胃动脉分离,结扎,将导管置入从肝右动脉分离的胃十二指肠动脉;C. 肝总动脉的三根分叉血管,结扎肝左动脉,导管置入胃十二指肠动脉。GD,胃十二指肠的; LH,左肝的; RH,右肝的; rLH,替代左肝的; rRH,替代右肝的; SPL,脾动脉.[改自Skitzki JJ, Chang AE. Hepatic artery chemotherapy for colorectal liver metastases: technical considerations and review of clinical trials. Surg Oncol 2002;11(3):126;with permission.]

四、术后的处理和监测

在行肝动脉灌注化疗术前,需检查放射性核素泵流量,评估肝脏的灌注情况。将放射性核素标记的硫胶体注入患者静脉内,然后经灌注泵注入放射性核素标记的聚合白蛋白。将灌注扫描图叠放在一起,比较肝内灌注是否均匀,以及肝外灌注情况。在一套正常的放射性核素标记的聚合白蛋白扫描后,一般在灌注泵置入 1~4 周开始肝动脉灌注化疗[13]。行肝动脉灌注化疗的患者需接受严格的临床表现评估、影像学检查以及实验室检查来检测治疗相关并发症和评估治疗反应(disease status)。通常来说,随访的项目主要有:每 2 周复查一次生化指标(谷草转氨酶,谷丙转氨酶,碱性磷酸酶,总胆红素),每 4 周评估一次临床表现和检测毒性反应,同时每 3~4 个月进行一次胸部、腹部和盆腔的 CT 扫描,监测病灶变化情况[39]。

五、并发症

早期行肝动脉灌注化疗的患者,肿瘤应答显著,但居高不下的并发症发生率限制了其在临床上的广泛应用。相关研究表明,并发症的发生率在 30%~79%[40-42]。不同于系统性化疗,较高的并发症发生率在一定程度上反映出,行肝动脉灌注化疗不仅受到化疗药物相关毒性的影响,还有可能受到手术设备的影响,如肝动脉灌注导管、植入泵相关并发症。

1. **技术相关并发症**

过去 40 多年,大量研究试图评估肝动脉灌注化疗相关并发症的发生率、危险因素和临床影响。到目前为止,最具综合性的一项研究由 Allen 等[37]在 2005 年发起,纳入了 544 例行灌注泵置入术的患者,随访期长达 15 年。在这项研究中,灌注泵相关并发症的发生率为 22%,其中与肝动脉系统相关的并发症(血栓、灌注不完全、肝外灌注、大出血)更为常见(发生率为 51%)。表 7-3 中以时间为分类标准,总结了各类并发症和需要采取补救措施的发生率。灌注泵置入过程中需采取补救措施的总发生率为 45%。依据并发症发生的时间分层,对比早期(<30 天)和晚期并发症(>30 天)发生率,发现晚期并发症发生率较高,而需要采取补救措施的发生率较低(30% vs 70%;$P<0.001$)。总体来说,有 12% 的患者因并发症导致泵失效,进而中止化疗。这项研究指出,导致灌注泵相关并发症的独立危险因素是,操作者未对胃十二指肠动脉插管和缺少手术经验。

表7-3 并发症具体类型、发生时间(自手术起<30天或>30天),以及
并发症发生在不同时间的灌注泵功能补救能力

并发症类型	数量	早期(<30天)		晚期(>30天)	
		数量	补救率(%)	数量	补救率(%)
泵故障	6	6	100	—	—
泵袋					
感染	14	4	50	10	40
血肿	1	1	100	—	—
泵移位	4	1	100	3	33
导管					
闭塞	11	—	—	11	36
移出	18	—	—	18	11
腐蚀	4	—	—	4	0
动脉					
大出血	1	1	100	—	—
栓塞	33	13	31	20	30
肝外灌注	16	9	100	7	57
不完全灌注	12	9	78	3	67
总计	120	44	70	76	30

引自 Allen PJ, et al. Technical complications and durability of hepatic artery infusion pumps for unresectable colorectal liver metastases: an institutional experience of 544 consecutive cases. J Am Coll Surg 2005;201(1):60; with permission.

2. 动脉血栓

已有文献报道,在灌注泵置入的过程中,会发生急性血栓和胃十二指肠或肝总动脉夹层。一项涵盖超过17个研究的系统性回顾表明,在置入灌注泵时,血栓发生率为6.6%[23]。血栓既可以在早期(<30天)形成也可以在晚期(>30天)形成。后者更为常见,并且一般与细胞毒性药物的慢性暴露、血管硬化以及继发性血栓有关。而早期血栓一般与导管位置不正确或血液湍流相关。排除时间因素,溶栓药物或抗凝药物的使用可使采取补救措施的发生率降至接近30%。

3. 肝外灌注或肝内灌注不完全

在所有患者中,肝脏灌注不完全的发生率约为2%,主要的原因是没有结扎未被发现的畸形肝动脉,或是在结扎叶动脉后衍生出并行的动脉。虽然灌注不完全不会对患者肝功能造成不利影响,但会降低肝动脉灌注化疗的抗肿瘤效应。一般来说,可以对大多数结扎叶动脉后灌注不完全的患者进行随访观察;每2~4周行影像学复查,几乎所有的扫描结果均显示灌注异

常[21,38]。对于明显的副动脉继发性灌注不全,可以通过栓塞相应动脉来解决。

肝外灌注的发生率为 2%~9%,可能由以下因素导致:导管位置不正确或并行的动脉远端超过了导管的尖端,从而导致胃、十二指肠或胰腺异常灌注。这类并发症可通过术后放射性核素标记的聚合白蛋白扫描,或化疗药物灌注发现。肝外灌注典型的临床表现有灌注后上腹疼痛或腹泻。这些症状可由溃疡或胰腺炎引起。在这种情况下,应停止灌注,将泵内药物排空,进行泵通畅性检查或内镜检查[12]。多数情况下,可通过栓塞可疑血管来补救。图 7-7 展示了异常放射性核素标记的聚合白蛋白扫描,肝门区有明显肝外灌注,行栓塞术后复查显示,上述问题得以解决。Sofocleous 等[43]评估了 473 例行灌注泵植入术的患者采用栓塞作为补救措施的情况。放射性核素标记的聚合白蛋白扫描提示,有 45 例(9.5%)患者出现了肝外灌注。在这些患者中,32 例(7%)行血管造影术发现了异常灌注,其中 8 例(25%)是因肝动脉血栓形成,或导管顶端移位而无需行血管栓塞术。另外 24 例患者行血管栓塞术,其中有 21 例手术成功(87.5%),需要采取临床补救措施的发生率为 79%。

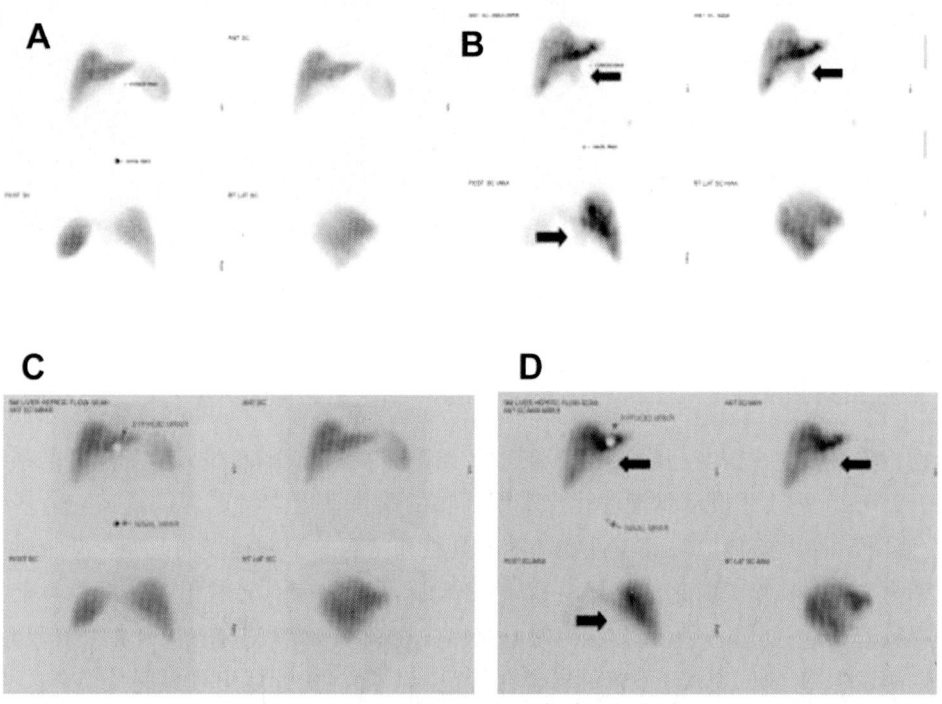

图 7-7 放射性核素异常流动研究

栓塞前:A. 基线锝标记硫胶体扫描。B. 锝标记大颗粒白蛋白(MAA)扫描,箭头指向灌注异常的位置。
栓塞后:C. 基线锝标记硫胶体扫描。D. 锝标记大颗粒白蛋白(MAA)扫描显示灌注异常结束,箭头指向异常灌注结束的位置

4. 灌注泵袋相关并发症

灌注泵袋相关并发症相对少见,但却会严重影响灌注系统的输送效率。泵袋感染发生率为 2%~3%[44]。一旦发生,可导致皮肤坏死、裂开和灌注泵挤出(图 7-8)。泵袋上的单纯蜂

窝织炎可口服抗生素治疗。然而考虑到灌注泵为异体,较严重的感染需行冲洗及静脉用抗生素。当感染无法控制、皮肤裂开或灌注泵移出时,需再次手术。这需要行开腹手术,切断导管,将旧的导管和新的灌注泵导管相连,同时搭建一个新的泵袋。灌注泵袋血肿的发生率不足1%,处理方法随着发生时间而有所不同。早期的血肿因进展较快,需立即再切开探查出血部位;对于迟发性血肿,需要先行影像学评估。较小的血肿可用细针穿刺吸出;较大的血肿需行常规血块清除术。

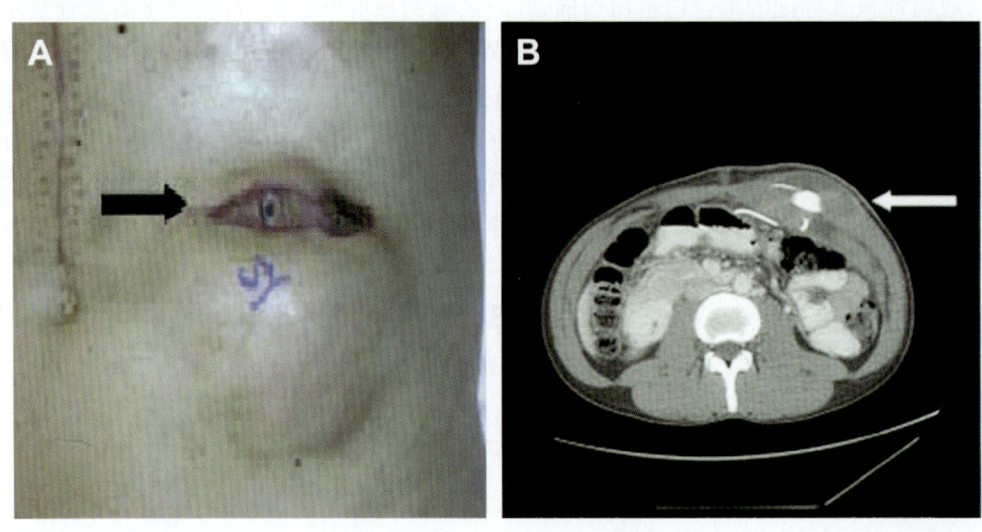

图7-8　A. 灌注泵袋感染和皮肤裂开(黑色箭头指示泵移出皮肤裂开);B. 灌注泵袋血肿(白色箭头)

5. 毒性相关并发症

药物相关并发症主要与药物的类型和剂量、给药方案、肝脏的首过效应和随后的系统性暴露相关。表7-1列出了肝动脉灌注化疗常用药物的药代动力学特点。以氟嘧啶为基础的化疗,最常使用5-FU或FUDR,其毒性特征随着肝脏和全身的暴露程度而改变。肝脏对5-FU的摄取率为20%~40%。因此,使用5-FU行肝动脉灌注化疗引起的相关并发症与全身化疗相似。胃肠道不适,如恶心、呕吐和腹泻等是最常见的不良反应,有超过30%的患者会出现。黏膜毒性的发生率较低,有接近3%的患者在行5-FU灌注化疗后出现黏膜反应[45]。发生严重毒性反应而对症治疗无法进行时,需考虑减少剂量或停止治疗。

FUDR几乎全部被肝脏摄取,从而限制了全身暴露剂量。因此,若使用FUDR灌注,首先观察到的毒性反应即为肝胆毒性。药物性肝炎较为常见,据报道,发生率根据定义的不同,在30%~70%之间波动。一般这种不良反应较轻,仅表现出生化指标的异常。

表7-4概括了随着FUDR剂量减少,AST、ALP和胆红素相应的变化情况。在遵从剂量-减小计划时,大多数患者的酶指标表现正常。

表7-4 FUDR肝动脉灌注剂量逐步减小

肝脏血液测试				FUDR剂量
AST	基础参考值	≤50 U/L	>50 U/L	
	当前值	0 to <3×ref	0 to <2×ref	100%
		3 to <4×ref	2 to <3×ref	80%
		4 to <5×ref	3 to <4×ref	50%
		≥5×ref	≥4×ref	不变
	停药后,达到以下值可重新开始	<4×ref	<3×ref	维持量的50%
ALP	基础参考值	≤90 U/L	>90 U/L	
	当前值	0 to <1.5×ref	0 to <1.2×ref	100%
		1.5 to <2×ref	1.2 to <1.5×ref	80%
		≥2×ref	≥1.5×ref	不变
	停药后,达到以下值可重新开始	<1.5×ref	<1.2×ref	维持量的25%
总胆红素	基础参考值	≤1.2 mg/dl	>1.2 mg/dl	
	当前值	0 to <1.5×ref	0 to <1.2×ref	100%
		1.5 to <2×ref	1.2 to <1.5×ref	50%
		≥2×ref	≥1.5×ref	不变
	停药后,达到以下值可重新开始	<1.5×ref	<1.2×ref	维持量的25%

缩写:ALP,碱性磷酸酶;AST,谷草转氨酶;ref,参考剂量。

摘自 Power DG, Kemeny NE. The role of floxuridine in metastatic liver disease. Mol Cancer Ther 2009;8(5):1021; with permission.

胆管硬化是肝动脉灌注化疗最严重的并发症,其发生率在1%~26%。与正常肝细胞不同,胆管细胞的血供主要来自肝动脉和胃十二指肠动脉的侧支。因此,在胃十二指肠放置导管后,胆管细胞会直接暴露于高浓度的化疗药物中。肝动脉灌注化疗相关的胆管硬化,是由缺血和化疗药物直接毒性的共同作用导致的[46]。胆管硬化几乎只出现在用FUDR行灌注化疗的患者,以FUDR行辅助化疗时,硬化更常见。在灌注化疗时加用地塞米松可降低胆管硬化发生率。在一个对比单用FUDR和联用FUDR+地塞米松的前瞻性临床研究中,胆管毒性发生率分别为30%和9%($P=0.07$)。此后,所有行FUDR灌注化疗的方案均加用了地塞米松。最近一项研究报道了系统性使用贝伐单抗和FUDR灌注联用后,胆管硬化的发生率显著增加,现已被禁用[47]。尽早发现胆管硬化十分重要。当减药或停药均无法使生化指标恢复正常,或仅有胆红素升高时,需及时行CT扫描,明确有无因复发病灶引起的压迫所致。当影像学提示胆管未受到外部压迫时,需进行磁共振胰胆管造影;当发现胆管局限性狭窄时,需经内镜逆行胰胆管造影,行支架植入术。即使已减药或停药,且行胆管支架植入术,胆管狭窄患者的生存率仍较低[46]。

六、行肝动脉灌注化疗患者的临床转归

1. 辅助肝动脉灌注化疗和可切除的结直肠癌肝转移

有70%~80%患者行结直肠癌肝转移病灶切除术后仍会复发,其中有50%的复发出现在肝脏。为了改善预后,可考虑在肝脏切除术后行辅助化疗。考虑到局部复发,在这种情况下行肝动脉灌注化疗具有应用价值。目前,多中心随机对照研究和回归分析评估了在直肠癌肝转移切除术后行肝动脉灌注化疗的临床应用价值。

Lorenz等[48]是首批开展术后行肝动脉灌注化疗方面临床研究的团队之一。在这项研究中,患者被随机分到手术组和手术+5-FU/LV(leucovorin,亚叶酸)组。两组总体无疾病生存期无统计学差异(手术+5-FU组为14.2个月,单手术组13.7个月),同时肝脏特异性总体无疾病生存期也无统计学差异(手术+5-FU组为21.6个月,单手术组24个月)。总体生存时间同样无统计学差异。然而,行肝动脉灌注化疗组的患者仅有30%接受了预定的治疗策略,使得研究效果不理想。这项研究出于安全性和有效性考虑而被过早终止了。德国一个小样本临床研究纳入了42例患者,这些患者被随机分到丝裂霉素C(mitomycin C,MMC)灌注+手术组或单手术组。两组之间的总生存率(MMC灌注+手术组25%,单手术组31%)和无疾病生存率(MMC灌注+手术组15%,单手术组23%)无统计学差异。在丝裂霉素C灌注+手术组的患者似乎更容易发生肝外转移,但这并没有统计学差异[49]。

在1999年,Kemeny等[12]进行了如下试验:结直肠癌肝转移患者行肝切除术后,被随机分到FUDR/DEX+5-FU/LV灌注组或单5-FU/LV灌注组。以既往治疗次数和转移瘤个数为分层标准。在治疗组,中位生存期为73个月,而对照组为60个月;累计2年生存率在灌注组中为86%,而系统性化疗组为74%($P=0.03$)。2年后,灌注组无肝内复发率高于系统性化疗组(90% vs 60%,$P<0.001$)。灌注组2年无疾病生存率为57%,而对照组为42%,无统计学差异($P=0.07$)。这项研究的主要缺陷在于原定的治疗方案改变太大。在治疗组,由于药物毒性导致减药,仅有26%的患者接受了超过原定治疗剂量1/2的量。尽管有这些不足,这项研究还是在一定程度上证明了FUDR/DEX+5-FU/LV治疗提高了对肝内病灶的控制,以及累计2年总生存率。这项研究的随访结果公布于2005年。此时,中位随访时间已达到10年[50]。FUDR/DEX+5-FU/LV灌注组的中位无疾病生存期为31.3个月,而单系统性化疗组为17.2个月($P=0.02$)。同时,相对单系统性化疗组(中位无肝脏复发时间为32.5个月),在FUDR/DEX+5-FU/LV结合组中,截止到2005年,仍未达到中位无肝脏复发时间,证明FUDR/DEX+5-FU/LV结合可显著提高中位无肝脏复发时间。FUDR/DEX+5-FU/LV灌注组中,中位总生存期是68个月,而系统性化疗组为59个月($P=0.10$)。FUDR/DEX+5-FU/LV灌注组累计总生存率为41%,而单系统性化疗组为27%。

一份来自希腊的随机对照研究,对比了在结直肠癌肝转移术后,肝动脉灌注化疗+系统性化疗-免疫治疗(MMC/FU灌注+MMC+IL-2)和单系统性MMC+IL-2治疗的疗效。在这

项研究中,肝动脉灌注化疗+系统性化疗组总体无疾病进展时间为46个月,而单系统性MMC+IL-2治疗组为19个月($P=0.006$)。前者的无肝内复发时间为79个月,后者为45个月($P=0.0001$)。相比单系统性MMC+IL-2治疗组,肝动脉灌注化疗+系统性化疗-免疫治疗组中位总生存期得到了显著提升(79个月 vs 66个月,$P=0.05$)。这些数据表明,将系统性化疗-免疫治疗和局部治疗结合,可提高无疾病生存期和总生存期。

在2002年,Kemeny等[51]报道了一项多中心研究:在低风险患者中(肿瘤数目为1~3个),对比FUDR+5-FU/LV灌注和单手术治疗。相比单手术组,FUDR灌注+5-FU/LV治疗组4年的无疾病生存率(46% vs 25%)和无肝脏复发率(67% vs 43%)均得到了提升。但两组之间就总生存期而言,无论是累计4年的总生存率,还是中位总生存期均无统计学差异。但在这项研究中,来自25个不同中心的患者只有109例达到了9年的随访周期。外科技术的提高,以及后续新疗法的使用导致研究结果不理想。此外,由于术前分组随机化,致使29例患者在手术时被剔出研究(18例灌注组患者,11例单手术组患者),最终的分析只剩下80例患者。同样,这项研究也无法有力说明生存期问题。

最近,有两个单组临床Ⅰ/Ⅱ期试验完成了新系统性化疗结合肝动脉灌注化疗的研究。在试验安全性/毒性阶段,首先将FUDR/DEX和伊立替康的结合剂量逐渐增加。当确定最大安全剂量(MTD)后,开始将MTD应用在24例患者身上。具体用药剂量为:伊立替康200mg/m²和0.12mg/kg FUDR×泵体积/流量。剂量限制性毒性反应为腹泻和中性粒细胞减少。在所有96例患者中,18个月无疾病生存率为47%,无肝脏复发率为88%,累计2年总生存率为89%。在27例接受MTD剂量的患者中,有1例患者在第16个月时出现了肝内复发。总的来说,组内有4例患者复发(1例肝内复发,3例肝外复发);1年无疾病进展生存率为91%[52]。另一个相似的Ⅰ期临床试验评估了FOLFOX[5-FU/LV/奥沙利铂(OX)]和FUDR/DEX结合使用的效果。MTD确立后,剂量限制性毒性反应包括腹泻和胆红素升高。4年的总生存率为88%,无疾病生存率为50%[53]。这两项试验证实,将FUDR/DEX灌注结合新的化疗方案应用于结直肠癌肝转移切除的患者,在安全性方面可行。尽管还不足以对预后下充分的结论,但这种将局部治疗和全身化疗相结合的治疗方案,为更大的Ⅲ期临床试验提供了循证医学证据。

到目前为止,还没有将新辅助系统性化疗和肝动脉灌注化疗结合的大规模随机Ⅲ期临床试验。但是,有关于正在进行的Ⅱ期临床试验的报道。Kemeny等[54]将73例患者随机分到FUDR/DEX灌注+系统性化疗+BEV组或者无BEV组,并对比了两组的预后。根据不同的临床危险因素进行分层。在BEV组,4年无疾病生存率和总生存率分别为37%和81%,而在无BEV组,分别为46%和85%,未发现统计学差异。在BEV组胆管毒性显著上升,其中有5例患者的胆红素上升至>3 mg/dl,并且有4例患者行胆道支架植入术;在无BEV组,无上述并发症出现。上述胆管毒性导致停用BEV。因此,可初步得出这样的结论:FUDR/DEX灌注+系统性化疗+BEV治疗结直肠癌肝转移患者,不仅无法显著提高无疾病生存率和总生存率,还会增加导管相关并发症,应该避免使用该方法。

一项单组Ⅱ期临床研究纳入了76例患者,旨在评估肝脏切除术后或者消融术后,联合应用FUDR/DEX灌注+系统性的奥沙利铂和卡培他滨的临床效用。有21例患者无法行既定的治疗方案,其余的55例患者正常进行。2年无疾病生存率为60%,而无肝脏复发率为76%,

总生存率为89%。就接受治疗的周期数而言,67%的患者接受了完整的6个疗程,这说明,这项治疗方案具有可耐受性和可接受性[55]。虽然只是Ⅱ期的临床试验,无法得出广泛的结论,但这项联合方案似乎是安全的,且复发率较低,生存率较高。

已经有一些回顾性临床研究的报道。Tomlinson等[56]回顾了612例接受切除术的结直肠癌肝转移患者。接受辅助FUDRA灌注的患者10年总生存率为38%,而那些未接受辅助治疗者为15%($P<0.0001$)。此外,Ito等[57]回顾了超过1000例行肝脏切除术的患者。在这些患者中,多变量分析提示,行HUDRG灌注可作为一项独立因素,可提高生存期(HUDR灌注68个月 vs 无灌注化疗50个月,$P<0.0001$)。另一份回顾性分析由MSKCC(Memorial Sloan Kettering Cancer Center)的House等[58]完成。他们回顾性分析了250例行切除术和新辅助化疗的结直肠癌肝转移患者,其中有125例患者接受了辅助的FUDR灌注治疗。结果表明,结合灌注化疗组无肝内复发率为79%,单系统性化疗组为55%($P<0.001$);联合灌注组5年无复发生存率为48%,单系统性化疗组为25%($P=0.01$);联合灌注组5年疾病特异性生存率为75%,单系统性化疗组为55%($P=0.01$)。最近,Goere等[59]进行了一项回顾性分析,纳入了98例高危患者(肿瘤数目>4个),对比了奥沙利铂灌注+系统性5-FU/LV($n=44$)治疗和单系统性5-FU/LV($n=54$)治疗。两组之间的总体3年无疾病生存率(灌注组33% vs 对照组5%,$P<0.0001$)和3年无肝脏复发率(灌注组49% vs 对照组21%,$P=0.0008$)有显著差异。两组之间的总生存率无统计学差异(3年总生存率:灌注组75% vs 对照组62%)。

以肝动脉灌注化疗为辅助化疗的一系列试验突出了一些争议性问题,阻碍了大规模的Ⅲ期临床试验的进行。首先,层出不穷的新型系统性化疗药物使得很难设定合适的对照组。此外,作为研究最广泛的辅助灌注药物FUDR,在美国之外的国家使用较少,使临床试验实施难度较大,无法广泛开展。另外,入选患者数目增长缓慢,导致试验进程缓慢,在试验开始承认的指南药物,在试验结束时已被停用。最后,手术技术的提高以及新的治疗手段如消融技术等,提高了行切除术后结直肠癌肝转移患者的预后,使得很难制定出试验组的治疗标准。然而,尽管缺少大规模的Ⅲ期临床试验,但辅助的肝动脉灌注术似乎可以提高患者的无疾病生存率和无肝脏复发率。而是否可以使总生存率显著获益,仍需进一步验证。

2. 不可切除的结直肠癌转移

(1)一线治疗方案(单肝动脉灌注化疗)

到目前为止,已经有10份随机对照试验研究评估了肝动脉灌注化疗对一线治疗不可手术切除的结直肠癌肝转移(UR-CRLM)患者的效果。由于这些研究在设计和实施方面存在显著的差异性,因而导致其相互矛盾或有不确定的结果。表7-5列举了这些试验,并对比其结果。

在1987—1990年,发表了5篇关于肝动脉灌注化疗治疗UR-CRLM的文献。Chang等[60]纳入64例患者,对比评估HUDR灌注治疗和系统性应用HUDR的效果。在灌注组,RR为62%,而对照组为17%($P<0.003$);中位总生存期在灌注组为17个月,对照组为12个月($P=0.27$),这项研究并未提示总生存率获益。同时,这项研究因在灌注组纳入了肝门区淋巴结转移阳性的患者而受到争议;而去除淋巴结因素后的亚组分析表明,灌注组2年总生存率为

47%,而对照组为13%($P=0.03$)。由MSKCC发起的更大规模的试验将162例患者随机分到FUDR肝动脉灌注组或系统性应用FUDR组。在行开腹手术时,由于出现了肝外病灶或可切除的病灶,有63例患者被剔除。在疾病出现进展时,允许联合使用试验灌注化疗和系统性化疗。在肝动脉灌注组,RR为50%,而对照组为20%($P=0.001$)。RR的提高不代表生存获益。然而,观察到联合治疗比率为60%,使生存分析变得困难。假如将联合治疗的患者排除在外,灌注组中位总生存期为18个月,而对照组为8个月[61]。第三个试验中,北加州癌症研究机构将143例患者随机分到FUDR灌注组或系统性应用FUDR组,主要的观察终点为RR或疾病进展时间(TTP)。在灌注组,RR为42%,对照组为6%($P=0.0001$)。灌注组疾病进展时间更长(13.2个月 vs 6.6个月,$P=0.009$),但中位总生存期在两组之间却无统计学差异(16.6个月 vs 16.1个月)[62]。在这项研究中,患者出现了较严重的毒性反应,治疗组有超过50%的患者未能接受预定治疗方案一半的剂量。在MSKCC的试验中,由于存在灌注治疗和系统治疗联合使用,生存期数据不能说明问题。

Wagman等[63]将56例UR-CRLM患者随机分到FUDR灌注组或系统性5-FU/LV组。结果表明,两组之间的RR(试验组55%,对照组20%)、疾病进展时间(试验组8.8个月,对照组7.5个月)或总生存期(试验组13.8个月,对照组11.6个月)均未观察到统计学差异。值得注意的是,在系统性化疗组中所应用的药物和先前的试验不同,为5-FU/LV而非FUDR。而以往试验已经证明,和5-FU/LV相比,FUDR会降低RR。同样,Mayo医疗中心将74例患者随机分到FUDR灌注组或系统性5-FU/LV组。结果显示,尽管试验组RR有所提高(试验组48%,对照组21%),疾病进展时间(试验组6.0个月,对照组5.0个月)与总生存期(试验组12.6个月,对照组10.5个月)均无统计学差异[64]。

Rougier等[65]对比了FUDR肝动脉灌注治疗和最佳支持治疗(BSC)或系统性应用5-FU的疗效。这项研究在疾病进展前允许联合使用。试验组RR为43%,对照组为9%。两组之间总生存期有统计学差异(试验组15个月 vs 对照组11个月,$P=0.02$)。在这项研究中,交叉率为30%并且未对对照组进行标准化处理,降低了试验结果的说服力。另一项相似的研究对比了FUDR灌注和最佳支持治疗对未接受治疗UR-CRLM患者的疗效,同样证明了肝动脉灌注可显著提高总生存期(试验组13.5个月 vs BSC 7.5个月,$P=0.03$)[66]。

2000年,德国研究者将168例UR-CRLM患者随机分到以下三组:5-FU/LV灌注组、FUDR组或系统性应用5-FU/LV,对应的疾病进展时间分别为9.2个月、6.6个月和5.9个月。结果显示,5-FU/LV灌注组和FUDR灌注组之间有统计学差异($P=0.033$)。虽然在5-FU/LV灌注组观察到生存获益的趋势,但总生存期无统计学差异。和其他实验结果相似的是,这项实验同样允许组与组联合治疗,降低了生存分析结果的可信度[67]。

2003年,一项最大规模的随机对照研究将290例患者分到5-FU/LV灌注组或系统性应用5-FU/LV组。两组之间的无进展生存期或总生存期均无统计学差异。然而,有37%的患者被分到灌注组后未接受治疗,同时有29%的患者由于置管失败被调至系统性治疗组。灌注组的中位疗程数为2,而系统性组为8.5。因此,试验研究者得出这样的结论:肝动脉灌注化疗并发症较高的发生率并未带来更多生存获益,因此不能将肝动脉灌注化疗应用于UR-CRLM患者[68]。

2006年公布的编号为CALGB 9481的临床研究,将135例UR-CRLM患者随机分到FUDR/LV/DEX灌注组或系统性使用5-FU/LV组。此试验主要以生存率为观察终点,不允许联合治疗,两组之间的RR存在显著差异(灌注组47% vs 对照组24%)。总体来说,两组之间的疾病进展时间无统计学差异。然而,灌注组肝脏的疾病进展时间却长于对照组(9.8个月 vs 7.3个月)。就总生存期而言,灌注组的中位总生存期为24.4个月,而对照组为20个月,两组之间的中位总生存期有统计学差异($P=0.003$)[69]。这项试验首次观察到,相比当时最有效的系统性应用5-FU/LV,肝动脉灌注化疗可使患者总生存期获益。

表7-5 不可切除的结直肠癌肝转移单肝动脉灌注化疗随机对照试验

作者[参考],年(组)	数量	治疗	应答率(%)	P值	无疾病进展生存期(月)	P值	总生存期(月)	P值
Chang等[50],1987(NCI)	64	HAIC FUDR	62	<0.003	—	—	17	0.72
		Systemic FUDR	17				12	
Kemeny等[61],1987(MSKCC)	99	HAIC FUDR	50	0.001	—	—	17	0.42
		Systemic FUDR	20				12	
Hohn等[62],1989(NCOG)	143	HAIC FUDR	42	0.0001	13.2	0.009	16.6	NS
		Systemic FUDR	6		6.6		16.1	
Wagman等[63],1990	56	HAI FUDR	55	NR	8.8	0.94	13.8	0.55
		Systemic 5FU/LV	20		7.5		11.6	
Martin等[64],1990(NCCTG)	74	HAIC FUDR	48	0.02	6.0	0.31	12.6	0.53
		Systemic 5-FU	21		5.0		10.5	
Rougier等[65],1992(France)	163	HAIC FUDR	43	NR			15	0.02
		BSCAK 5-FU	9				11	
Allen-Mersh等[66],1994(UK-HAPT)	100	HAIC FUDR					13.5	0.03
		BSC					7.5	
Lorenz等[67],2000(德国合作组)	168	HAIC 5-FU/LV			9.2	0.03	18.7	0.09(HAIC 5-FU)
		Systemic 5-FU			6.6		17.6	
Kerr等[68],2003(EORTC)	290	HAIC 5-FU/LV	—	—	7.7	0.27	14.4	0.79
		Systemic 5-FU	—	—	6.7		14.8	
Kemeny等[69],2006(CALGB)	135	HAIC/FUDR/DEX/LV	47	0.012	5.3	0.95	24.4	0.003
		Systemic 5-FU/LV	24		6.8		20.0	

加粗数值为显著值。

BSC:最佳支持治疗;CALGB,癌症与白血病组B;DEX,地塞米松;EORTC,欧洲癌症研究和治疗组织;HAIC,肝动脉灌注化疗;LV,亚叶酸钙;MSKCC,Sloan Kettering纪念癌症中心;NCCTG,北部中心癌症治疗组;NCI,美国国家癌症研究所;NCOG,北加州肿瘤组;NR,未报道;NS,非显著;UK-HAPT,肝动脉泵试验(英国)

首个此类临床试验的meta分析报道于1996年,包含了1994年前的随机对照研究(表7-5)。合并数据后,在不同的治疗方案之间,RR存在显著统计学差异。与系统性化疗组(5-FU

或 FUDR) RR 14% 相比,灌注组(5-FU 或 FUDR)为 41%[风险比(OR) 0.25,95% 置信区间(CI)0.16~0.40]。

对所有的数据分析后表明,相对于系统性化疗组,肝动脉灌注化疗可使患者获益($P=0.0009$)。然而,把无治疗对照组试验排除后,生存获益并不明显($P=0.14$)[70]。一项 2007 年更新后的 meta 分析包含了表 7-5 中所有的随机对照试验[71]。合并数据后,RR 与之前的 meta 分析相同(灌注组 42.9% vs 系统性化疗组 18.4%,$P<0.0001$)。之前 meta 分析观察到的较小总生存期获益并未体现出来:相比对照组的中位总生存期 12.4 个月,灌注组为 15.9 个月[(风险比(hazard ratio) 0.90,95% CI 0.76~1.07;$P=0.24$]。累积分析这些数据表明,单肝动脉灌注化疗(不联用系统性化疗)可降低肿瘤 RR,但这似乎并未转化为生存获益。

(2)二线治疗方案(肝动脉灌注化疗+系统性化疗)

UR-CRLM 患者行一线治疗方案失败后预后较差。即使采用新的化疗方案,RR 最高才能达到 20%,中位总生存期为 9~12 个月[72]。尽管缺乏生存获益,及早行肝动脉灌注化疗仍可延缓肝内疾病进展,并且治疗失败往往是因为系统性疾病。为了解决这一问题,研究者进行了大量将肝动脉灌注化疗与系统性化疗结合的临床试验。

一项研究将 84 例患者随机分到 FUDR 灌注+系统性应用 5-FU/LV 组或单系统性应用 5-FU/LV 组,两组之间生存时间无明显统计学差异,1 年总生存期在联合用药组为 46%,而对照组为 53%。在联合用药组还观察到毒性反应增强,无生存获益并存在潜在的危险[73]。从那时起,有一些Ⅰ期临床试验便开始评估 FUDR 灌注联合新的化疗方案的效果,相对于标准的 5-FU/LV 方案,新的联合用药方案(Ox,伊立替康)可提高 RR。一项Ⅰ期临床试验将 FUDR 灌注联合系统性应用伊立替康,治疗 46 例曾接受过治疗的患者,并未发现药物毒性有所增加。试验结果表明,RR 为 74%,中位整体疾病进展时间为 8.1 个月,肝内疾病进展时间为 8.5 个月。中位总生存期为 17.2 个月[74]。另一项Ⅰ期临床研究将双药联合 FUDR 灌注,双药分别为 Ox+伊立替康或 Ox+5-FU/LV(FOLFOX),同样导致 RR 较低和总生存期较长。在 FUDR 灌注+FOLFOX 组,RR 为 87%,而在 Ox+伊立替康+FUDR 灌注组,RR 为 90%。中位总生存期分别为 22 个月和 36 个月[75]。这些研究回顾了 39 例曾接受系统性应用 Ox 治疗又接受 FUDR 灌注+伊立替康患者的治疗情况。在这 39 例患者中,有 33 例曾经历 1~2 个治疗方案失败。肝内疾病进展时间为 8.6 个月,而肝外疾病进展时间为 6.5 个月。治疗负荷较大的患者 RR 为 44%,中位总生存期为 20 个月,转变为可切除病灶的概率为 18%。

考虑到许多国家无法使用 FUDR 作为灌注药物,Ox 灌注化疗成为替代选择。一项来自法国的Ⅰ期临床试验,纳入了 44 例行一线化疗方案失败的 UR-CRLM 患者,并就其评估 Ox 灌注+系统性应用 5-FU/LV 的疗效。先前治疗失败的次数在 1~5 次,平均为 2 次。中位总生存期为 16 个月,无进展生存期为 7 个月,总体 RR 为 55%。有 17 例行 FOLFIRI(5-FU/LV/伊立替康)方案失败的患者和 12 例行 FOLFOX 失败的患者对此方案部分应答。有 7 例(18%)由不可切除病灶转变为可切除病灶,进而接受了外科手术治疗[76]。之后,研究者又在另外 28 例未接受过 Ox 治疗的患者中评估此方案(Ox 灌注+5-FU/LV)的疗效。在这批患者中,RR 为 64%,中位总生存期为 27 个月,无进展生存期为 27 个月[77]。尽管试验规模小且为回顾性研究,但结果还是比较令人满意,肝动脉灌注化疗联合新的系统性化疗药物,可改善一线治疗方案失败的 UR-CRLM 患者的 RR 和生存时间。

(3)从不可切除转变为可切除

针对结直肠癌肝转移,尽管新的化疗药物层出不穷,但 RR 仍在 30%~40%,中位总生存期也仅为 20 个月[78]。手术切除为唯一能治愈结直肠癌肝转移的方法。因此,最近有几项研究旨在将不可切除的病灶转变为可切除病灶。最近一项来自 MSKCC 的研究纳入了 49 例 UR-CRLM 患者(73% >5 个肿瘤,98% 的患者肝左右叶均有病灶),并评估其 FUDR 灌注+伊立替康/Ox 的疗效。结果表明,总体 RR 为 92%,其中 8% 的患者完全应答,84% 的患者部分应答。49 例患者中有 23 例病灶由不可切除转变为可切除(47%)。那些接受肝切除术的患者,中位无疾病进展生存期为 7.6 个月。MSKCC 开展的另一项研究中,有 39 例病灶不可切除的患者接受了 FUDR/DEX 灌注+伊立替康治疗。结果发现,RR 为 44%,有 7 例患者病灶转变为可切除。此外,由 MSKCC 开展的一项回顾性分析中,纳入了 373 例接受 FUDR 灌注+系统性化疗的 UR-CRLM 患者。其中有 297 例患者(79%)曾接受过系统性化疗。93 例(25%)患者病灶转变为可切除,并接受了切除术,其中一些还接受了消融术。未接受切除术的患者,中位总生存期为 16 个月,而接受了肝切除术的患者为 59 个月($P<0.001$)[79]。尽管这些患者的肿瘤负荷较大,且接受了明显的预处理,仍有 25% 患者病灶变为可切除,并接受相关切除术。这些说明,FUDR 灌注联合新的系统性化疗方案是一种有效的治疗方案。

在法国,由于无法使用 FUDR 行肝动脉灌注化疗,因而 Ox 灌注广泛应用于临床。前文中已提及一些小的临床试验将 Ox 灌注联合系统性化疗应用于不可切除病灶,其转换为可切除的概率为 18%。一项回顾性分析纳入了 87 例接受 Ox 灌注+系统性应用 5-FU/LV 患者,其结果为:21 例患者(24%)接受了根治性切除术。总随访时间为 63 个月,在切除组,5 年总生存率为 56%,而对照组则为 0($P<0.0001$)[80]。这表明,与 FUDR 灌注+系统性化疗的结果相似,Ox 灌注+系统性化疗可使超过 20% 不可切除病灶转变为可切除病灶,进而带来长期生存获益。

七、肝动脉灌注化疗和原发性肝恶性肿瘤

原发性肝恶性肿瘤(PLC)包括肝内胆管细胞癌(ICC)和肝细胞癌(HCC)。大多数 PLC 患者诊断时已为晚期,从而失去了根治性手术的机会。PLC 的中位总生存期不足 12 个月。在北美,迄今为止,几乎没有关于 PLC 行肝动脉灌注化疗的临床试验。2009 年,Jarnagin 等[81]报道了一项Ⅱ期单组临床研究,这项研究纳入了 34 例 PLC 患者(26 例不可切除的 ICC 患者,8 例晚期 HCC 患者)。毒性反应发生率为 14.7%,导管相关并发症发生率为 24%。RR 为 47%,肝内应答时间持续 24 个月。14 例患者(41%)疾病稳定(SD),3 例患者(9%)疾病进展(PD)。疾病控制率(PR + SD)为 88%。ICC 的总体 RR 为 54%,而 HCC 的 RR 为 25%。在随后的 25 个月,有 33 例患者出现疾病进展,21 例患者(61.8%)出现肝内病灶进展(18 例肝内病灶进展,3 例肝内肝外均有进展)。在这 33 例患者中,有 21 例最初疾病进展部位在肝外器官。DSS

分层反应如下:PR 35.1 个月,SD 28.6 个月,PD 9.8 个月。总体无进展生存期为 7.4 个月,肝脏特异性无进展生存期为 10.3 个月。MSKCC 另一项临床试验纳入了 56 例 PLC 患者,其中 22 例患者(18 例 ICC,4 例 HCC)接受 FUDR/DEX 灌注+BEV,其余 34 例接受单 FUDR/DEX 灌注。ICC 患者中,有 7 例 PR(39%),11 例 SD(61%);在 PR 患者中,中位应答时间为 11 个月,SD 患者为 6 个月。所有的 HCC 患者均为 SD,中位应答时间为 9 个月。在 BEV 组,中位无进展生存期为 8.5 个月,对照组为 7.5 个月;在 BEV 组,肝内无进展生存期为 11 个月,对照组为 10 个月。在 BEV 组,中位总生存期为 31 个月,对照组为 30 个月。在这项试验中,接受 BEV 治疗的患者出现了严重的胆管毒性;22 例中有 5 例出现了胆管毒性,3 例(14%)行胆道支架置入术。而在对照组,34 例患者仅有 2 例出现胆管毒性,且无需胆道支架置入[82]。基于这些发现,出于安全性的考虑,将 BEV 行停药处理。最近针对 ICC 患者,报道了一项改进的临床试验研究。这项研究共纳入了 44 例接受肝动脉灌注化疗的 ICC 患者,有 22 例患者接受单 FUDR/DEX 灌注,18 例患者接受 FUDR/DEX + BEV。中位随访期达 29 个月,有 93% 已死亡。总体 PR 为 48%,SD 为 50%,出现应答后,3 例患者接受切除手术。进展首先出现在肝内的占 55%,肝外的占 43%,同时出现的占 2%。单 FUDR 组,中位总生存期为 29 个月,联合用药组为 28 个月。有 10 例患者 3 年后仍然存活,5 年后有 5 例存活。这些生存期较长(>3 年)的患者中,相对生存期少于 3 年的患者,其肝脏特异性无进展生存期更长(13 个月 vs 9 个月)[83],说明肝内控制较好的患者可能有更长的总生存期。对于病灶不可切除的 PLC 患者,尤其是 ICC 患者,行肝动脉 FUDR/DEX 灌注化疗是安全的,可带来较长的生存时间。大多数有关 PLC,尤其是 HCC 的临床试验,主要在日本和亚洲其他国家进行,由于 HCC 在这些国家发病率很高,且病因学和北美地区有明显的差别,这些结论在非亚洲地区不具有普遍适用性。

八、肝动脉灌注化疗和非结直肠癌肝转移

很少有研究关注非结直肠癌肝转移的肝动脉灌注化疗。然而,已有几个将肝动脉灌注化疗应用于高度侵袭性恶性肿瘤的临床研究。目前对于眼黑色素瘤肝转移还没有有效的治疗方法,中位生存期不足 5 个月。有研究者建议,将肝动脉灌注化疗应用于此类疾病,并且已经有几项临床试验评估此方案的可行性。一项来自法国的单组前瞻性临床试验对行减瘤术后的眼黑色素瘤肝转移患者行福莫司汀灌注治疗。对于治疗的耐受性而言,有 2 例患者因肝脏毒性而停药,有 9 例患者在中位 10 个周期后,出现导管相关并发症而停止灌注。4 例(13%)患者完全应答,8 例(27%)部分应答。总体来讲,RR 为 40%,应答持续时间为 11 个月。中位总生存期在无应答患者中为 10 个月,而在应答患者中为 20 个月[84]。Melichar 等[85]也进行了一项回顾性研究,对 10 例已接受系统性化疗的眼黑色素瘤肝转移患者行多药肝动脉灌注化疗。有 2 例患者 PR,4 例患者 SD,4 例患者 PD。中位总生存期为 16 个月,所有 PD 的患者均在 1 年内死亡。由于眼黑色素瘤肝转移的病灶呈粟粒样分布,其他治疗方案在理论上效果不理想,因此肝动脉灌注化疗是较好的治疗方案。到目前为止,由于循证医学证据不足,这种方案尚没有大规模应用于临床。

最近,一项Ⅰ期临床试验选取了多种类型肝转移的恶性肿瘤患者,并评估应用顺铂灌注+系统性应用脂质体阿霉素治疗的疗效[86]。此项试验纳入了30例患者[11例乳腺癌患者,8例结直肠癌患者,4例眼黑色素瘤患者和7例其他的肿瘤患者(HCC/胃癌/胰腺癌/头颈肿瘤/神经内分泌肿瘤/皮肤黑色素瘤/平滑肌肉瘤)]。这项研究设计的初衷是为了评估安全性和毒性,并同时报道临床结果。在疾病控制方面,4例(17%)患者PR,7例(29%)SD。对于乳腺癌患者,3例(27%)PR,5例SD(45%)。中位总生存期为7.5个月。乳腺癌患者中位总生存期为8.5个月,而其他的癌症为5.3个月[86]。此治疗方案似乎是安全的,且能改善RR,但是仍需要更多的临床数据支持才能得出肯定结论。

九、总结

肝动脉灌注化疗是一种局部的抗肿瘤疗法,应用于临床的时间已有数十年,既可针对原发性肝恶性肿瘤,也可针对继发性肝恶性肿瘤。导管置入和通过输液泵持续泵入药物的技术已逐渐成熟。同时,导管相关并发症已可减少至最低限度。对于UR-CRLM患者和需要行辅助化疗的患者来说,肝动脉灌注化疗可降低RR,然而,还未发现总生存期获益。将肝动脉灌注化疗同新的抗肿瘤药物相结合,在使UR-CRLM转变为可切除结直肠癌方面,似乎有着很好的应用前景。然而,仍需注意显著的药物毒性反应。因此,需要进一步临床研究的支持。在北美地区,只有少数评估肝动脉灌注对于PLC疗效的临床试验。虽然试验数量较少,但肝动脉灌注疗法似乎是安全的,已有证据支持此疗法可改善RR和生存时间。为了能得出确定的结论,需要进行更大规模、更长时间随访,以及将新的抗肿瘤药物和靶向药物疗效对比的临床试验。已有少数临床试验评估了将肝动脉灌注疗法应用于不可切除结直肠癌的疗效。由于试验数量较少,且存在显著异质性,仍未得出确定结论。仍有学者担心,肝动脉灌注化疗会引发相关并发症,并怀疑总体的生存获益是否存在。因此,肝动脉灌注化疗治疗原发或继发性肝恶性肿瘤的临床应用仍存在争议。

参考文献

[1] Breedis C, Young G. The blood supply of neoplasms in the liver. Am J Pathol 1954;30(5):969-77.

[2] Sullivan RD, Norcross JW, Watkins E Jr. Chemotherapy of metastatic liver cancer by prolonged hepatic-artery infusion. N Engl J Med 1964;270:321-7.

[3] Cady B. Hepatic arterial patency and complications after catheterization for infusion chemotherapy. Ann Surg 1973;178(2):156-61.

[4] Ensminger WD, Gyves JW. Clinical pharmacology of hepatic arterial chemotherapy. Semin Oncol 1983;10(2):176-82.

[5] Ensminger WD. Regional chemotherapy. Semin Oncol 1993;20(1):3-11.

[6] Burrows JH, Talley RW, Drake EH, et al. Infusion of fluorinated pyrimidines into hepatic artery for treatment of metastatic carcinoma of liver. Cancer 1967;20(11):1886-92.

[7] Clarkson B, Young C, Dierick W, et al. Effects of continuous hepatic artery infusion of antimetabolites on

primary and metastatic cancer of the liver. Cancer 1962;15: 472 – 88.

[8] Ensminger WD, et al. A clinical – pharmacological evaluation of hepatic arterial infusions of 5 – fluoro – 20 – deoxyuridine and 5 – fluorouracil. Cancer Res 1978;38(11 Pt 1):3784 – 92.

[9] Ensminger WD, Rosowsky A, Raso V, et al. Hepatic arterial BCNU: a pilot clinicalpharmacologic study in patients with liver tumors. Cancer Treat Rep 1978;62(10): 1509 – 12.

[10] Kelsen DP, Hoffman J, Alcock N, et al. Pharmacokinetics of cisplatin regional hepatic infusions. Am J Clin Oncol 1982;5(2):173 – 8.

[11] Garnick MB, Ensminger WD, Israel M. A clinical – pharmacological evaluation of hepatic arterial infusion of adriamycin. Cancer Res 1979;39(10):4105 – 10.

[12] Kemeny N, Huang Y, Cohen AM, et al. Hepatic arterial infusion of chemotherapy after resection of hepatic metastases from colorectal cancer. N Engl J Med 1999; 341(27):2039 – 48.

[13] Kingham TP, D'Angelica M, Kemeny NE. Role of intra – arterial hepatic chemotherapy in the treatment of colorectal cancer metastases. J Surg Oncol 2010;102(8):988 – 95.

[14] Arru M, Aldrighetti L, Gremmo F, et al. Arterial devices for regional hepatic chemotherapy: transaxillary versus laparotomic access. J Vasc Access 2000;1(3):93 – 9.

[15] Urbach DR, Herron DM, Khajanchee YS, et al. Laparoscopic hepatic artery infusion pump placement. Arch Surg 2001;136(6):700 – 4.

[16] Franklin ME Jr, Gonzalez JJ Jr. Laparoscopic placement of hepatic artery catheter for regional chemotherapy infusion: technique, benefits, and complications. Surg Laparosc Endosc Percutan Tech 2002;12(6): 398 – 407.

[17] Franklin M, Trevino J, Hernandez – Oaknin H, et al. Laparoscopic hepatic artery catheterization for regional chemotherapy: is this the best current option for liver metastatic disease? Surg Endosc 2006;20(4): 554 – 8.

[18] Hellan M, Pigazzi A. Robotic – assisted placement of a hepatic artery infusion catheter for regional chemotherapy. Surg Endosc 2008;22(2):548 – 51.

[19] Blackshear PJ, Rohde TD, Dorman FD, et al. An implantable pump for long – term intravascular drug infusion. Med Instrum 1981;15(4):226 – 8.

[20] Buchwald H, Grage TB, Vassilopoulos PP, et al. Intraarterial infusion chemotherapy for hepatic carcinoma using a totally implantable infusion pump. Cancer 1980;45(5):866 – 9.

[21] Heinrich S, Petrowsky H, Schwinnen I, et al. Technical complications of continuous intra – arterial chemotherapy with 5 – fluorodeoxyuridine and 5 – fluorouracil for colorectal liver metastases. Surgery 2003;133(1):40 – 8.

[22] Fordy C, Burke D, Earlam S, et al. Treatment interruptions and complications with two continuous hepatic artery floxuridine infusion systems in colorectal liver metastases. Br J Cancer 1995;72(4):1023 – 5.

[23] Bacchetti S, Pasqual E, Crozzolo E, et al. Intra – arterial hepatic chemotherapy for unresectable colorectal liver metastases: a review of medical devices complications in 3172 patients. Med Devices (Auckl) 2009; 2:31 – 40.

[24] Portal vein chemotherapy for colorectal cancer: a meta – analysis of 4000 patients in 10 studies. Liver Infusion Meta – analysis Group. J Natl Cancer Inst 1997;89(7): 497 – 505.

[25] James RD, on behalf of the AXIS collaborators. Intraportal 5FU (PVI) and perioperative radiotherapy

(RT) in the adjuvant treatment of colorectal cancer (CRCa)—3681 patients randomised in the UK Coordinating Committee on Cancer Research (UKCCCR) AXIS trial. Proc Am Soc Clin Oncol 1999;18:1013 [abstract].

[26] Labianca R, Boffi L, Marsoni S, et al. A randomized trial of intraportal (IP) versus systemic (SY) versus IP 1 SY adjuvant chemotherapy in patients (pts) with resected Dukes B – C colon carcinoma (CC). Proc Am Soc Clin Oncol 1999;18: 1014 [abstract].

[27] Rougier P, Sahmoud T, Nitti D, et al. Adjuvant portal – vein infusion of fluorouracil and heparin in colorectal cancer: a randomised trial. European Organisation for Research and Treatment of Cancer Gastrointestinal Tract Cancer Cooperative Group, the Gruppo Interdisciplinare Valutazione Interventi in Oncologia, and the Japanese Foundation for Cancer Research. Lancet 1998;351(9117): 1677 – 81.

[28] Laffer U, Maibach R, Metzger U, et al. Randomized trial of adjuvant perioperative chemotherapy in radically resected colorectal cancer (SAKK 40/87). Proc Am Soc Clin Oncol 17:983, [abstract].

[29] Cohen AD, Kemeny NE. An update on hepatic arterial infusion chemotherapy for colorectal cancer. Oncologist 2003;8(6):553 – 66.

[30] Skitzki JJ, Chang AE. Hepatic artery chemotherapy for colorectal liver metastases: technical considerations and review of clinical trials. Surg Oncol 2002; 11(3):123 – 35.

[31] Kemeny MM. The surgical aspects of the totally implantable hepatic artery infusion pump. Arch Surg 2001;136(3):348 – 52.

[32] Saba L, Mallarini G. Multidetector row CT angiography in the evaluation of the hepatic artery and its anatomical variants. Clin Radiol 2008;63(3):312 – 21.

[33] Grobmyer SR, Fong Y, D'Angelica M, et al. Diagnostic laparoscopy prior to planned hepatic resection for colorectal metastases. Arch Surg 2004;139(12): 1326 – 30.

[34] Michels NA. Newer anatomy of the liver and its variant blood supply and collateral circulation. Am J Surg 1966;112(3):337 – 47.

[35] Kemeny MM, Hogan JM, Goldberg DA, et al. Continuous hepatic artery infusion with an implantable pump: problems with hepatic artery anomalies. Surgery 1986;99(4):501 – 4.

[36] Rayner AA, Kerlan RK, Stagg RJ, et al. Total hepatic arterial perfusion after occlusion of variant lobar vessels: implications for hepatic arterial chemotherapy. Surgery 1986;99(6):708 – 15.

[37] Allen PJ, Nissan A, Picon AI, et al. Technical complications and durability of hepatic artery infusion pumps for unresectable colorectal liver metastases: an institutional experience of 544 consecutive cases. J Am Coll Surg 2005;201(1):57 – 65.

[38] Curley SA, Chase JL, Roh MS, et al. Technical considerations and complications associated with the placement of 180 implantable hepatic arterial infusion devices. Surgery 1993;114(5):928 – 35.

[39] Kemeny N, Seiter K, Niedzwiecki D, et al. A randomized trial of intrahepatic infusion of fluorodeoxyuridine with dexamethasone versus fluorodeoxyuridine alone in the treatment of metastatic colorectal cancer. Cancer 1992;69(2):327 – 34.

[40] Patt YZ, Mavligit GM, Chuang VP, et al. Percutaneous hepatic arterial infusion (HAI) of mitomycin C and floxuridine (FUDR): an effective treatment for metastatic colorectal carcinoma in the liver. Cancer 1980;46(2):261 – 5.

[41] Kemeny N, Daly J, Oderman P, et al. Hepatic artery pump infusion: toxicity and results in patients with

metastatic colorectal carcinoma. J Clin Oncol 1984;2(6):595-600.

[42] Niederhuber JE, Ensminger W, Gyves J, et al. Regional chemotherapy of colorectal cancer metastatic to the liver. Cancer 1984;53(6):1336-43.

[43] Sofocleous CT, Schubert J, Kemeny N, et al. Arterial embolization for salvage of hepatic artery infusion pumps. J Vasc Interv Radiol 2006;17(5):801-6.

[44] Roybal JJ, Feliberti EC, Rouse L, et al. Pump removal in infected patients with hepatic chemotherapy pumps: when is it necessary? Am Surg 2006;72(10):880-4.

[45] Barnett KT, Malafa MP. Complications of hepatic artery infusion: a review of 4580 reported cases. Int J Gastrointest Cancer 2001;30(3):147-60.

[46] Ito K, Ito H, Kemeny NE, et al. Biliary sclerosis after hepatic arterial infusion pump chemotherapy for patients with colorectal cancer liver metastasis: incidence, clinical features, and risk factors. Ann Surg Oncol 2012;19(5):1609-17.

[47] Cercek A, D'Angelica M, Power D, et al. Floxuridine hepatic arterial infusion associated biliary toxicity is increased by concurrent administration of systemic bevacizumab. Ann Surg Oncol 2014;21(2):479-86.

[48] Lorenz M, Muller HH, Schramm H, et al. Randomized trial of surgery versus surgery followed by adjuvant hepatic arterial infusion with 5-fluorouracil and folinic acid for liver metastases of colorectal cancer. German Cooperative on Liver Metastases (Arbeitsgruppe Lebermetastasen). Ann Surg 1998;228(6):756-62.

[49] Rudroff C, Altendorf-Hoffmann A, Stangl R, et al. Prospective randomised trial on adjuvant hepatic-artery infusion chemotherapy after R0 resection of colorectal liver metastases. Langenbecks Arch Surg 1999;384(3):243-9.

[50] Kemeny NE, Gonen M. Hepatic arterial infusion after liver resection. N Engl J Med 2005;352(7):734-5.

[51] Kemeny MM, Adak S, Gray B, et al. Combined-modality treatment for resectable metastatic colorectal carcinoma to the liver: surgical resection of hepatic metastases in combination with continuous infusion of chemotherapy - an intergroup study. J Clin Oncol 2002;20(6):1499-505.

[52] Kemeny N, Jarnagin W, Gonen M, et al. Phase I/II study of hepatic arterial therapy with floxuridine and dexamethasone in combination with intravenous irinotecan as adjuvant treatment after resection of hepatic metastases from colorectal cancer. J Clin Oncol 2003;21(17):3303-9.

[53] Kemeny N, Capanu M, D'Angelica M, et al. Phase I trial of adjuvant hepatic arterial infusion (HAI) with floxuridine (FUDR) and dexamethasone plus systemic oxaliplatin, 5-fluorouracil and leucovorin in patients with resected liver metastases from colorectal cancer. Ann Oncol 2009;20(7):1236-41.

[54] Kemeny NE, Jarnagin WR, Capanu M, et al. Randomized phase II trial of adjuvant hepatic arterial infusion and systemic chemotherapy with or without bevacizumab in patients with resected hepatic metastases from colorectal cancer. J Clin Oncol 2011;29(7):884-9.

[55] Alberts SR, Roh MS, Mahoney MR, et al. Alternating systemic and hepatic artery infusion therapy for resected liver metastases from colorectal cancer: a North Central Cancer Treatment Group (NCCTG)/National Surgical Adjuvant Breast and Bowel Project (NSABP) phase II intergroup trial, N9945/CI-66. J Clin Oncol 2010;28(5):853-8.

[56] Tomlinson J, Jarnagin W, DeMatteo R, et al. Actual 10-year survival after resection of colorectal liver metastases. J Clin Oncol 2007;25:4575-82.

[57] Ito H, Are C, Gonen M, et al. Effect of postoperative morbidity on long-term survival after hepatic resection for metastatic colorectal cancer. Ann Surg 2008; 247(6):994-1002.

[58] House MG, Kemeny NE, Gonen M, et al. Comparison of adjuvant systemic chemotherapy with or without hepatic arterial infusional chemotherapy after hepatic resection for metastatic colorectal cancer. Ann Surg 2011;254(6):851-6.

[59] Goere D, Benhaim L, Bonnet S, et al. Adjuvant chemotherapy after resection of colorectal liver metastases in patients at high risk of hepatic recurrence: a comparative study between hepatic arterial infusion of oxaliplatin and modern systemic chemotherapy. Ann Surg 2013;257(1):114-20.

[60] Chang AE, Schneider PD, Sugarbaker PH, et al. A prospective randomized trial of regional versus systemic continuous 5-fluorodeoxyuridine chemotherapy in the treatment of colorectal liver metastases. Ann Surg 1987;206(6):685-93.

[61] Kemeny N, Daly J, Reichman B, et al. Intrahepatic or systemic infusion of fluorodeoxyuridine in patients with liver metastases from colorectal carcinoma. A randomized trial. Ann Intern Med 1987;107(4):459-65.

[62] Hohn DC, Stagg RJ, Friedman MA, et al. A randomized trial of continuous intravenous versus hepatic intraarterial floxuridine in patients with colorectal cancer metastatic to the liver: the Northern California Oncology Group trial. J Clin Oncol 1989;7(11):1646-54.

[63] Wagman LD, Kemeny MM, Leong L, et al. A prospective, randomized evaluation of the treatment of colorectal cancer metastatic to the liver. J Clin Oncol 1990; 8(11):1885-93.

[64] Martin JK Jr, O'Connell MJ, Wieand HS, et al. Intra-arterial floxuridine vs systemic fluorouracil for hepatic metastases from colorectal cancer. A randomized trial. Arch Surg 1990;125(8):1022-7.

[65] Rougier P, Laplanche A, Huguier M, et al. Hepatic arterial infusion of floxuridine in patients with liver metastases from colorectal carcinoma: long-term results of a prospective randomized trial. J Clin Oncol 1992;10(7):1112-8.

[66] Allen-Mersh TG, Earlam S, Fordy C, et al. Quality of life and survival with continuous hepatic-artery floxuridine infusion for colorectal liver metastases. Lancet 1994;344(8932):1255-60.

[67] Lorenz M, Muller HH. Randomized, multicenter trial of fluorouracil plus leucovorin administered either via hepatic arterial or intravenous infusion versus as adjuvant treatment after resection of hepatic metastases from colorectal cancer. J Clin Oncol 2003;21(17):3303-9.

[68] Kerr DJ, McArdle CS, Ledermann J, et al. Intrahepatic arterial versus intravenous fluorouracil and folinic acid for colorectal cancer liver metastases: a multicentre randomised trial. Lancet 2003;361(9355):368-73.

[69] Kemeny NE, Niedzwiecki D, Hollis DR, et al. Hepatic arterial infusion versus systemic therapy for hepatic metastases from colorectal cancer: a randomized trial of efficacy, quality of life, and molecular markers (CALGB 9481). J Clin Oncol 2006;24(9):1395-403.

[70] Reappraisal of hepatic arterial infusion in the treatment of nonresectable liver metastases from colorectal cancer. Meta-Analysis Group in Cancer. J Natl Cancer Inst 1996;88(5):252-8.

[71] Mocellin S, Pilati P, Lise M, et al. Meta-analysis of hepatic arterial infusion for unresectable liver me-

［72］ Kemeny N. The management of resectable and unresectable liver metastases from colorectal cancer. Curr Opin Oncol 2010;22(4):364-73.

［73］ Allen-Mersh TG, Glover C, Fordy C, et al. Randomized trial of regional plus systemic fluorinated pyrimidine compared with systemic fluorinated pyrimidine in treatment of colorectal liver metastases. Eur J Surg Oncol 2000;26(5):468-73.

［74］ Kemeny N, Gonen M, Sullivan D, et al. Phase I study of hepatic arterial infusion of floxuridine and dexamethasone with systemic irinotecan for unresectable hepatic metastases from colorectal cancer. J Clin Oncol 2001;19(10):2687-95.

［75］ Kemeny N, Jarnagin W, Paty P, et al. Phase I trial of systemic oxaliplatin combination chemotherapy with hepatic arterial infusion in patients with unresectable liver metastases from colorectal cancer. J Clin Oncol 2005;23(22):4888-96.

［76］ Boige V, Malka D, Elias D, et al. Hepatic arterial infusion of oxaliplatin and intravenous LV5FU2 in unresectable liver metastases from colorectal cancer after systemic chemotherapy failure. Ann Surg Oncol 2008;15(1):219-26.

［77］ Ducreux M, Ychou M, Laplanche A, et al. Hepatic arterial oxaliplatin infusion plus intravenous chemotherapy in colorectal cancer with inoperable hepatic metastases: a trial of the gastrointestinal group of the Federation Nationale des Centres de Lutte Contre le Cancer. J Clin Oncol 2005;23(22):4881-7.

［78］ Power DG, Kemeny NE. Chemotherapy for the conversion of unresectable colorectal cancer liver metastases to resection. Crit Rev Oncol Hematol 2011;79(3): 251-64.

［79］ Ammori JB, Kemeny NE, Fong Y, et al. Conversion to complete resection and/or ablation using hepatic artery infusional chemotherapy in patients with unresectable liver metastases from colorectal cancer: a decade of experience at a single institution. Ann Surg Oncol 2013;20(9):2901-7.

［80］ Goere D, Deshaies I, de Baere T, et al. Prolonged survival of initially unresectable hepatic colorectal cancer patients treated with hepatic arterial infusion of oxaliplatin followed by radical surgery of metastases. Ann Surg 2010;251(4): 686-91.

［81］ Jarnagin WR, Schwartz LH, Gultekin DH, et al. Regional chemotherapy for unresectable primary liver cancer: results of a phase II clinical trial and assessment of DCE-MRI as a biomarker of survival. Ann Oncol 2009;20(9):1589-95.

［82］ Kemeny NE, Schwartz L, Gonen M, et al. Treating primary liver cancer with hepatic arterial infusion of floxuridine and dexamethasone: does the addition of systemic bevacizumab improve results? Oncology 2011;80(3-4):153-9.

［83］ Konstantinidis IT, Do RK, Gultekin DH, et al. Regional chemotherapy for unresectable intrahepatic cholangiocarcinoma: a potential role for dynamic magnetic resonance imaging as an imaging biomarker and a survival update from two prospective clinical trials. Ann Surg Oncol 2014;21(8):2675-83.

［84］ Leyvraz S, Spataro V, Bauer J, et al. Treatment of ocular melanoma metastatic to the liver by hepatic arterial chemotherapy. J Clin Oncol 1997;15(7):2589-95.

［85］ Melichar B, Voboril Z, Lojik M, et al. Liver metastases from uveal melanoma: clinical experience of hepatic arterial infusion of cisplatin, vinblastine and dacarbazine. Hepatogastroenterology 2009;56(93): 1157-62.

[86] Tsimberidou AM, Moulder S, Fu S, et al. Phase I clinical trial of hepatic arterial infusion of cisplatin in combination with intravenous liposomal doxorubicin in patients with advanced cancer and dominant liver involvement. Cancer Chemother Pharmacol 2010;66(6):1087-93.

第八章 肝动脉化疗栓塞术治疗原发性肝癌及结直肠癌肝转移

John T. Miura, md[a], T. Clark Gamblin, MD, Ms[b,*]

【关键词】
- 肝脏;肝细胞癌;肝内胆管细胞癌
- 结直肠癌肝转移;肝动脉化疗栓塞术
- 药物洗脱微球肝动脉化疗栓塞术
- 局部治疗

> **要点**
> - 对于无法手术切除的肝恶性肿瘤或其他方式无法治疗的顽固性恶性肿瘤,肝动脉栓塞化疗是可行的治疗选择。
> - 与过去的经动脉治疗相比较,目前进行的 TACE 治疗具有更高的安全性和有效性。
> - 化疗栓塞可用于治疗肿瘤不可切除但肝功能正常的患者。最佳的化疗栓塞治疗方案仍需进一步的前瞻性研究。

一、简介

在过去的 20 年里,治疗原发性肝恶性肿瘤和转移性肝脏肿瘤的新方法不断出现。虽然手术切除是肝恶性肿瘤患者长期生存的最佳治疗方法,但是 70% 的患者在发现时已错过了根治性手术治疗的最佳时机。肝移植是另一个有效根治性治疗方法,但是可供移植器官的匮乏,限

声明:无。

[a] Division of Surgical Oncology, Medical College of Wisconsin, 9200 West Wisconsin Avenue, Milwaukee, WI 53226, USA; [b] Division of Surgical Oncology, Department of Surgery, Medical College of Wisconsin, 9200 West Wisconsin Avenue, Milwaukee, WI 53226, USA

* Corresponding author.
E-mail address: tcgamblin@mcw.edu

制了这种方式的使用。相反,大多数患者通常依靠姑息疗法,其目的同手术切除一样,是为了提高患者生活质量,延长生存期。由于肝脏独特的双血供特征,以肝动脉化疗栓塞为主的局部治疗已成为治疗肝脏恶性肿瘤的主要方法。正常肝实质血供主要由门静脉系统提供,而肝脏肿瘤则主要由肝动脉系统供血,此为肝动脉化疗栓塞术疗法的基本原理[1,2]。

在20世纪70年代末提出肝细胞癌(HCC)肝动脉化疗栓塞术治疗后,随其不断发展,已成为针对肝癌等恶性肿瘤,包括肝内胆管细胞癌(ICC)和结直肠癌肝转移(CRLM)不可或缺的治疗方法[3-5]。虽然有各种技术,如肝动脉栓塞术(transcatheter arterial embolization,TAE)、肝动脉化疗灌注术、钇-90放射性栓塞术及经肝动脉手术治疗的方法,但经肝动脉化学栓塞术(TACE)仍然是不可手术切除肝恶性肿瘤使用最广泛的局部治疗方式。在本章节中,我们根据目前的循证医学证据,对有关TACE和药物洗脱微球(DEB)TACE针对HCC、ICC和CRLM的治疗效果进行回顾和总结。

二、肝动脉化疗栓塞术的准则

TACE疗法的优点在于,其通过选择性破坏为肿瘤供血的动脉,输注高浓度的细胞毒性剂至富血肝肿瘤病灶,可减少对正常肝细胞的损害[6,7]。栓塞材料结合化疗药物有协同抗肿瘤的效果,肿瘤供血动脉栓塞后可出现肿瘤缺血性坏死,另一方面还可延长化疗药物的释放时间。此外,使用栓塞剂与化疗药物结合有利于降低全身药物水平,从而降低毒性。

1. 患者选择

经肝动脉治疗肝恶性肿瘤的适应证在不断扩大。TACE患者评估通常包括肝功能、门脉高压、肝动脉解剖、肿瘤的大小和分布,以及合并症和身体功能状况。相对禁忌证如门静脉癌栓形成的情况下,局部TACE治疗可通过侧支血管入肝进行[8,9]。目前对于肝癌治疗,巨块型或多结节肿瘤不合并血管侵犯,无肝外病灶,非失代偿性肝病(Child-Pugh A/B级),以及良好体力活动状态[东部肿瘤协作组(ECOG)性能状态]的患者,肝病研究协会(AASLD)推荐TACE作为一线非根治性治疗方法[10]。虽无正式的指南说明,但TACE禁忌证一般包括:年龄大于70~80岁,胆红素水平大于3mg/dl,肿瘤大于10cm,胆管阻塞以及肿瘤体积超过肝脏的50%[11-14]。技术禁忌证包括无法治愈的动静脉瘘[11]。TACE治疗其他无法切除的肝恶性肿瘤的适应证与肝细胞癌类似。另外,TACE也用于其他临床治疗方案的辅助治疗。TACE可作为术前辅助治疗,如在手术切除/肝移植前,降低肿瘤分期,还可补救治疗耐药肿瘤肝动脉化疗栓塞[15]。

TACE目前仍然是最广泛进行的经肝动脉治疗方法。一般在适度镇静下进行。该过程通过导管注射化疗药物和栓塞材料混合剂至肝脏肿瘤的动脉供血血管(图8-1)。目前,已有多种细胞毒性剂用于TACE治疗。然而,阿霉素、顺铂、表柔比星、米托蒽醌、丝裂霉素和苯乙烯马来酸新制癌菌素(SMANCS)仍然是最常见的TACE单药化疗药物[16]。三联用药(顺铂、阿霉素和丝裂霉素)栓塞疗法亦有报道[17]。

细胞毒性药物是在碘化油(一种油性造影剂)的辅助下,作为载体携带药物进入局部肿瘤病灶内[18]。此过程通常伴随着肿瘤血管的物理栓塞,栓塞剂为球形或非球形。明胶海绵颗粒为最常用的栓塞剂。用于栓塞肿瘤动脉的其他材料包括聚乙烯醇(PVA)、淀粉微球或弹簧圈[16]。通常血管栓塞成功的定义为,二级或三级肝动脉分支肿瘤供血动脉的造影剂淤滞[19]。

2. 药物洗脱微球-肝动脉化疗栓塞(DEB-TACE)

DEB-TACE 是一种类似于常规 TACE 疗法的替代技术,药物洗脱微球是一种高吸收性聚乙烯醇微球,当与细胞毒性药物混合后,细胞毒性化合物与微球以磺酸酯键聚合。栓塞后,DEB 以受控的方式将细胞毒性剂在几天内缓慢释放。DEB 中最常用的细胞毒性剂包括阿霉素、奥沙利铂、伊立替康。研究报道[20],与传统 TACE 相比较,DEB-TACE 具有更有利于治疗的药代动力学,并可降低全身毒性。

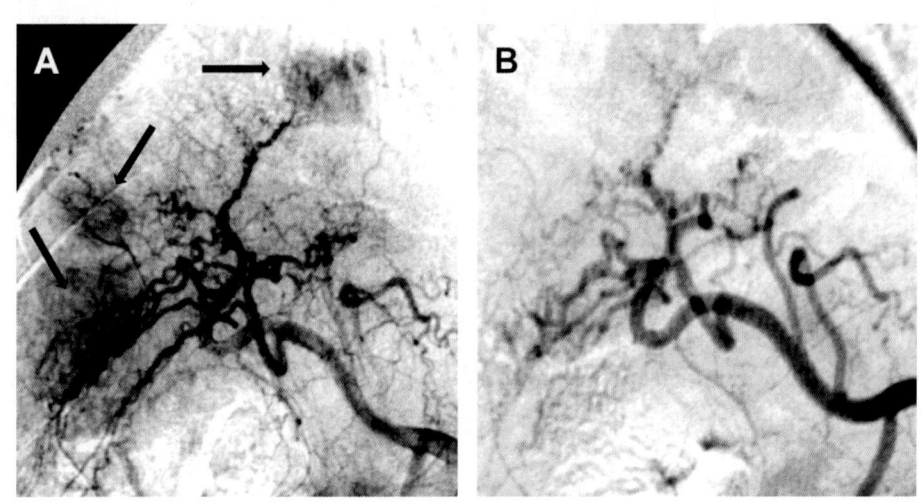

图 8-1 肝动脉化疗栓塞

A. 选择性动脉造影显示,肝动脉分支有 3 处富血管肿瘤结节(箭头);B. 阿霉素碘油乳剂和明胶海绵栓塞递送后,造影完成显示肿瘤血管不存在。(Courtesy of D. Geller, MD, Pittsburgh, PA.)

3. 对治疗的应答评估

虽然评价肿瘤治疗与发展的主要指标是总生存期,但疾病进展时间和肿瘤应答率仍然是治疗效果的重要评估指标[21]。世界卫生组织规范实体瘤疗效评价标准(RECIST)的初衷是为了评估化疗药物对肿瘤的作用情况[22,23]。随后临床上亦采用此评价标准来评估局部治疗的效果。然而由于该标准无法评估超过解剖大小的肿瘤存活情况,对疗效评估产生了一定的误导[24]。2008 年,世界卫生组织修订了 RECIST 准则,称为 RECIST 修订准则(mRECIST),把在对比增强影像学检查时肿瘤动脉增强情况作为附加准则,来评估肿瘤对治疗的应答程度[25]。

根据 EASL 和 EORTC 近期发布的研究指南,治疗应答评估应基于对比增强影像学检查的 mRECIST 标准(图 8-2)[26]。此外,建议治疗后的初次影像学评估在首次治疗 4 周后进行。TACE 和 DEB-TACE 直接造成的肿瘤坏死可由 mRECIST 标准准确表现出来,最近的研究也已证实其与生存结果的相关性[27,28]。

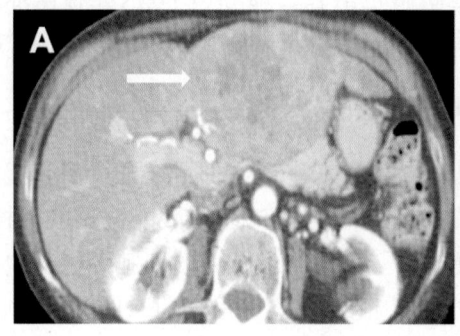
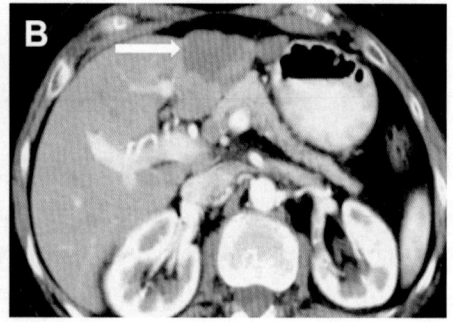

图 8-2　HCC 患者经 TACE 治疗，mRECIST 完全应答
A. 预处理对比增强计算机断层扫描(CT)显示,富血管肿瘤累及段 Ll/LLL(箭头);B. TACE 3 个月后,CT 扫描显示肿瘤不再增强而体积减小(箭头)。(Courtesy of D. Geller, MD, Pittsburgh, PA.)

4. 毒副作用/并发症

TACE 和 DEB-TACE 治疗相关并发症的总发生率和严重程度存在极大波动。其中以栓塞术后综合征最为常见(发生率 60%~80%),包括急性腹痛、恶心、发热、疲劳、转氨酶升高。然而,它不是一种并发症,而是一种治疗预期内的副作用[29]。而发生严重并发症的患者达 10%,TACE 术后 30 天死亡率为 2%~4%[8,30,31]。肝脓肿和胆汁性肝硬化是最常见的主要并发症[32,33]。其他并发症包括肝功能衰竭、胆汁瘤、缺血性胆囊炎、胃肠出血/溃疡、血管损伤、肺栓塞,但这些并不常见(发生率<1%)[31,34]。

虽然 DEB-TACE 和 TACE 毒性特征相似,但有关 DEB-TACE 药物的不良事件报道较少[35-37]。最近,一系列由 Malagari 等[36]进行的研究,对用阿霉素 DEB-TACE(DEBDOX)治疗的 237 例病例相关并发症进行了评价。根据 NCICTC 对不良事件的标准,4 级和 5 级并发症发生率分别为 5.48%和 1.26%。此外,无围术期死亡,而 30 天死亡率仅为 1.26%。尽管是一个新的、不断发展的技术,但 DEB-TACE 在安全性方面表现优秀。

三、肝细胞癌

肝细胞癌是全球范围内致死率排名第三的恶性肿瘤。肝细胞癌是一种复杂的疾病,一直给医学界带来巨大挑战[10,38]。有关肝癌发生发展原因的研究已经非常成熟(乙肝病毒,饮酒,代谢紊乱包括非酒精性脂肪肝等),但仍难以通过有效的监控手段在肝癌发生的早期及时发现[39]。因此,根治性治疗(如手术切除、肝移植、局部消融治疗)只能用于早期肝癌患者,而只有小部分初诊为肝细胞癌的患者可行根治性治疗,超过 70% 患者在发现肝癌时已经发展为中晚期肝癌[巴塞罗那临床肝癌分期(BCLC)B/C 期],缩小了可以接受有效治疗患者的选择范围[40]。

1. 肝癌的 TACE 治疗

TACE 治疗是中期肝癌(BCLC - B 期):多结节病灶、无血管侵犯或肝外转移灶的标准治疗[10,26]。然而,最初的研究将 TACE 的作用与保守治疗对比评估,得出一个模棱两可的结果(表 8-1)[41-43]。直到 2002 年,两个开创性的随机对照试验(RCT)结果发布,显示经 TACE 治疗的肝癌患者总生存期显著提高。Llovet 等[44]在研究中,将 112 例不可手术切除的肝细胞癌和肝硬化患者(Child - Pugh 分级 A／B 类)随机分配到接受阿霉素为主的 TACE 治疗组或保守的姑息治疗(症状管理)组。研究报告指出,接受 TACE 治疗的患者 1 年和 2 年生存率(分别为 82% 和 63%)与保守治疗组(63% 和 27%,$P = 0.009$)相比,有显著提高。此外,在多变量模型分析中,治疗方法与生存有关(95% CI,0.25~0.81,$P = 0.02$,OR 0.45)。同样,Lo 等[45]报道,在不可手术切除的肝细胞癌患者中,与对症治疗相比,使用顺铂为基础的 TACE 治疗提高了患者生存率。共有 40 例患者接受 TACE 治疗,其 1 年和 2 年生存率(分别为 57% 和 31%)与对照组(32% 和 11%,$P = 0.002$)相比,有显著提高。虽然两个研究均显示 TACE 治疗可带来生存获益,但与 Lo 等的试验相比,Llovet 等的试验显示出更大生存获益,这是因为后者在选取患者时更加严格。Llovet 等人招募的大多数患者有代偿性肝病(70% Child - Pugh 分级 A 级),具有良好的体力活动状态(80% ECOG 体力活动状态 0),这可能是对照组患者 2 年生存率为 27% 的原因。与此相反,Lo 等人以更宽松的入选标准纳入了晚期患者(57% 为 ECOG

表 8-1 不可切除肝细胞癌患者接受 TACE 或 DEB - TACE 治疗试验生存总结

作者,时间	患者数量	研究设计	治疗方案	中位生存期(月)	总生存率		
					1 年(%)	2 年(%)	3 年(%)
TACE							
Pelletier 等[41],1990	42	RCT	Doxorubicin	NR	24	NR	NR
Trinchet 等[42],1995	96	RCT	Cisplatin	NR	62	37.8	NR
Llovet 等[44],2002	112	RCT	Doxorubicin	28.7[a]	82	63	29
Lo 等[45],2002	80	RCT	Cisplatin	NR	57	31	26
Brown 等[46],2008	209	RC	Cisplatin, Doxorubicin, mitomycin C	15.5	NR	NR	NR
Georgiades 等[17],2006	172	PC	Cisplatin, doxorubicin, mitomycin C	18.3	NR	NR	NR
Sahara 等[51],2012	51	RCT	Epirubicin vs ECMF	21 19	85 95	76 65	NR
DEB - TACE							
Burrel 等[55],2012	104	RC	Doxorubicin	48.6	89.9	66.3	54.2
Malagari 等[56],2013	45	RC	Doxorubicin	NR	NR	NR	62.2[b]

缩写:5 - FU,5 - 氟尿嘧啶;ECMF,表柔比星;Cisplatin,丝裂霉素 C;NR,未报道;PC,前瞻性队列研究;RC,回顾性队列研究;RCT,随机对照试验;[a]平均总生存率;[b] 5 年总生存率

评分1/2/3,27%出现门静脉受累)。尽管两项研究结果存在变量上的差异,但是这些试验第一次证明了TACE可带来潜在生存获益,这对治疗不可手术切除的肝细胞癌患者具有重要意义。

多项前瞻性和回顾性临床试验[17,46]肯定了TACE在肝癌治疗中的作用。最近,在一个大型回顾性分析研究中,Brown等[46]总结其超过15年的TACE治疗结果。研究中的209例患者中位总生存期为15.5个月。另外,两项meta分析也已证实TACE的疗效[2]。2003年,一项研究评估了14个将TACE/TAE治疗与最佳支持治疗或他莫昔芬(对照组)治疗[14]作对比的随机临床试验。相比对照组,TACE/TAE 2年生存率显著改善(41% vs 27%;$P=0.17$)。此外,TACE与最佳支持治疗的敏感性分析也显示,TACE可带来明显生存获益(OR 0.42;95% CI 0.20~0.88)。另一项由Mrelli等[16]进行的meta分析也显示,相比非手术治疗,TACE/TAE可明显降低死亡率(OR 0.705;95% CI 0.499~0.994;$P=0.0026$)。这些研究结果证明,TACE已成为中期肝癌患者(BCLC-B)的标准治疗方法。

尽管已为TACE治疗肝细胞癌建立了化疗方案,但是何为最优化疗方案仍无定论,无论阿霉素和表柔比星还是顺铂,多项研究均未显示出显著生存差异[48-50]。最近一项随机对照试验[51]对63例患者表柔比星与多剂化疗药物(表柔比星,顺铂,丝裂霉素C和5-氟尿嘧啶)治疗结果进行对比。结果显示,两种方案间的生存获益差异无法确定。相比之下,一项回顾性研究评估了肝细胞癌患者使用阿霉素或顺铂/阿霉素/丝裂霉素C(CDM)的疗效,结果显示,CDM-TACE组具有较高的肿瘤应答率和较长无疾病进展生存时间[52]。化疗药物相关结果的多变性导致TACE缺乏统一的细胞毒性最佳治疗方案。

2. DEB-TACE

与传统的TACE相比,DEB-TACE是化疗栓塞术中一项新兴创新技术。早期临床试验证明,DEB-TACE具有良好的药代动力学特性以及较低的药物峰值血浆释放浓度,可降低与治疗相关的毒副作用[20,53]。随后的Ⅱ期随机临床对照研究,PRECISION V,比较了阿霉素DEB-TACE疗效与常规TACE的安全性及有效性[54]。虽然这项研究未能显示两者间总生存期和客观应答率的差异,但是在Child-Pugh B,ECOG 1双叶肿瘤患者分组分析中,DEB-TACE治疗组的客观应答率较TACE显著提高($P=0.038$)。另外,DEB-TACE相对于常规TACE治疗,患者严重肝毒性显著降低,从而提高其耐受性($P<0.001$)。

多项回顾性研究肯定了DEB-TACE在肝细胞癌治疗中的作用。2012年,Burrel等[55]评估不可手术切除的中期肝癌患者(BCLC-A/B)采取DEB-TACE治疗的生存期。实验最终纳入104例患者,其中位生存期为48.6个月,5年总生存率为38.3%。Malagari等[56]进行了回顾性研究,患者5年总生存率62.2%。生存获益的改善、相关毒性的降低表明,与常规TACE肝细胞癌治疗相比,DEB-TACE可能是一种更优的选择。

3. **联合治疗策略**

所有的TACE治疗方案面临的共同挑战是治疗持续时间。肿瘤的高复发率及疾病进展仍然是限制TACE总体疗效的主要因素[44,45]。2002年,由Llovet等进行的随机对照试验显示,行 TACE 治疗后,只有 35% 的患者在 6 个月后仍存在持续应答。肿瘤高复发的一个潜在原因是 TACE 治疗后肿瘤微环境紊乱。研究已证实,在 TACE 术后引发的栓塞缺氧使诱导因子 1α 上调,继而增加了血管内皮生长因子(VEGF)和血小板衍生生长因子受体的表达,导致肿瘤血管再生[57,58]。鉴于此,TACE 联合抗血管生成靶向剂的治疗策略,有望提升总生存期。

索拉非尼是一种多激酶抑制剂,通过靶向作用于 VEGF-2 受体,抑制血管生成,研究已证实,与安慰剂治疗晚期肝细胞癌相比,其可提高总生存期(10.7 个月)[59]。2011 年,第一批 II 期试验结果发表[60],其目的是评估 DEB-TACE 联合索拉非尼治疗晚期肝癌的安全性和有效性。虽然大多数患者在试验观察中至少出现了 1 级 3~4 种毒性反应,但是毒性反应大都较轻(1~2 级 83% vs 3~4 级 17%)。此外,初步的效率试验数据显示,按照 RECIST 标准,疾病控制率可达 95%。但关于 TACE 与索拉非尼联合治疗的多中心回顾性 II、III 期临床试验已进行,其结论并不一致[61-64]。一份 meta 分析共纳入了 17 项研究结果,旨在评估 TACE 联合索拉非尼治疗的安全性和有效性,其中只有 3 项为随机对照试验[65]。研究者报告指出,与单 TACE 相比,TACE 联合索拉非尼治疗组的疾病进展时间明显改善[风险比(HR) 0.76;$P < 0.001$;95% CI 0.66~0.89],但是总生存率并未改善(HR 0.81;95% CI 0.65~1.01;$P = 0.061$)。在这些试验中,两种治疗方案和纳入标准均存在多变性,这降低了研究对联合治疗方案生存获益的评估能力。尽管关于索拉非尼联合 TACE 治疗目前文献报道的结果模棱两可,但是设计更加严格的 III 期临床研究已在进行,希望能得出更有说服力的结果[66]。

4. 扩大治疗适应证/未来的发展方向

根据 AASLD 指南,肝细胞癌合并门静脉癌栓是 TACE 手术禁忌证。然而,近年来治疗适应证的扩大,促使研究开始评估门静脉癌栓条件下的 TACE 治疗[9,67]。由 Georgiades 等[9]设计的前瞻性研究纳入 32 例不可切除的肝细胞癌合并门静脉癌栓患者,依次进行肝动脉化疗栓塞治疗。报告结果显示,其安全性以及生存结果优于以往行最佳支持护理的对照组。研究人员得出结论,在适当选择患者的前提下,门静脉癌栓不应该作为 TACE 的绝对禁忌证。

虽然切除和移植是肝细胞癌患者获得长期生存的最好治疗方案,但是 TACE 可作为其辅助治疗联合使用。一项由 Luo 等[68]开展的前瞻性研究评价了 TACE 作为辅助治疗应用于切除术前的疗效。共有 168 例大肿瘤(>5 cm)或多结节可切除肝细胞癌患者,随机分到单手术切除或联合治疗组。联合治疗组的 1 年、3 年、5 年总生存率分别为 92%、67% 和 50%,明显高于单手术切除组,说明联合治疗大肿瘤或多结节可切除肝细胞癌更加有效。

此外,TACE 可降低癌症分期,使患者能够进行肝脏移植[69]。2008 年,一系列病例显示,研究中 23.7% 的患者采用 TACE 治疗后符合可进行肝移植的米兰标准[70]。平均随访 19.6 个月后,94.1% 的患者成功接受肝移植并存活。研究报道,移植成功的患者可达到与美国癌症联合委员会 II 期患者类似的生存结果。

四、肝内胆管癌

肝内胆管癌是发病率排名第二的原发性肝脏恶性肿瘤,仅次于肝细胞癌。其较罕见,但进展迅速,总体预后不良(未经治疗的患者中位总生存期 3~8 个月)[71]。手术切除是最好的治疗手段。然而,与肝细胞癌相似,大多数(50%~70%)患者在初诊时已为晚期,从而错过了手术切除的时机[72]。姑息治疗包括系统性化疗和外部放射治疗,但是作用有限[73,74]。近年来,由于其良好的安全性和有效性[75],TACE 成为 ICC 的一个新治疗模式,但大部分文献主要集中在肝细胞癌,只有少数是针对 ICC(表 8-2)。

1. 肝内胆管细胞癌的 TACE 治疗

2005 年,Burger 等[76]报道了不可切除的 ICC 患者进行 TACE 治疗的安全性和有效性。这项研究中的 17 例患者都接受了 TACE 治疗,包括顺铂、阿霉素和丝裂霉素-C。与既往接受最佳支持治疗的对照组相比,TACE 治疗的患者获得 23 个月的中位生存期。治疗过程中大部分人群耐受良好,肝功能情况和体力活动状态分别保持在 88% 和 82%。

2012 年,Vogl 等[77]开展了目前评估 TACE 治疗 ICC 规模最大的队列研究。这项研究的主要目的是比较 4 种方案的有效性:①丝裂霉素 C;②吉西他滨;③吉西他滨联合丝裂霉素 C;④丝裂霉素 C、吉西他滨与顺铂。从 TACE 治疗开始,115 例患者的平均生存期是 13 个月。研究报道,治疗组之间平均生存期无显著统计学差异。目前的研究已经证实,TACE 可有效治疗不可手术切除的 ICC。

表 8-2 不可切除肝内胆管癌行 TACE 或 DEB-TACE 治疗试验生存总结

作者,时间	患者数量	研究设计	治疗方案	中位生存期(月)	总生存率 1年(%)	2年(%)	3年(%)
TACE							
Burger 等[76], 2005	17	PC	Cis, doxorubicin, mito	23	NR	NR	NR
Gusani 等[92], 2008	42	PC	Gem, cis, ox, or gem/cis combo	9.1	NR	NR	NR
Kiefer 等[93], 2011	62	PC	Cis, doxorubicin, mito	15	61	27	8
Park 等[94], 2011	72	RC	Cis	12.2	51	12	NR
Vogl 等[77], 2012	115	RC	Mito or gem or mito-cis or gem-cis	13	52	29	10
DEB-TACE							
Aliberti 等[78], 2008	11	RC	Doxorubicin	13	NR	NR	NR
Poggi 等[95], 2009	9	RC	Ox DEB-TACE + systemic gem-ox	30	NR	NR	NR
Kuhlman 等[79], 2012	36	PC	Irinotecan DEB-TACE vs Mito TACE	11.7 5.7	NR	NR	NR

cis:顺铂;gem:吉西他滨;mito:丝裂霉素 C;NR:未报道;OX:奥沙利铂;PC:前瞻性队列研究;RC:回顾性队列研究

2. DEB-TACE 治疗 ICC

2008年,Aliberti 等[78]首先对 DEB-TACE 治疗 ICC 进行报道。在这项研究中,11例不可切除的 ICC 患者用阿霉素 DEB-TACE 治疗,RECIST 标准的应答率为100%,获得了13个月的中位生存期。DEB-TACE 治疗过程中,患者的耐受性良好,无严重并发症发生。

然而,与 TACE 比较研究结果仍未有定论。最近,Khulman 等[79]一项前瞻性单中心研究评估了丝裂霉素 C-TACE 和伊立替康 DEB-TACE 的疗效,并将其与既往吉西他滨和奥沙利铂系统性化疗进行对比。DEB-TACE 组中位总生存期是11.7个月,TACE 组为5.7个月,全身化疗组为11.7个月。尽管研究得出的结论显示 DEB-TACE 疗效与全身化疗相当,但是肿瘤的异质性特征也会导致生存期差异。关于 TACE 及 DEB-TACE 治疗 ICC 的研究仍在进行中,但目前的证据表明,与最佳支持治疗相比,前两种治疗能带来更多生存获益。仍需进一步研究评估这些新技术的有效性。

五、结直肠癌肝转移

肝脏是结直肠癌最常转移的部位。目前的证据表明,尽管有转移性病灶,大约50%的孤立结直肠癌(CRLM)患者手术切除后可获得5年生存期[80]。然而,只有25%的患者可进行手术切除,TACE/DEB-TACE 为无法进行手术切除的患者提供选择[81]。

1. TACE 治疗 CRLM

TACE 治疗 CRLM 首先在20世纪90年代初报道,结果喜人[82,83]。然而,多项后续研究的结果却模棱两可(表8-3)。最近,专家达成共识,认为由于各研究之间缺乏标准化治疗方案[84],现有证据对 TACE 治疗 CRLM 的疗效评估仍然有限。

2009年由 Vogl 等[85]进行的研究是目前规模最大的队列研究。此研究为Ⅰ/Ⅱ期试验,研究了包括丝裂霉素 C、丝裂霉素 C+吉西他滨、丝裂霉素 C+伊立替康在内的不同药物组合TACE 治疗不可切除 CRLM 的疗效。共有463例不可手术切除的 CRLM 患者进行了4周为1个疗程的 TACE 序贯治疗,见表8-3。62.9%的患者实现了局部肿瘤控制(PR:14.7%,SD:48.2%),1年和2年生存率分别为62%和28%,肝转移诊断后,平均生存期为38个月。另外一项回顾性研究纳入121例患者,用顺铂、阿霉素、丝裂霉素 CTACE 治疗,其1年和2年生存率分别为85%和55%[86]。而据报道,使用全身化疗方案的 FOLFOX(5-氟尿嘧啶、甲酰四氢叶酸和奥沙利铂)或 FOLFIRI(叶酸、氟尿嘧啶和伊立替康)1年和2年生存率分别为55%和33%,这显示,TACE 在 CRLM 治疗上具有极大的潜在治疗效果[87-89]。

表8-3 不可切除结直肠癌肝转移行TACE或DEB-TACE治疗试验生存总结

作者,时间	患者数量	研究设计	治疗方案	中位生存期(月)	总生存率 1年(%)	2年(%)	3年(%)
TACE							
Lang and Brown[82], 1993	46	PC	Doxorubicin	NR	65	22	15
Sanz-Altamira 等[96], 1997	40	PC	5-Fluorouracil, mitomycin C	10	NR	NR	NR
Tellez 等[97], 1998	30	PC	Cisplatin, doxorubicin, mitomycin C	8.6	20	NR	NR
Hong 等[98], 2009	21	RC	Cisplatin, doxorubicin, mitomycin C	7.7	43	10	NR
Vogl 等[85], 2009	463	PC	Mitomycin C; mitomycin C + gemcitabine; mitomycin C + irinotecan	14	62	28	NR
Albert 等[86], 2011	121	RC	Cisplatin, doxorubicin, mitomycin C	9	36	13	4
DEB-TACE							
Bower 等[99], 2010	55	PC	Irinotecan	12	NR	NR	NR
Martin 等[90], 2011	55	PC	Irinotecan	19	75	NR	NR
Fiorentini 等[91], 2012	36	RCT	Irinotecan	22	NR	NR	NR
Narayanan 等[100], 2013	28	RC	Irinotecan	13.3	NR	NR	NR

缩略词：NR，未报道；PC，前瞻性队列研究；RC，回顾性队列研究. ª来自首次TACE治疗

2. DEB-TACE 治疗 CRLM

类似于其他恶性肿瘤,DEB-TACE治疗CRLM的作用较小,但在不断发展。若干Ⅱ期临床试验报道,在DEB-TACE治疗后,安全性较高且获得了较高的肿瘤应答率。最近,一项前瞻性研究[90]纳入了55例全身化疗失败的CRLM患者,继续接受伊立替康-DEB-TACE治疗,肿瘤应答率达到75%。中位生存期为19个月,1年生存率为75%。并发症发生率为28%,但是大部分较轻。由此可见,DEB-TACE具有明显优势。

唯一一项Ⅲ期随机对照试验[91]纳入74例不可手术切除的CRLM患者,随机分配接受伊立替康DEB-TACE与系统性FOLFIRI全身化疗。DEB-TACE组的总生存期(22个月)较FOLFIRI全身化疗组(15个月,$P=0.031$)显著提升。DEB-TACE肿瘤应答率为68.6%,而FOLFIRI只有20%。相对FOLFIRI组,DEB-TACE组可保证较长时间的生活质量(3 vs 8个月,$P<0.001$)。虽然仍然需要进一步的前瞻性研究来评估其疗效,但现有证据已表明,在治疗不可切除CRLM患者方面,DEB-TACE可替代标准化疗,且确实有效。

六、总结

在治疗不可切除肝恶性肿瘤方面,TACE仍然是应用最广泛的经肝动脉局部治疗手段。

随着医疗科技的进步,TACE 也进一步提高了其安全性和有效性,扩大了适应证范围。虽然最初只是一种姑息性治疗,但 TACE 现已被证明是一种可行的治疗选择。TACE 的主要缺陷依然是治疗反应持久性。因此,需要进一步的前瞻性研究来评估不同方案 TACE 及联合治疗策略,从而提高患者的生存率和生活质量。

参考文献

[1] Breedis C, Young G. The blood supply of neoplasms in the liver. Am J Pathol 1954;30(5):969-77.

[2] Lucke B, Breedis C, Woo ZP, et al. Differential growth of metastatic tumors in liver and lung: experiments with rabbit V2 carcinoma. Cancer Res 1952;12(10):734-8.

[3] Tadavarthy SM, Knight L, Ovitt TW, et al. Therapeutic transcatheter arterial embolization. Radiology 1974;112(1):13-6.

[4] Yamada R, Nakatsuka H, Nakamura K, et al. Hepatic artery embolization in 32 patients with unresectable hepatoma. Osaka City Med J 1980;26(2):81-96.

[5] Wheeler PG, Melia W, Dubbins P, et al. Non-operative arterial embolisation in primary liver tumours. Br Med J 1979;2(6184):242-4.

[6] Bruix J, Sala M, Llovet JM. Chemoembolization for hepatocellular carcinoma. Gastroenterology 2004;127(5 Suppl 1):S179-88.

[7] Vogl TJ, Naguib NN, Nour-Eldin NE, et al. Review on transarterial chemoembolization in hepatocellular carcinoma: palliative, combined, neoadjuvant, bridging, and symptomatic indications. Eur J Radiol 2009;72(3):505-16.

[8] Brown DB, Nikolic B, Covey AM, et al. Quality improvement guidelines for transhepatic arterial chemoembolization, embolization, and chemotherapeutic infusion for hepatic malignancy. J Vasc Interv Radiol 2012;23(3):287-94.

[9] Georgiades CS, Hong K, D'Angelo M, et al. Safety and efficacy of transarterial chemoembolization in patients with unresectable hepatocellular carcinoma and portal vein thrombosis. J Vasc Interv Radiol 2005;16(12):1653-9.

[10] Bruix J, Sherman M, American Association for the Study of Liver Diseases. Management of hepatocellular carcinoma: an update. Hepatology 2011;53(3):1020-2.

[11] Raoul JL, Sangro B, Forner A, et al. Evolving strategies for the management of intermediate-stage hepatocellular carcinoma: available evidence and expert opinion on the use of transarterial chemoembolization. Cancer Treat Rev 2011;37(3):212-20.

[12] Befeler AS. Chemoembolization and bland embolization: a critical appraisal. Clin Liver Dis 2005;9(2):287-300, vii.

[13] Kettenbach J, Stadler A, Katzler IV, et al. Drug-loaded microspheres for the treatment of liver cancer: review of current results. Cardiovasc Intervent Radiol 2008;31(3):468-76.

[14] Lau WY, Yu SC, Lai EC, et al. Transarterial chemoembolization for hepatocellular carcinoma. J Am Coll Surg 2006;202(1):155-68.

[15] Xing M, Kooby DA, El-Rayes BF, et al. Locoregional therapies for metastatic colorectal carcinoma to the liver-an evidence-based review. J Surg Oncol 2014;110(2):182-96.

[16] Marelli L, Stigliano R, Triantos C, et al. Transarterial therapy for hepatocellular carcinoma: which technique is more effective? A systematic review of cohort and randomized studies. Cardiovasc Intervent Radiol 2007;30(1):6-25.

[17] Georgiades CS, Liapi E, Frangakis C, et al. Prognostic accuracy of 12 liver staging systems in patients with unresectable hepatocellular carcinoma treated with transarterial chemoembolization. J Vasc Interv Radiol 2006;17(10):1619-24.

[18] Nakakuma K, Tashiro S, Hiraoka T, et al. Studies on anticancer treatment with an oily anticancer drug injected into the ligated feeding hepatic artery for liver cancer. Cancer 1983;52(12):2193-200.

[19] Lencioni R, Petruzzi P, Crocetti L. Chemoembolization of hepatocellular carcinoma. Semin Intervent Radiol 2013;30(1):3-11.

[20] Varela M, Real MI, Burrel M, et al. Chemoembolization of hepatocellular carcinoma with drug eluting beads: efficacy and doxorubicin pharmacokinetics. J Hepatol 2007;46(3):474-81.

[21] Lencioni R, Llovet JM. Modified RECIST (mRECIST) assessment for hepatocellular carcinoma. Semin Liver Dis 2010;30(1):52-60.

[22] Miller AB, Hoogstraten B, Staquet M, et al. Reporting results of cancer treatment. Cancer 1981;47(1):207-14.

[23] Therasse P, Arbuck SG, Eisenhauer EA, et al. New guidelines to evaluate the response to treatment in solid tumors. European Organization for Research and Treatment of Cancer, National Cancer Institute of the United States, National Cancer Institute of Canada. J Natl Cancer Inst 2000;92(3):205-16.

[24] Forner A, Ayuso C, Varela M, et al. Evaluation of tumor response after locoregional therapies in hepatocellular carcinoma: are response evaluation criteria in solid tumors reliable? Cancer 2009;115(3):616-23.

[25] Llovet JM, Di Bisceglie AM, Bruix J, et al. Design and endpoints of clinical trials in hepatocellular carcinoma. J Natl Cancer Inst 2008;100(10):698-711.

[26] European Association for the Study of The Liver, European Organisation for Research and Treatment of Cancer. EASL-EORTC clinical practice guidelines: management of hepatocellular carcinoma. J Hepatol 2012;56(4):908-43.

[27] Gillmore R, Stuart S, Kirkwood A, et al. EASL and mRECIST responses are independent prognostic factors for survival in hepatocellular cancer patients treated with transarterial embolization. J Hepatol 2011;55(6):1309-16.

[28] Shim JH, Lee HC, Kim SO, et al. Which response criteria best help predict survival of patients with hepatocellular carcinoma following chemoembolization? A validation study of old and new models. Radiology 2012;262(2):708-18.

[29] Leung DA, Goin JE, Sickles C, et al. Determinants of postembolization syndrome after hepatic chemoembolization. J Vasc Interv Radiol 2001;12(3):321-6.

[30] Sakamoto I, Aso N, Nagaoki K, et al. Complications associated with transcatheter arterial embolization for hepatic tumors. Radiographics 1998;18(3):605-19.

[31] Chung JW, Park JH, Han JK, et al. Hepatic tumors: predisposing factors for complications of transcatheter oily chemoembolization. Radiology 1996;198(1):33-40.

[32] Yu JS, Kim KW, Jeong MG, et al. Predisposing factors of bile duct injury after transcatheter arterial che-

moembolization (TACE) for hepatic malignancy. Cardiovasc Intervent Radiol 2002;25(4):270-4.

[33] Kim HK, Chung YH, Song BC, et al. Ischemic bile duct injury as a serious complication after transarterial chemoembolization in patients with hepatocellular carcinoma. J Clin Gastroenterol 2001;32(5):423-7.

[34] Xia J, Ren Z, Ye S, et al. Study of severe and rare complications of transarterial chemoembolization (TACE) for liver cancer. Eur J Radiol 2006;59(3):407-12.

[35] Vogl TJ, Lammer J, Lencioni R, et al. Liver, gastrointestinal, and cardiac toxicity in intermediate hepatocellular carcinoma treated with PRECISION TACE with drug-eluting beads: results from the PRECISION V randomized trial. AJR Am J Roentgenol 2011;197(4):W562-70.

[36] Malagari K, Pomoni M, Spyridopoulos TN, et al. Safety profile of sequential transcatheter chemoembolization with DC Bead: results of 237 hepatocellular carcinoma (HCC) patients. Cardiovasc Intervent Radiol 2011;34(4):774-85.

[37] Prajapati HJ, Dhanasekaran R, El-Rayes BF, et al. Safety and efficacy of doxorubicin drug-eluting bead transarterial chemoembolization in patients with advanced hepatocellular carcinoma. J Vasc Interv Radiol 2013;24(3):307-15.

[38] Ferlay J, Shin HR, Bray F, et al. Estimates of worldwide burden of cancer in 2008: GLOBOCAN 2008. Int J Cancer 2010;127(12):2893-917.

[39] Lencioni R. Chemoembolization for hepatocellular carcinoma. Semin Oncol 2012;39(4):503-9.

[40] Llovet JM, Burroughs A, Bruix J. Hepatocellular carcinoma. Lancet 2003; 362(9399):1907-17.

[41] Pelletier G, Roche A, Ink O, et al. A randomized trial of hepatic arterial chemoembolization in patients with unresectable hepatocellular carcinoma. J Hepatol 1990;11(2):181-4.

[42] Trinchet JC, Rached AA, Beaugrand M, et al. A comparison of lipiodol chemoembolization and conservative treatment for unresectable hepatocellular carcinoma. Groupe d'Etude et de Traitement du Carcinome Hépatocellulaire. N Engl J Med 1995;332(19):1256-61.

[43] Bruix J, Llovet JM, Castells A, et al. Transarterial embolization versus symptomatic treatment in patients with advanced hepatocellular carcinoma: results of a randomized, controlled trial in a single institution. Hepatology 1998;27(6):1578-83.

[44] Llovet JM, Real MI, Montaña X, et al. Arterial embolisation or chemoembolisation versus symptomatic treatment in patients with unresectable hepatocellular carcinoma: a randomised controlled trial. Lancet 2002;359(9319):1734-9.

[45] Lo CM, Ngan H, Tso WK, et al. Randomized controlled trial of transarterial lipiodol chemoembolization for unresectable hepatocellular carcinoma. Hepatology 2002;35(5):1164-71.

[46] Brown DB, Chapman WC, Cook RD, et al. Chemoembolization of hepatocellular carcinoma: patient status at presentation and outcome over 15 years at a single center. AJR Am J Roentgenol 2008;190(3):608-15.

[47] Llovet JM, Bruix J. Systematic review of randomized trials for unresectable hepatocellular carcinoma: chemoembolization improves survival. Hepatology 2003;37(2):429-42.

[48] Kasugai H, Kojima J, Tatsuta M, et al. Treatment of hepatocellular carcinoma by transcatheter arterial embolization combined with intraarterial infusion of a mixture of cisplatin and ethiodized oil. Gastroenterology 1989;97(4):965-71.

[49] Kawai S, Tani M, Okamura J, et al. Prospective and randomized trial of lipiodoltranscatheter arterial che-

moembolization for treatment of hepatocellular carcinoma: a comparison of epirubicin and doxorubicin (second cooperative study). The Cooperative Study Group for Liver Cancer Treatment of Japan. Semin Oncol 1997;24(2 Suppl 6). S6 – 38 – S6 – 45.

[50] Watanabe S, Nishioka M, Ohta Y, et al. Prospective and randomized controlled study of chemoembolization therapy in patients with advanced hepatocellular carcinoma. Cooperative Study Group for Liver Cancer Treatment in Shikoku area. Cancer Chemother Pharmacol 1994;33(Suppl):S93 – 6.

[51] Sahara S, Kawai N, Sato M, et al. Prospective evaluation of transcatheter arterial chemoembolization (TACE) with multiple anti – cancer drugs (epirubicin, cisplatin, mitomycin c, 5 – fluorouracil) compared with TACE with epirubicin for treatment of hepatocellular carcinoma. Cardiovasc Intervent Radiol 2012;35(6):1363 –71.

[52] Petruzzi NJ, Frangos AJ, Fenkel JM, et al. Single – center comparison of three chemoembolization regimens for hepatocellular carcinoma. J Vasc Interv Radiol 2013;24(2):266 – 73.

[53] Poon RT, Tso WK, Pang RW, et al. A phase I/II trial of chemoembolization for hepatocellular carcinoma using a novel intra – arterial drug – eluting bead. Clin Gastroenterol Hepatol 2007;5(9):1100 – 8.

[54] Lammer J, Malagari K, Vogl T, et al. Prospective randomized study of doxorubicin – eluting – bead embolization in the treatment of hepatocellular carcinoma: results of the PRECISION V study. Cardiovasc Intervent Radiol 2010; 33(1):41 – 52.

[55] Burrel M, Reig M, Forner A, et al. Survival of patients with hepatocellular carcinoma treated by transarterial chemoembolisation (TACE) using drug eluting beads. Implications for clinical practice and trial design. J Hepatol 2012;56(6):1330 – 5.

[56] Malagari K, Pomoni M, Sotirchos VS, et al. Long term recurrence analysis post drug eluting bead (DEB) chemoembolization for hepatocellular carcinoma (HCC). Hepatogastroenterology 2013;60(126):1413 – 9.

[57] Li X, Feng GS, Zheng CS, et al. Expression of plasma vascular endothelial growth factor in patients with hepatocellular carcinoma and effect of transcatheter arterial chemoembolization therapy on plasma vascular endothelial growth factor level. World J Gastroenterol 2004;10(19):2878 – 82.

[58] Wang B, Xu H, Gao ZQ, et al. Increased expression of vascular endothelial growth factor in hepatocellular carcinoma after transcatheter arterial chemoembolization. Acta Radiol 2008;49(5):523 – 9.

[59] Llovet JM, Ricci S, Mazzaferro V, et al. Sorafenib in advanced hepatocellular carcinoma. N Engl J Med 2008;359(4):378 – 90.

[60] Pawlik TM, Reyes DK, Cosgrove D, et al. Phase II trial of sorafenib combined with concurrent transarterial chemoembolization with drug – eluting beads for hepatocellular carcinoma. J Clin Oncol 2011;29(30):3960 – 7.

[61] Park JW, Koh YH, Kim HB, et al. Phase II study of concurrent transarterial chemoembolization and sorafenib in patients with unresectable hepatocellular carcinoma. J Hepatol 2012;56(6):1336 – 42.

[62] Sansonno D, Lauletta G, Russi S, et al. Transarterial chemoembolization plus sorafenib: a sequential therapeutic scheme for HCV – related intermediate – stage hepatocellular carcinoma: a randomized clinical trial. Oncologist 2012;17(3):359 – 66.

[63] Kudo M, Imanaka K, Chida N, et al. Phase III study of sorafenib after transarterial chemoembolisation in Japanese and Korean patients with unresectable hepatocellular carcinoma. Eur J Cancer 2011;47(14):2117

-27.

[64] Zhao Y, Wang WJ, Guan S, et al. Sorafenib combined with transarterial chemoembolization for the treatment of advanced hepatocellular carcinoma: a largescale multicenter study of 222 patients. Ann Oncol 2013;24(7):1786-92.

[65] Liu L, Chen H, Wang M, et al. Combination therapy of sorafenib and TACE for unresectable HCC: a systematic review and meta-analysis. PLoS One 2014; 9(3):e91124.

[66] Hoffmann K, Glimm H, Radeleff B, et al. Prospective, randomized, double-blind, multi-center, phase III clinical study on transarterial chemoembolization (TACE) combined with sorafenib versus TACE plus placebo in patients with hepatocellular cancer before liver transplantation - HeiLivCa [ISRCTN24081794]. BMC Cancer 2008;8:349.

[67] Chung GE, Lee JH, Kim HY, et al. Transarterial chemoembolization can be safely performed in patients with hepatocellular carcinoma invading the main portal vein and may improve the overall survival. Radiology 2011;258(2): 627-34.

[68] Luo J, Peng ZW, Guo RP, et al. Hepatic resection versus transarterial lipiodol chemoembolization as the initial treatment for large, multiple, and resectable hepatocellular carcinomas: a prospective nonrandomized analysis. Radiology 2011;259(1):286-95.

[69] Heckman JT, Devera MB, Marsh JW, et al. Bridging locoregional therapy for hepatocellular carcinoma prior to liver transplantation. Ann Surg Oncol 2008; 15(11):3169-77.

[70] Chapman WC, Majella Doyle MB, Stuart JE, et al. Outcomes of neoadjuvant transarterial chemoembolization to downstage hepatocellular carcinoma before liver transplantation. Ann Surg 2008;248(4):617-25.

[71] Shaib Y, El-Serag HB. The epidemiology of cholangiocarcinoma. Semin Liver Dis 2004;24(2):115-25.

[72] Yamamoto M, Ariizumi S. Surgical outcomes of intrahepatic cholangiocarcinoma. Surg Today 2011;41(7):896-902.

[73] Ben-Josef E, Normolle D, Ensminger WD, et al. Phase II trial of high-dose conformal radiation therapy with concurrent hepatic artery floxuridine for unresectable intrahepatic malignancies. J Clin Oncol 2005; 23(34):8739-47.

[74] Valle J, Wasan H, Palmer DH, et al. Cisplatin plus gemcitabine versus gemcitabine for biliary tract cancer. N Engl J Med 2010;362(14):1273-81.

[75] Maithel SK, Gamblin TC, Kamel I, et al. Multidisciplinary approaches to intrahepatic cholangiocarcinoma. Cancer 2013;119(22):3929-42.

[76] Burger I, Hong K, Schulick R, et al. Transcatheter arterial chemoembolization in unresectable cholangiocarcinoma: initial experience in a single institution. J Vasc Interv Radiol 2005;16(3):353-61.

[77] Vogl TJ, Naguib NN, Nour-Eldin NE, et al. Transarterial chemoembolization in the treatment of patients with unresectable cholangiocarcinoma: results and prognostic factors governing treatment success. Int J Cancer 2012;131(3): 733-40.

[78] Aliberti C, Benea G, Tilli M, et al. Chemoembolization (TACE) of unresectable intrahepatic cholangiocarcinoma with slow-release doxorubicin-eluting beads: preliminary results. Cardiovasc Intervent Radiol 2008;31(5):883-8.

[79] Kuhlmann JB, Euringer W, Spangenberg HC, et al. Treatment of unresectable cholangiocarcinoma: conventional transarterial chemoembolization compared with drug eluting bead – transarterial chemoembolization and systemic chemotherapy. Eur J Gastroenterol Hepatol 2012;24(4):437 – 43.

[80] Seo SI, Lim SB, Yoon YS, et al. Comparison of recurrence patterns between 5 years and >5 years after curative operations in colorectal cancer patients. J Surg Oncol 2013;108(1):9 – 13.

[81] Geoghegan JG, Scheele J. Treatment of colorectal liver metastases. Br J Surg 1999;86(2):158 – 69.

[82] Lang EK, Brown CL. Colorectal metastases to the liver: selective chemoembolization. Radiology 1993;189(2):417 – 22.

[83] Martinelli DJ, Wadler S, Bakal CW, et al. Utility of embolization or chemoembolization as second – line treatment in patients with advanced or recurrent colorectal carcinoma. Cancer 1994;74(6):1706 – 12.

[84] Abdalla EK, Bauer TW, Chun YS, et al. Locoregional surgical and interventional therapies for advanced colorectal cancer liver metastases: expert consensus statements. HPB (Oxford) 2013;15(2):119 – 30.

[85] Vogl TJ, Gruber T, Balzer JO, et al. Repeated transarterial chemoembolization in the treatment of liver metastases of colorectal cancer: prospective study. Radiology 2009;250(1):281 – 9.

[86] Albert M, Kiefer MV, Sun W, et al. Chemoembolization of colorectal liver metastases with cisplatin, doxorubicin, mitomycin C, ethiodol, and polyvinyl alcohol. Cancer 2011;117(2):343 – 52.

[87] Douillard JY, Cunningham D, Roth AD, et al. Irinotecan combined with fluorouracil compared with fluorouracil alone as first – line treatment for metastatic colorectal cancer: a multicentre randomised trial. Lancet 2000;355(9209):1041 – 7.

[88] de Gramont A, Figer A, Seymour M, et al. Leucovorin and fluorouracil with or without oxaliplatin as first – line treatment in advanced colorectal cancer. J Clin Oncol 2000;18(16):2938 – 47.

[89] Saltz LB, Cox JV, Blanke C, et al. Irinotecan plus fluorouracil and leucovorin for metastatic colorectal cancer. Irinotecan Study Group. N Engl J Med 2000;343(13):905 – 14.

[90] Martin RC, Joshi J, Robbins K, et al. Hepatic intra – arterial injection of drugeluting bead, irinotecan (DEBIRI) in unresectable colorectal liver metastases refractory to systemic chemotherapy: results of multi – institutional study. Ann Surg Oncol 2011;18(1):192 – 8.

[91] Fiorentini G, Aliberti C, Tilli M, et al. Intra – arterial infusion of irinotecan – loaded drug – eluting beads (DEBIRI) versus intravenous therapy (FOLFIRI) for hepatic metastases from colorectal cancer: final results of a phase III study. Anticancer Res 2012;32(4):1387 – 95.

[92] Gusani NJ, Balaa FK, Steel JL, et al. Treatment of unresectable cholangiocarcinoma with gemcitabine – based transcatheter arterial chemoembolization (TACE): a single – institution experience. J Gastrointest Surg 2008;12(1):129 – 37.

[93] Kiefer MV, Albert M, McNally M, et al. Chemoembolization of intrahepatic cholangiocarcinoma with cisplatinum, doxorubicin, mitomycin C, ethiodol, and polyvinyl alcohol: a 2 – center study. Cancer 2011;117(7):1498 – 505.

[94] Park SY, Kim JH, Yoon HJ, et al. Transarterial chemoembolization versus supportive therapy in the palliative treatment of unresectable intrahepatic cholangiocarcinoma. Clin Radiol 2011;66(4):322 – 8.

[95] Poggi G, Amatu A, Montagna B, et al. OEM – TACE: a new therapeutic approach in unresectable intrahepatic cholangiocarcinoma. Cardiovasc Intervent Radiol 2009;32(6):1187 – 92.

[96] Sanz – Altamira PM, Spence LD, Huberman MS, et al. Selective chemoembolization in the management

of hepatic metastases in refractory colorectal carcinoma: a phase II trial. Dis Colon Rectum 1997;40(7): 770 - 5.

[97] Tellez C, Benson AB, Lyster MT, et al. Phase II trial of chemoembolization for the treatment of metastatic colorectal carcinoma to the liver and review of the literature. Cancer 1998;82(7):1250 - 9.

[98] Hong K, McBride JD, Georgiades CS, et al. Salvage therapy for liver - dominant colorectal metastatic adenocarcinoma: comparison between transcatheter arterial chemoembolization versus yttrium - 90 radioembolization. J Vasc Interv Radiol 2009;20(3):360 - 7.

[99] Bower M, Metzger T, Robbins K, et al. Surgical downstaging and neo - adjuvant therapy in metastatic colorectal carcinoma with irinotecan drug - eluting beads: a multi - institutional study. HPB (Oxford) 2010;12(1):31 - 6.

[100] Narayanan G, Barbery K, Suthar R, et al. Transarterial chemoembolization using DEBIRI for treatment of hepatic metastases from colorectal cancer. Anticancer Res 2013;33(5):2077 - 83.

第九章 钇-90选择性体内放射治疗

Edward W. Lee, MD, PhD[a,*], Avnesh S. Thakor, MD, PhD[b],
Bashir A. Tafti, MD[a], David M. Liu, MD[b]

【关键词】

Y-90；选择性体内放射治疗；肝；恶性肿瘤

要点

- 多个前瞻性Ⅱ期、Ⅲ期和回顾性研究证实，选择性内放射疗法（SIRT）在治疗原发性肝细胞癌（HCC）和转移性结直肠癌（CRM）中有更高的安全性、有效性和耐受性。
- SIRT可用于缩小HCC病灶，以便进行下一步治疗，如肝脏移植或肝脏切除术。
- 在治疗化疗难治性转移性结直肠癌中，SIRT已经显示出生存获益。
- 相比肝动脉栓塞化疗，SIRT的并发症患者更易耐受。

一、简介

全世界有数百万原发性肝癌和转移性肝癌患者[1-3]，而不可切除的肝脏肿瘤（原发性和继发性）缺乏权威疗法[4]。公认的肝癌治愈方法包括手术切除和肝移植，其成功概率很小，且仅适用于约10%的患者[5-8]。微创治疗如消融和肝动脉化疗栓塞（TACE），传统上用于治疗部分早期患者，或作为不可切除患者的姑息性治疗。即使有这么多的治疗方法，但各种治疗的方式不同，导致技术、患者的选择和临床疗效（特别是栓塞治疗）都受到限制。

作者无其他声明。

[a] Interventional Radiology, Department of Radiology, UCLA Medical Center, David Geffen School of Medicine, Los Angeles, CA, USA; [b] Interventional Radiology, Department of Radiology, University of British Columbia Medical Center, Vancouver, British Columbia, Canada

* Corresponding author. Division of Interventional Radiology, Department of Radiology, Ronald Reagan Medical Center at UCLA, David Geffen School of Medicine at UCLA, 757 Westwood Plaza, Suite 2125, Los Angeles, CA 90095-743730.

E-mail address: EdwardLee@mednet.ucla.edu

肝细胞癌(HCC)发病率在癌症中排名第6。致HCC的危险因素包括病毒性肝炎(乙型肝炎病毒和丙型肝炎病毒)、酗酒、非酒精性脂肪肝、摄入受黄曲霉素污染的食物、肥胖、糖尿病和遗传(如血色病)。

以碘油为基础的TACE可有效治疗早、中期HCC[9],但是对于晚期患者的疗效仍存在争议。尚没有前瞻性随机对比研究来证实出现转移后TACE的疗效。在接受调查的人群中(回顾性或单臂前瞻性试验),大部分出现神经内分泌疾病(一种恶劣条件下发生及预后不良的变异表现)。少数小型前瞻性研究(在不同的临床条件下)证实,伊立替康药物洗脱珠治疗可让早期CRM人群受益。

使用选择性内放射治疗(SIRT)CRM和HCC患者已有较严格规范。CRM患者人群Ⅲ期一级数据,和针对HCC患者的大型前瞻性和回顾性队列研究证实,SIRT具有更高的安全性、有效性和耐受性[11-15]。

1. 放射性栓塞的历史和进展

虽然放射治疗已被证明有益于各种恶性肿瘤的治疗,但不包括肝恶性肿瘤。因为肝脏对于射线的相对低耐受性,致使外放射治疗并不能成为肝肿瘤的常规治疗[16]。肝脏仅能耐受30~50Gy范围内的射线,过高会出现辐射性肝病(RILD)[16]。但通常需要90~100Gy或更高的剂量才能对肝肿瘤产生治疗作用。放射性栓塞的出现使放射治疗应用的局限性得以解决[16,17]。放射性栓塞或SIRT都是通过导管选择性地进入为肝脏肿瘤供血的肝动脉分支,并注入放射性微粒,而微粒可滞留在微血管处持续发挥作用[18]。利用这种技术,肝病灶局部辐射剂量可高达150Gy,从而持续杀伤肿瘤细胞,而其余正常肝脏组织则受影响不大,这大大降低了RILD的发病率[19,20]。

放射性栓塞治疗理论基于肝脏的血管解剖结构,肝脏肿瘤的血供大部分来源于肝动脉,而正常肝实质则大部分来源于门静脉[17]。此外,肝脏肿瘤常常会有一些来源于肝动脉分支的新生微血管,这些微血管甚至比正常肝实质中的微血管更为密集[21]。基于这种解剖学结构,经肝动脉给药治疗肝肿瘤显然是一个非常有效的方法,因为这将减少细胞毒性药物对正常肝实质的损伤[21]。经过数十年的发展,在治疗肝病方面,这种方式已变得更加安全、有效。目前TACE已成为一种广泛使用的治疗原发性肝细胞癌和转移性肝癌的方法,它的疗效显著,但也存在明显的副作用,如肝毒性[22,23]。

SIRT的作用机制与化疗栓塞有着本质的不同。化疗栓塞是对肿瘤供血血管进行栓塞/阻断,从而使化疗药物最大剂量滞留并作用于肿瘤内产生的缺血性环境。相反,SIRT需要血流量和氧,因为这样β射线才能对水分子进行电离从而产生自由基。临床应用钇-90(Y-90)微球治疗肝脏肿瘤的历史可追溯至20世纪60年代初[24]。这种微球中嵌入钇的同位素Y-90,可以放射出β射线[4]。Y-90半衰期为63小时,每次裂变发放的能量平均为0.937MeV,所放射出的β射线可引起约2.5mm范围内的细胞坏死[4]。这些特性使Y-90尤其适用于体内放射治疗[4]。

目前,经FDA批准,已有两种产品应用于临床放射性栓塞治疗。TheraSphere,一种玻璃微球(BTG Medical,PA;FDA于1999年批准用于肝癌),具有较高的平均放射活性,直径范围

20~30μm[25,26]。平均放射活性是指每一个微球的 Y-90 放射剂量。由于每个微球中的玻璃颗粒放射剂量约 2500Bq，所以每次治疗仅需要 100~200 万微球[19]。SIR-Sphere 颗粒（Sirtex，澳大利亚；美国 FDA 于 2002 年批准用于结直肠癌肝转移）由树脂制成，具有较低的比重，直径 20~60μm。每个树脂微球颗粒的放射剂量约 50Bq，所以每次治疗用量为 4000~6000 万微球。TheraSphere 对肝肿瘤无明显栓塞作用，而 SIRSphere 用量较多，可产生轻微栓塞作用[19,26]。

在临床中，由于 SIRSphere 微球用量更多，所以它们在肿瘤中可分布得更均匀，放射范围覆盖整个肿瘤。而 TheraSphere 微球具有较高的平均放射活性和较大的直径，会在肿瘤中出现微聚集现象（颗粒优先在肿瘤的周边积累）。微粒聚集带来的局部过高辐射剂量会导致肝实质裂开、肝叶水肿或其余肝组织代偿性肥大。每个微球都有自己的云量，通过各微球云量累积，可达到等量为 100~1000Gy 的致死剂量，这就是内放射性治疗肿瘤的机制。

每种微球的放射活性总量（电离辐射剂量）可根据体表面积（BSA）或分区模型来估计。最近有一项研究表明，根据 CT 估算的非肿瘤区域肝脏体积与体表面积直接关联，并可由此估算 SIRT 所用树脂微球的放射活性量[27]。常用单室模型估算 SIRT 所用玻璃微球量（仅是根据肝脏大小，而与瘤灶大小无关）。之前也曾使用过双室模型（既考虑瘤灶大小，也考虑正常肝组织大小），其优势在于，可以更为精确地估算传递至瘤灶的放射剂量。室模型估算内放射剂量，既保证了可造成肿瘤细胞死亡的最大剂量，又降低了患者出现 RILD 的风险，这对于残肝较少的患者尤为重要[28,29]。不建议仅根据影像学判断出的肿瘤大小来进行经验性用量选择[30]。

2. 放射栓塞技术

一般来说，预期寿命为 3 个月的不可切除（原发或转移性肝脏肿瘤）患者，或者那些肝肿瘤严重影响生存期的患者，是放射性栓塞治疗的适应对象[31]。有转移性病灶的未经临床试验选择的病例，必须是在行一线化疗者，或一线化疗失败者[31]。禁忌证包括患者肿瘤负荷严重，残肝不能耐受放射治疗[31]。不可逆转的高血清总胆红素水平（大于 2mg/dl）是相对禁忌证[31]。与化疗栓塞治疗不同，门静脉癌栓形成并非禁忌，因为 SIRT 栓塞作用很小。

在进行放射性栓塞治疗前应评估患者的肝肾功能，还应检测肿瘤标志物水平（例如，肝癌标志物甲胎蛋白，胆管癌标志物 CA19-9，结直肠癌标志物 CEA）[31]。此外，肝内的靶肿瘤灶及体内的其他肿瘤灶均应进行胸部、腹部、骨盆等处的 3 期增强 CT 或钆增强 MRI 扫描评估[31]。通过 CT 或 MRI 数据的三维分析，在治疗前计算肝内肿瘤体积、总肝脏体积及肝功能储备（图 9-1）。

经评估，确定患者肝内肿瘤和临床表现适合放射性栓塞治疗后，患者还应在治疗前 1~3 周接受肝血管造影（SIRT 前的预映射过程）（图 9-2）[31]，这对于治疗前进行剂量估算至关重要[31]。而且造影还可以显示肝总动脉、肠系膜上动脉、腹腔内其他动脉的走向[31]。如果发现变异解剖结构，可以通过栓塞或放置抗反流导管进行封堵，以避免放射性颗粒分流到胃肠等器官造成辐射伤害（包括辐射诱发的胰腺炎或胃炎）。除了血管造影，还要使用 ^{99m}Tc 标记的颗粒蛋白（MAA）对肝肺分流进行评估（图 9-3）[31,32]。在这个核医学试验中，首先将 MAA 注入动

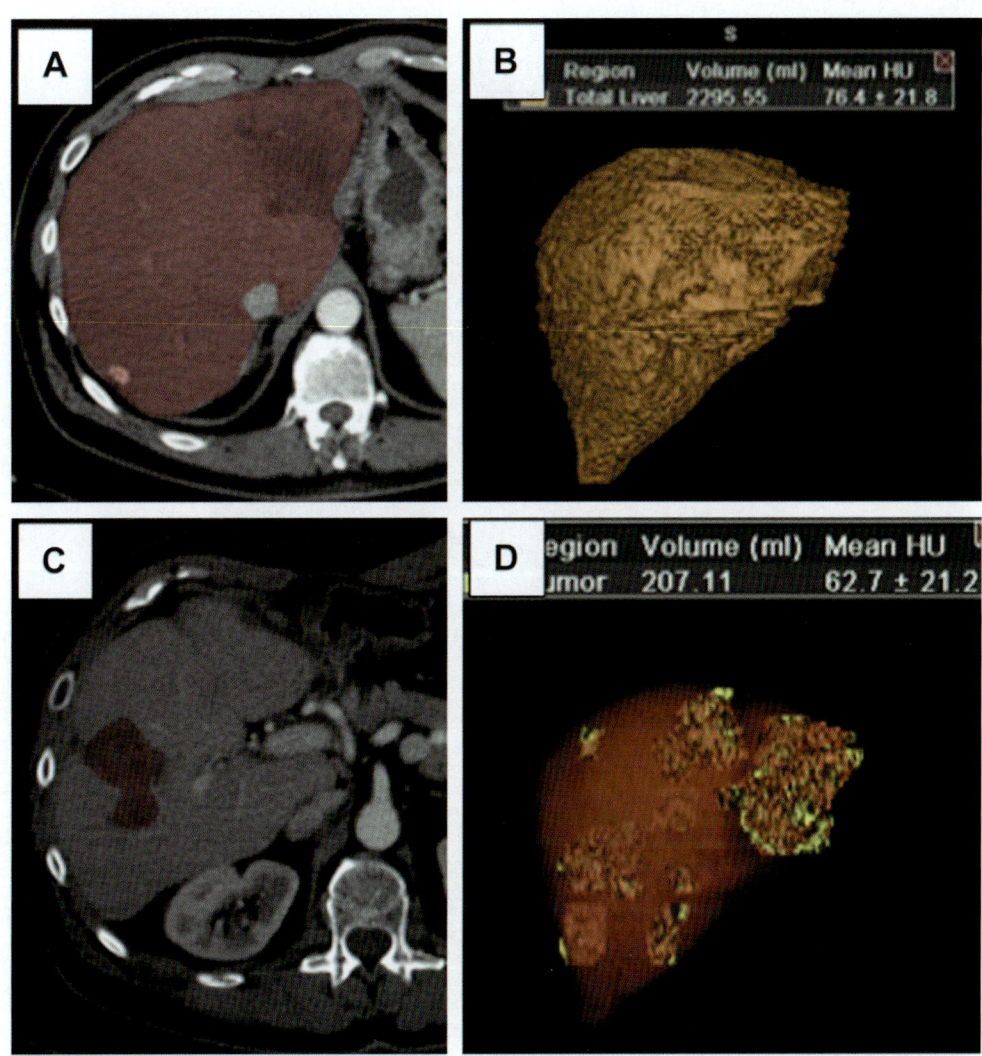

图 9-1　SIRT 治疗前,2D 和 3D 总肝体积分析(A,B),治疗前使用 CT 估算肿瘤体积(C,D)。这些数值将用于 SIRT 微球剂量估算

脉内,然后在随后的几个小时内进行单光子发射 CT(SPECT)扫描或胸部和腹部的 CT 平扫[33]。如果扫描分析显示肺部和/或胃肠道的辐射剂量暴露大于 30Gy,那患者术后出现肝外毒性,特别是放射性肺炎等致命并发症的风险将大大增加,这是一个相对禁忌证。不过,也可通过栓塞观察到分流,或术前进行 TACE,减少肝外毒性,但必须再进行一次 MAA 扫描来确认栓塞后分流是否减少。

进行 SIRT 治疗时,同样须通过肝血管造影并同之前的预映射造影对比,再次确认血管解剖结构,并确保微球注射剂滞留于最佳位置。确认之后,勾选进入供应靶肿瘤灶的肝叶或肝段血管,并根据不同厂家各自的注射装置和技术说明进行微球注射。完成放射性微球注射后,应将患者移到核医学科室,进行 SPECT 或胸部和腹部平面扫描,以确认 SIRT 微球滞留在最佳位

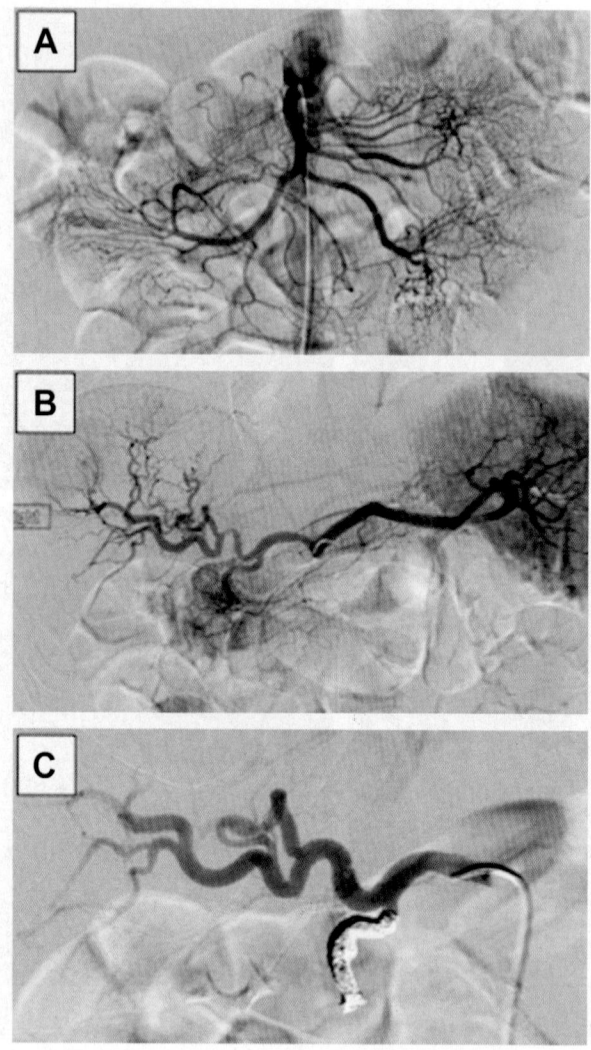

图9-2 SIRT治疗前,肠系膜上动脉(A)和腹腔动脉造影(B),显示肝脏和肝脏肿瘤血管解剖结构,并寻找变异解剖结构,如:替代右或左肝动脉。此次血管造影还要识别胃动脉和胃十二指肠动脉(C),并对其实施预防性栓塞处理,以免放射对胃和胰腺造成伤害

置(图9-4)。如果患者需连续行 SIRT 治疗,应在第一次治疗后约1个月内对残肝和患者全身功能进行对症治疗。

放射性栓塞治疗后,应在1、3和6个月时,进行肝脏3期 CT 或对比增强 MRI 扫描,以便监测肝脏和肝肿瘤情况[34,35]。术后1个月,影像学最常见的是肿瘤坏死区域减弱或栓塞区域强化,这是由于肝内出现水肿、充血或者组织微栓塞[34,35]所致。早期 CT 影像学并不能准确反映放射性栓塞的有效性,因为这些变化大部分是可逆的,或部分可逆,或具有自限性。因此,还需要在3~6个月时进行 CT 扫描评估瘤灶变化[34,35]。此外,对于少血管性肿瘤患者,可行

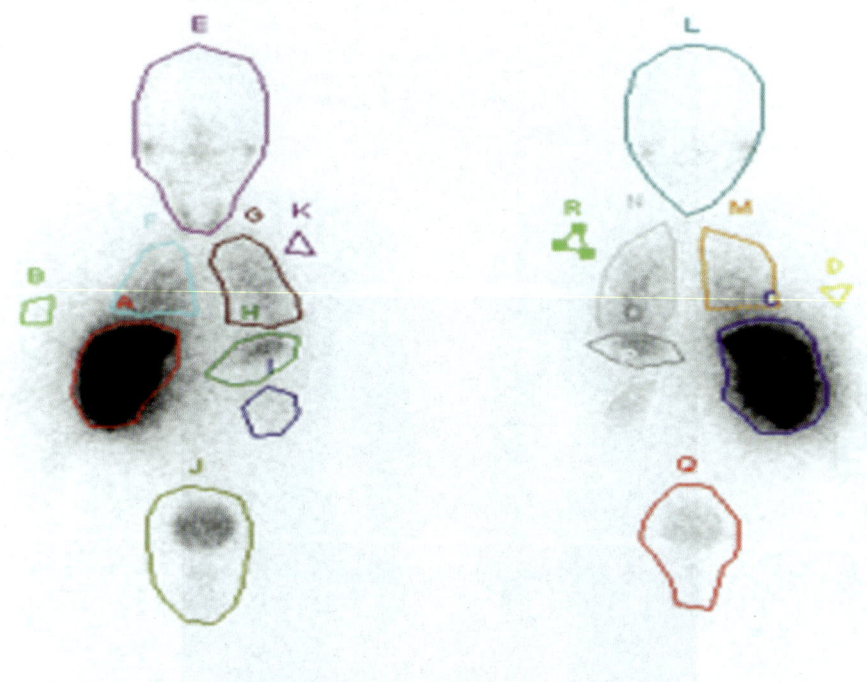

图 9-3 注入 ^{99m}Tc 标记的颗粒蛋白后,全身平面扫描。根据肺部和肝部颗粒蛋白分布判断肺部分流量

PET 成像,它可以跟踪治疗后变化,并显示治疗区域减弱的代谢活性[36]。

二、临床应用

1. 肝细胞癌

全世界每年 HCC 新诊断病例超过 125 万,死亡病例超过 50 万[6,37]。HCC 是世界第六常见恶性肿瘤,也是导致恶性肿瘤死亡的第三常见诱因[1,6]。可以明确的是,HCC 正影响着全世界数百万患者的生命。尽管现在内外科治疗不断取得新进展,HCC 的治疗效果仍未能令人满意[4]。随机对照试验证明,局部治疗可以提高试验患者的生存期。然而,TACE 和经动脉栓塞术(TAE)有可能诱发肝功能衰竭,特别是对于门静脉癌栓形成,致使门静脉血流不能供应肝脏的患者,以及那些多发子灶、大肿瘤肝癌患者[38]。在过去的十年中,人们对 SIRT 治疗 HCC 的疗效进行了大量的研究(表 9-1)。其中较为突出的是 Salem 等[39]所进行的队列研究,其纳入 291 例 HCC 患者,进行了共 526 次 SIRT 治疗(平均每人 1.8 次)。应答率和生存率是评估疗效的两个重要指标。根据世界卫生组织(WHO)标准,治疗应答率为 42%,根据欧洲肝脏病协会(EASL)标准为 57%[39]。Child-Pugh 分级 A 级患者,术后平均生存期约 17.2 个月,B 级患者平均为 7.7 个月[39],而治疗过程中 30 天内死亡率为 3%[39]。在欧洲,Sangro 和 Inarrai-

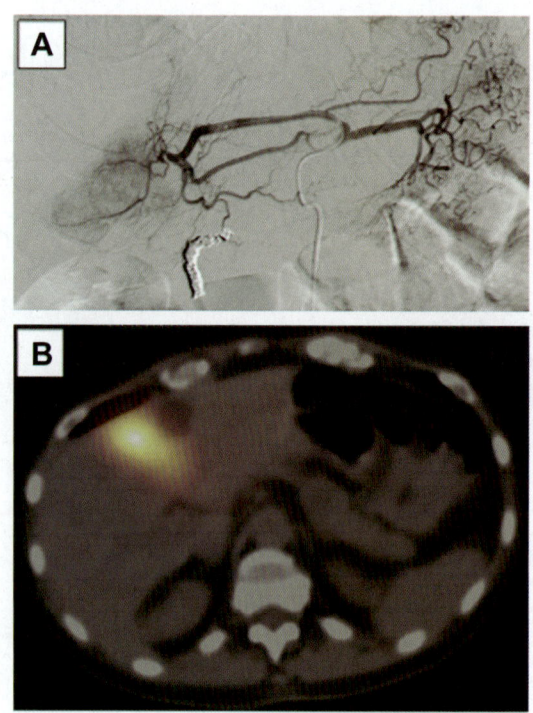

图9-4 A. 通过胃左动脉,向替代肝左动脉注射SIRT微球。血管造影显示出一处血管染色,由SIRT治疗后SPECT CT检测出,并与之相关。B. 此SPECT CT可成功确认治疗区域SIRT微球的分布情况。

raegui[40]研究了8个医疗中心的325例患者,其中位生存期为12.8个月(82% CP-A级,18% CP-B级,24%单发,76%多发)。Mazzaferro等[41]研究了52例接受放射性栓塞的肝癌患者,发现9.6%患者出现完全应答,而40.4%患者出现客观整体应答。他们还发现,该治疗具有良好的治疗耐受性,患者30天死亡率、90天死亡率分别为0和3.8%[41]。

表9-1 SIRT治疗HCC主要研究总结

研究人员	数量	治疗方案	总应答率(%)	生存期
SIRT一线或二线治疗中晚期HCC				
D'Avola	35	SIRT	NR	16个月
	43	传统治疗	NR	8个月
Salem	291	SIRT	42(WHO)	17个月(Child A)
			57(EASL)	8个月(Child B)
Sangro	325	SIRT	NR	12.8个月
		BCLC A		24.4个月

续表

研究人员	数量	治疗方案	总应答率（%）	生存期
		BCLC B		16.9 个月
		BCLC C		10.0 个月
		Child A		14.9 个月
		Child B		10.3 个月
Inarrairaegui	72	SIRT	94	13 个月
Lau	18	SIRT（>120 Gy）	100	14 个月
Chow	35	SIRT then sorafenib	79	11.8 个月
		BCLC B	100	18.3 个月
		BCLC C	68	8.8 个月
Inarrairaegui	25	PVT 情况下，SIRT 治疗	67	10 个月
Sangro	183	PVT 情况下，SIRT 治疗	NR	
		主静脉 PVT		10.8 个月
		静脉分支 PVT		7.4 个月

缩略词：BCLC，巴塞罗那分期；EASL，欧洲肝脏病学协会；PVT，门静脉栓塞；WHO，世界卫生组织

SIRT 可缩小肝癌病灶，为肝脏切除术或肝移植等进一步治疗做准备。Inarrairaegui 等人[42]研究了 21 例行放射性栓塞治疗延缓肿瘤进展的患者。其中 6 例经治疗后病灶较稳定，并可接受肝脏切除术或肝移植等进一步治疗。正如所预期的，这几例患者表现出良好的总体生存获益。Vouche 等[43]在 2013 年也进行了类似的研究，他们对 83 例患者采用 SIRT 治疗，为辐射肝叶切除术做准备[43]。治疗后，5 例患者行根治性右叶切除术，6 例患者进行了肝移植手术。

人们对常规 TACE 和 SIRT 的疗效进行了对比研究。最大规模的一项研究是 Salem 等[44]对 245 例肝癌患者行栓塞化疗（122 例）或放射性栓塞（123 例）治疗进行的对比研究。其中，放射性栓塞治疗组应答率为 49%，而化疗栓塞组应答率为 36%[44]。放射性栓塞治疗组术后疾病进展时间较长，为 13.3 个月，而化疗栓塞组术后进展时间为 8.4 个月，但两组的中位生存期无显著统计学差异[44]。Lance 等[45]对 73 例不可手术切除的 HCC 患者做了上述两组疗效比较的研究，同样发现两组中位生存时间无显著统计学差异。然而，Salem 等[44]和 Lance 等[45]的研究中均发现，在 TACE 组中出现栓塞后综合征的情况更为突出，并需要住院治疗。人们对如何改善 SIRT 治疗后的生活质量也做了相关研究。Steel 等[46]对接受肝动脉灌注顺铂或 SIRT 治疗的 HCC 患者做了健康相关的调查研究。术后短期内，放射性栓塞治疗组在局部功能性评估及整体健康性评估均获得较高评分。术后 6 个月，SIRT 组依然在局部功能性评估中获得较高评分，但两组疗法在整体健康性评估方面并未出现显著性差异[46]。Salem 等[47]还对 29 例接受 SIRT 和 27 例接受 TACE 治疗的原发性肝癌患者进行了生活质量调查研究。他们发现，接受 SIRT 的患者在生活质量评分上高于接受 TACE 的患者[47]。

2. 肝脏转移性肿瘤

HCC 影响较广,而肝脏也是结直肠、神经内分泌腺体、乳房、肾脏等原发性瘤灶的易转移部位[14,48-51]。这主要与肝脏的双重血供有关,它既接受肝动脉的灌注,也接受胃肠道回流血液的门静脉灌注[52]。

3. 结直肠癌

结直肠癌(CRC)在美国是第三常见的恶性肿瘤,也是致死率第二高的恶性肿瘤[2]。每年约有 10 万结肠癌新发病例和 4 万直肠癌新发病例。在 CRC 患者中,因为肝脏是肝静脉系统、门静脉和胃肠道静脉的血液过滤器,所以约 60% 患者可出现肝转移[50]。而且,肝转移常常是导致 CRC 死亡的主要原因[52]。

人们对单放射性栓塞及其与常规一线或二线化疗药物联合的疗法进行了大量研究(表 9-2)。比较突出的是 Sharma 等[14]所做的 I 期临床试验。他们对 22 例不可切除的结直肠癌肝转移患者进行研究,这些患者均接受了 SIRT 联合全身化疗。第一个周期,患者接受奥沙利铂/氟尿嘧啶(FU)/亚叶酸(LV)联合化疗,而第二个周期,患者接受 FU/LV 联合 SIRT 治疗。然后,在 4~12 周期,患者接受奥沙利铂、亚叶酸和氟尿嘧啶(FOLFOX4)联合治疗。其中 18 例患者出现部分应答,2 例患者疾病稳定,中位疾病进展时间为 12.3 个月[14]。Kosmider 等[53]更进一步地研究了 SIRT 联合全身化疗的效果。他们的研究纳入了 19 例不可切除的结直肠癌肝转移患者,其中 7 例患者给予 FU、LV 和放射性栓塞联合治疗,而 12 例患者接受 FOLFOX 方案联合放射性栓塞治疗。两组总应答率为 84%,有 2 例患者完全应答,14 例患者部分应答[53]。Chu 等[54]对 140 例接受放射性栓塞联合全身化疗的结直肠癌肝转移患者进行研究。他们发现,1% 患者完全应答,31% 患者部分应答,而 31% 患者疾病稳定。总体上,37% 患者出现疾病进展。对比历史研究数据,他们发现,联合全身化疗可显著增加放射性栓塞治疗的效果。

表 9-2 SIRT 治疗结直肠癌肝转移主要研究总结

研究人员	数量	治疗方案	总应答率(%)	生存期/率
SIRT 一线治疗结直肠癌肝转移				
II 期/III 期		单 FOLFOX4	27~59	16.2~20.7 个月
Gray	74	SIRT + HAC	44	39%(2 年)
		单 HAC	18	29%(2 年)
Van Hazel	21	SIRT + 5-FU/LV	91	29.4 个月
		单 5-FU/LV	0	12.8 个月
Sharma	20	SIRT + FOLFOX4	90	NR
Kosmider	19	SIRT + FOLFOX4 ± 5-FU/LV	84	29.4 个月 37.8 个月(L)

续表

研究人员	数量	治疗方案	总应答率（%）	生存期/率
Tie	31	SIRT + FQLFOX4 ±5 - FU/LV	91	30.7个月（L）
SIRT 二线治疗结直肠癌肝转移				
Ⅱ期/Ⅲ期		Irinotecan	4~13	6.4~10个月
		Irinotecan + cetuximab	16~27	8.6~10.7个月
		Panitumumab	9~14	6.3~9.3
Lim	30	SIRT + 5 - FU/LV（70%）	33	NR
Van Hazel	25	SIRT + irinotecan	48	12.2个月
Cove - Smith	33	SIRT + FOLFIRI or FOLFOX - based chemo	38	17.0个月
SIRT 补救治疗化疗难治性结直肠癌肝转移				
Hedlisz	44	SIRT + 5 - FU	86	10.0个月
		5 - FU	35	7.3个月
Seidensticker	29	SIRT	58	8.3个月
	29	支持治疗	0	3.5个月
Bester	224	SIRT	NR	11.9个月
	29	传统治疗		6.6个月
Cosimelli	50	SIRT	48	12.6个月
Sofocleous	19	SIRT	71	16个月
Kennedy	606	SIRT	NR	9.6个月
Coldwell	25	SIRT KRAS wt	NR	NR
		SIRT KRAS	NR	7.0个月
Leoni	51	SIRT	53	10.5个月
Cianni	41	SIRT	82	11.8个月
Jakobs	41	SIRT	78	10.5个月
Nace	51	SIRT	77	10.2个月

缩略词：FOLFIRI，亚叶酸钙 + 5 - FU + 伊立替康；HAC，肝动脉灌注化疗；KRAS，基因名称；NR，未报道；Tx，治疗；wt，野生型

此外，SIRT 也是难治性、转移性 CRC 患者的姑息治疗选择。Cosimelli 等[55]对 50 例全身化疗失败患者进行了放射性栓塞治疗的Ⅱ期临床试验研究。他们使用 RECIST 标准（实体瘤疗效评价标准），其中 2% 患者完全应答，22% 患者部分应答，24% 患者疾病稳定[55]。与早前的联合治疗研究的结果相类似，44% 患者最后还是出现了疾病进展[55]。总的中位生存期为 12.6 个月，2 年生存率为 19.6%[55]。同样，Nace 等[56]对 51 例不可切除的结直肠癌肝转移患

者进行一线和二线化疗联合 SIRT 治疗,最后也出现进展。采用 RECIST 标准,Nace 等[56]的研究中,77%患者部分应答或疾病稳定。总中位生存期为 10.2 个月。一项Ⅲ期临床试验纳入了 46 例接受 SIRT 联合化疗、难治性 CRC 肝转移患者。所有 46 例患者此前曾进行一线化疗,但均未适当应答。这些患者被随机分到单 5-FU 或 5-FU 联合放射性栓塞两个治疗组。其中,单 5-FU 组疾病进展时间为 2.1 个月,联合组为 5.5 个月,但两组的总生存率无显著统计学差异。值得注意的是,仍缺乏准确评估 SIRT 治疗后肿瘤学疗效的标准。常用的有影像学应答标准,如 WHO 标准、RECIST 标准或 MRECIST 标准。Keppke 等提出,MRECIST 标准可以更准确地评估 SIRT 疗效。

SIRT 也可作为一种急救治疗手段。2011 年,Beste 等[57]对 339 例化疗难治性、转移性 CRC 患者接受 SIRT 治疗及保守姑息治疗的疗效进行研究。报告显示,接受 SIRT 治疗的患者有 63% 的应答率。保守姑息治疗组中位生存期为 6 个月,而 SIRT 治疗后中位生存期为 12 个月[57]。Seidensticker 等[58]的研究也得出了类似的结论,其中,SIRT 补救治疗组的中位生存期为 8.3 个月,而保守治疗组为 3.5 个月[58]。

4. 神经内分泌肿瘤

神经内分泌肿瘤比较少见,发病率在 0.002%~0.003%[2,59]。它们易发于人体内分泌腺体,常见于胃肠道和肺部。某些特定类型的肿瘤,如类癌、胰岛细胞瘤、神经节瘤、嗜铬细胞瘤以及甲状腺髓样癌中较为常见[2,59]。这些肿瘤通常无明显症状,只有肿瘤增大和/或激素分泌过多才会导致明显的变化[59]。类癌可导致血清素过量的症状,如腹泻、皮肤潮红、支气管痉挛,特别是当其转移至肝脏时[59]。对于转移性神经内分泌肿瘤患者,50%~95%最终会出现肝转移,5 年内死亡率为 80%[60]。手术切除且尽可能多的切除肿瘤组织是目前治疗的首选方法。然而,90%患者存在有多个较大病灶,手术切除效果并不理想。即使进行手术切除,其 5 年生存率仍只有 60%~80%[61]。而神经内分泌肿瘤肝转移患者进行肝移植后,5 年生存率为 26%~47%[62]。对于不可切除的神经内分泌转移瘤,已证实治疗方案包括:药物治疗,如生长抑素类似物治疗;消融疗法,如冷冻治疗或射频消融(RFA);全身化疗、TAE;TACE[63-65]。

已证实 SIRT 也可在神经内分泌肿瘤肝转移阶段发挥作用(表 9-3)。在一项由 Cao 等[66]进行的前瞻性研究中,51 例神经内分泌肿瘤肝转移患者进行放射性栓塞治疗。其中,6 例患者完全应答,14 例患者部分应答,14 例患者疾病稳定,17 例患者疾病进展。总中位生存期为 36 个月,而 3 年生存率为 89%[66]。Memon 等[59]对 40 例接受 SIRT 治疗的神经内分泌肿瘤肝转移患者进行研究,也得出类似结论。他们使用的中位放射剂量为 113Gy,根据 WHO 标准进行评估,1.2%患者完全应答,62.7%患者部分应答[59]。若根据 EASL 标准进行评估,则完全应答率提高到 20.5%[59]。Paprottka 等[67]对 42 例难治性神经内分泌肿瘤肝转移患者进行 SIRT 疗效研究,并得到了积极的结果。经过 3 个月的 SIRT 治疗,部分应答率为 22.5%,疾病稳定率为 75%,而疾病进展率为 2.5%[67]。Shaheen 等[68]对 25 例神经内分泌肿瘤肝转移患者(NETLM)使用放射性栓塞玻璃微球进行治疗。他们发现,根据 RECIST 标准评估,单期放射性栓塞治疗,病灶坏死率为 48%[68]。此外,对比 SIRT 治疗后应答患者和无应答患者的基本情况,他们发现,已行手术切除的患者再进行 SIRT 治疗可获得较明显的应答[68]。他们还发现,双叶肝脏病变或病变累及大部分肝脏的患者对 SIRT 治疗应答较差[68]。在对 42 例 NETLM 患者分别进行玻璃或树脂 SIRT 微球放射性栓塞后，Rhee 等[51]发现，92% 玻璃微球组患者出现部分应答或疾病稳定，而 94% 树脂微球组患者出现部分应答或疾病稳定[51]。

表 9-3 SIRT 治疗 NETLM 主要研究总结

研究人员	数量	治疗方案	总应答率（%）	生存期/率
SIRT 治疗化疗难治性 NETLM 混合队列研究				
Kennedy	148	SIRT	86	70 个月
King	34	SIRT + 5-FU	64.7（症状缓解 = 55%）	35 个月
Saxena	48	SIRT + 5-FU	77	35 个月
Cao	58	SIRT + 5-FU	66	36 个月
Rhee	42	SIRT	94	28 个月
Jakobs	25	SIRT	96（症状缓解 = 92%）	96%（1 年）
Coldwell	84	SIRT	100（症状缓解 = 80%）	NR
Ezziddin	23	SIRT	91（症状缓解 = 80%）	29 个月
Paprottka	42	SIRT	97（症状缓解 = 95%）	95%（16 个月）

在研究 34 例接受放射性栓塞不可切除的 NETLM 患者中，因神经内分泌肿瘤过度分泌而引发症状时，King 等[69]发现，根据 RECIST 标准评估，18% 患者出现完全应答，32% 患者部分应答。治疗 3 个月后，神经内分泌症状缓解率达 55%，6 个月后，神经内分泌症状缓解率达 50%。在前面介绍的 Memon 的研究中，还讨论了 SIRT 栓塞对改善神经内分泌症状的作用。研究显示，84% 患者原有临床症状显著缓解。

5. 胆管癌

肝内胆管癌（IHCC）是第二常见的原发肝脏恶性肿瘤。在过去 20 年里，虽然整体发病率非常低，但在持续上升。IHCC 死亡率很高，中位生存期为 3~8 个月。由于 IHCC 患者病情普遍进展较快，所以不适合手术切除或肝移植[70]。但因为胆管癌细胞对辐射较敏感[71,72]，一些对肝内胆管细胞癌患者进行 SIRT 治疗的研究获得了较为满意的结果[73,74]。

最近 2 项前瞻性、非随机研究报告，SIRT 治疗肝内胆管癌具有有效性和可行性[73,74]。在研究中，Mouli 等[73]对 46 例不可切除的肝内胆管细胞癌进行 SIRT 治疗。其中，根据 WHO 评估标准，总应答率是 98%（根据 EASL 标准则是 100%），11% 患者分期下降，可进行肝脏移植或手术切除。总体而言，中位生存期为 14.6 个月。肝外部位 IHCC 患者中位生存期略长，约为 15.6 个月。Rafi 等[74]的研究也得出类似的结果，总应答率是 79%，中位生存期为 15 个月。

三、并发症

虽然 SIRT 可能是某些肝脏肿瘤有效的治疗方法，但随着治疗的进行，也会出现一些并发症。放射性栓塞后综合征在治疗后的几天至几周内出现,症状通常包括轻度腹痛、轻度恶心、呕吐和低热[26]。总体来看,20%~55%患者会出现放射性栓塞后综合征。在 Mulcahy 等[50]的研究发现,61%患者出现疲劳,21%患者出现恶心,25%患者出现腹痛。此外,因为 SIRT 微球发出的辐射也影响正常肝实质和胆道系统,肝损伤和胆道功能障碍也是常见的并发症。Sangro 等[75]对25例患者的研究中,20%患者在治疗后数周出现由于肝损害导致的并发症,包括黄疸和腹水。高并发症发生率可能与全肝大范围栓塞治疗有关。而一般情况下,SIRT 治疗后 RILD 的发生率为0~4%[75-77]。关于胆道并发症,Atassi 等[78]研究发现,SIRT 治疗后影像学检查显示,327 例患者中,有33例出现胆道损害相关并发症。总体而言,胆道损害相关并发症发生率不超过10%[78]。就胃肠并发症而言,Carretero 等[79]发现,78例患者中3例出现胃和小肠损伤。由于进行 SIRT 时会对分支血管造影,并进行栓塞来预期控制,所以胃肠道的损伤很可能与无法识别的胃和十二指肠侧支循环、分流放射剂量有关[79]。Andrews 等[5]研究发现,有4例患者出现胃炎和十二指肠炎,这与胃肠道中放射性栓塞微球沉积有关。另一种可能出现的并发症是放射性肺炎,常见于 MAA 扫描时分流血液流向肺部的患者[80,81]。SIRT 治疗后,出现放射性肺炎的发生率低于1%[80,81]。放射性栓塞治疗也会导致一过性淋巴细胞减少,大多数患者的淋巴细胞数会下降25%,甚至更多[82,83]。但并未证明淋巴细胞数的降低可导致患者出现感染。

四、总结

经研究证明,对于某些不可切除的肝脏肿瘤患者,放射性栓塞治疗具有缩小肿瘤和延长生存期的作用。虽然这是一种新兴的疗法,但越来越多的证据表明,相比其他现有疗法(例如 TAE、TACE、RFA),在治疗和提高患者生活质量方面,放射性栓塞治疗与前者疗效相当或更为有效。无论是原发性肝癌或者转移性肝癌中不可手术切除的患者,SIRT 均可提供一种疗效确切且可改善生存期的治疗方案。对于某些不可切除或移植的患者,SIRT 还可以通过缩小肿瘤或减少肿瘤数目使患者疾病分期下降,从而可接受肝脏切除术或肝移植。特别是对于结直肠癌肝转移患者,已证实,SIRT 作为有效的治疗选择,可联合化疗药物作为首选治疗,而对化疗失败的肿瘤患者为次选治疗方案,对于需要补救治疗的患者,也是一种有效的姑息治疗方案。最后,SIRT 在 NETLM 治疗上也显示出良好的效果,尤其对于已行手术切除的患者,或者病灶局限于一个肝叶的小肝癌患者。

SIRT 治疗具有上述优点和疗效的同时,也伴随其固有的并发症。然而,最近的证据显示,未来几年,SIRT 将在某些不可切除肝癌患者的治疗上发挥重要的作用。

参考文献

[1] Parkin DM, Bray F, Ferlay J, et al. Global cancer statistics, 2002. CA Cancer J Clin 2005;55:74-108.
[2] Siegel R, Naishadham D, Jemal A. Cancer statistics, 2013. CA Cancer J Clin 2013;63:11-30. Available at: http://apps.who.int/bookorders/anglais/detart1.jsp?codlan51&codcol576&codcch531&content51.

[3] Stewart BW, Wild CP. World Cancer Report 2014, vol. 13. World Health Organization; 2014.

[4] Andrews JC, Walker SC, Ackermann RJ, et al. Hepatic radioembolization with yttrium-90 containing glass microspheres: preliminary results and clinical follow-up. J Nucl Med 1994;35:1637-44.

[5] Bentrem DJ, Dematteo RP, Blumgart LH. Surgical therapy for metastatic disease to the liver. Annu Rev Med 2005;56:139-56.

[6] Bosch FX, Ribes J, Borras J. Epidemiology of primary liver cancer. Semin Liver Dis 1999;19:271-85. http://dx.doi.org/10.1055/s-2007-1007117.

[7] Chamberlain MN, Gray BN, Heggie JC, et al. Hepatic metastases-a physiological approach to treatment. Br J Surg 1983;70:596-8.

[8] Llovet JM, Ricci S, Mazzaferro V, et al. Sorafenib in advanced hepatocellular carcinoma. N Engl J Med 2008;359:378-90. http://dx.doi.org/10.1056/NEJMoa 0708857.

[9] Llovet JM, Real MI, Montana X, et al. Arterial embolisation or chemoembolisation versus symptomatic treatment in patients with unresectable hepatocellular carcinoma: a randomised controlled trial. Lancet 2002;359:1734-9. http://dx.doi.org/10.1016/S0140-6736(02)08649-X.

[10] Aliberti C, Tilli M, Benea G, et al. Trans-arterial chemoembolization (TACE) of liver metastases from colorectal cancer using irinotecan-eluting beads: preliminary results. Anticancer Res 2006;26:3793-5.

[11] Hendlisz A, Van den Eynde M, Peeters M, et al. Phase III trial comparing protracted intravenous fluorouracil infusion alone or with yttrium-90 resin microspheres radioembolization for liver-limited metastatic colorectal cancer refractory to standard chemotherapy. J Clin Oncol 2010;28:3687-94. http://dx.doi.org/10.1200/JCO.2010.28.5643 JCO.2010.28.5643.

[12] Kulik LM, Atassi B, van Holsbeeck L, et al. Yttrium-90 microspheres (Thera-Sphere) treatment of unresectable hepatocellular carcinoma: downstaging to resection, RFA and bridge to transplantation. J Surg Oncol 2006;94:572-86. http://dx.doi.org/10.1002/jso.20609.

[13] Sangro B, Carpanese L, Cianni R, et al. Survival after yttrium-90 resin microsphere radioembolization of hepatocellular carcinoma across Barcelona clinic liver cancer stages: a European evaluation. Hepatology 2011;54:868-78. http://dx.doi.org/10.1002/hep.24451.

[14] Sharma RA, Van Hazel GA, Morgan B, et al. Radioembolization of liver metastases from colorectal cancer using yttrium-90 microspheres with concomitant systemic oxaliplatin, fluorouracil, and leucovorin chemotherapy. J Clin Oncol 2007;25:1099-106. http://dx.doi.org/10.1200/jco.2006.08.7916.

[15] Vouche M, Habib A, Ward TJ, et al. Unresectable solitary hepatocellular carcinoma not amenable to radiofrequency ablation: multicenter radiologypathology correlation and survival of radiation segmentectomy. Hepatology 2014. http://dx.doi.org/10.1002/hep.27057.

[16] Dawson LA, Normolle D, Balter JM, et al. Analysis of radiation-induced liver disease using the Lyman NTCP model. Int J Radiat Oncol Biol Phys 2002;58:1318-9 [author reply: 1319-20].

[17] Goin JE, et al. Treatment of unresectable hepatocellular carcinoma with intrahepatic yttrium 90 microspheres: a risk-stratification analysis. J Vasc Interv Radiol 2005;16(2 Pt 1):195-203.

[18] Price TJ, Townsend A. Yttrium 90 microsphere selective internal radiation treatment of hepatic colorectal metastases. Arch Surg 2007;143:675-82.

[19] Kennedy AS, Nutting C, Coldwell D, et al. Pathologic response and microdosimetry of (90)Y microspheres in man: review of four explanted whole livers. Int J Radiat Oncol Biol Phys 2004;60:1552-63.

[20] Yorke ED, Jackson A, Fox RA, et al. Can current models explain the lack of liver complications in Y-90 microsphere therapy? Clin Cancer Res 1999;5:3024s-30s.

[21] Sato KT, Omary Ra, Takehana C, et al. The role of tumor vascularity in predicting survival after yttrium-90 radioembolization for liver metastases. J Vasc Interv Radiol 2009;20:1564-9. http://dx.doi.org/10.1016/j.jvir.2009.08.013.

[22] A comparison of lipiodol chemoembolization and conservative treatment for unresectable hepatocellular carcinoma. Groupe d'Etude et de Traitement du Carcinome Hepatocellulaire. N Engl J Med 1995;332:1256-61. http://dx.doi.org/10.1056/NEJM199505113321903.

[23] Peynircioglu B, Cil B, Bozkurt F, et al. Radioembolization for the treatment of unresectable liver cancer: initial experience at a single center. Diagn Interv Radiol 2010;16:70-8. http://dx.doi.org/10.4261/1305-3825.DIR.2693-09.1.

[24] Irving A. Radioactive isotopes for cancer therapy adjuvant. Arch Surg 1964;89:244-9.

[25] Vente AD. Microspheres for radioembolization of liver malignancies. Expert Rev Med Devices 2010;7:581-3.

[26] Riaz A, Lewandowski RJ, Kulik LM, et al. Complications following radioembolization with yttrium-90 microspheres: a comprehensive literature review. J Vasc IntervRadiol 2009;20:1121-30. http://dx.doi.org/10.1016/j.jvir.2009.05.030 S1051-0443(09)00578-8 [quiz: 1131].

[27] Urata K, Kawasaki S, Matsunami H, et al. Calculation of child and adult standard liver volume for liver transplantation. Hepatology 1995;21:1317-21.

[28] Ho S, Lau WY, Leung TW, et al. Partition model for estimating radiation doses from yttrium-90 microspheres in treating hepatic tumours. Eur J Nucl Med 1996;23:947-52.

[29] Kao YH, Hock Tan AE, Burgmans MC, et al. Image-guided personalized predictive dosimetry by artery-specific SPECT/CT partition modeling for safe and effective 90Y radioembolization. J Nucl Med 2012;53:559-66. http://dx.doi.org/10.2967/jnumed.111.097469.

[30] Ackerman NB, Lien WM, Kondi ES, et al. The blood supply of experimental liver metastases. I. The distribution of hepatic artery and portal vein blood to "small" and "large" tumors. Surgery 1969;66:1067-72.

[31] Kennedy A, Nag S, Salem R, et al. Recommendations for radioembolization of hepatic malignancies using yttrium-90 microsphere brachytherapy: a consensus panel report from the radioembolization brachytherapy oncology consortium. Int J Radiat Oncol Biol Phys 2007;68:13-23. http://dx.doi.org/10.1016/j.ijrobp.2006.11.060.

[32] Ahmadzadehfar H, Sabet A, Biermann K, et al. The significance of 99mTc-MAA SPECT/CT liver perfusion imaging in treatment planning for 90Y-microsphere selective internal radiation treatment. J Nucl Med 2010;51:1206-12. http://dx.doi.org/10.2967/jnumed.109.074559.

[33] Lambert B, Mertens J, Sturm EJ, et al. 99mTc-labelled macroaggregated albumin (MAA) scintigraphy for planning treatment with 90Y microspheres. Eur J Nucl Med Mol Imaging 2010;37:2328-33. http://dx.doi.org/10.1007/s00259-010-1566-2.

[34] Marn CS, Andrews JC, Francis IR, et al. Hepatic parenchymal changes after intraarterial Y-90 therapy: CT findings. Radiology 1993;187:125-8.

[35] Murthy R, Xiong H, Nunez R, et al. Yttrium 90 resin microspheres for the treatment of unresectable colorectal hepatic metastases after failure of multiple chemotherapy regimens: preliminary results. J Vasc Interv Radiol 2005;16:937-45. http://dx.doi.org/10.1097/01.RVI.0000161142.12822.66. pii:16/7/937.

[36] Lewandowski R, Thurston KG, Goin J, et al. 90Y microsphere (TheraSphere) treatment for unresectable colorectal cancer metastases of the liver: response to treatment at targeted doses of 135-150 gy as measured by [18F] Fluorodeoxyglucose positron emission tomography and computed tomographic imaging. J Vasc Interv Radiol 2005;16:1641-51.

[37] El-Serag HB. Hepatocellular carcinoma and hepatitis C in the United States. Hepatology 2002;36:S74-83. http://dx.doi.org/10.1053/jhep.2002.36807.

[38] Sangro B, Bilbao JI, Boan J, et al. Radioembolization using 90Y-resin microspheres for patients with advanced hepatocellular carcinoma. Int J Radiat Oncol Biol Phys 2006;66:792-800.

[39] Salem R, Lewandowski RJ, Mulcahy MF, et al. Radioembolization for hepatocellular carcinoma using Yttrium-90 microspheres: a comprehensive report of long-term outcomes. Gastroenterology 2010;138:52-64. http://dx.doi.org/10.1053/j.gastro.2009.09.006.

[40] Sangro B, Inarrairaegui M. Radioembolization for hepatocellular carcinoma: evidence-based answers to frequently asked questions. J Nucl Med Radiat Ther 2011;01:1-6. http://dx.doi.org/10.4172/2155-9619.1000110.

[41] Mazzaferro V, Sposito C, Bhoori S, et al. Yttrium-90 radioembolization for intermediate-advanced hepatocellular carcinoma: a phase 2 study. Hepatology 2013;57:1826-37. http://dx.doi.org/10.1002/hep.26014.

[42] Inarrairaegui M, Pardo F, Bilbao JI, et al. Response to radioembolization with yttrium-90 resin microspheres may allow surgical treatment with curative intent and prolonged survival in previously unresectable hepatocellular carcinoma. Eur J Surg Oncol 2012;38:594-601. http://dx.doi.org/10.1016/j.ejso.2012.02.189.

[43] Vouche M, Lewandowski RJ, Atassi R, et al. Radiation lobectomy: time-dependent analysis of future liver remnant volume in unresectable liver cancer as a bridge to resection. J Hepatol 2013. http://dx.doi.org/10.1016/j.jhep.2013.06.015.

[44] Salem R, Lewandowski RJ, Kulik L, et al. Radioembolization results in longer timeto-progression and reduced toxicity compared with chemoembolization in patients with hepatocellular carcinoma. Gastroenterology 2011;140:497-507.e492. http://dx.doi.org/10.1053/j.gastro.2010.10.049 S0016-5085(10)01587-8.

[45] Lance C, McLennan G, Obuchowski N, et al. Comparative analysis of the safety and efficacy of transcatheter arterial chemoembolization and yttrium-90 radioembolization in patients with unresectable hepatocellular carcinoma. J Vasc Interv Radiol 2011;22:1697-705. http://dx.doi.org/10.1016/j.jvir.2011.08.013.

[46] Steel J, Baum A, Carr B. Quality of life in patients diagnosed with primary hepatocellular carcinoma: hepatic arterial infusion of Cisplatin versus 90-Yttrium microspheres (Therasphere). Psychooncology 2004;13(2):73-9.

[47] Salem R, Gilbertsen M, Butt Z, et al. Increased quality of life among hepatocellular carcinoma patients treated with radioembolization, compared with chemoembolization. Clin Gastroenterol Hepatol 2013. ht-

tp://dx. doi. org/10. 1016/j. cgh. 2013. 04. 028.

[48] Abdelmaksoud MH, Louie JD, Hwang GL, et al. Yttrium - 90 radioembolization of renal cell carcinoma metastatic to the liver. J Vasc Interv Radiol 2012;23:323 - 30. e321. http://dx. doi. org/10. 1016/j. jvir. 2011. 11. 007.

[49] Jakobs TF, Hoffmann RT, Fischer T, et al. Radioembolization in patients with hepatic metastases from breast cancer. J Vasc Interv Radiol 2008;19:683 - 90. http://dx. doi. org/10. 1016/j. jvir. 2008. 01. 009.

[50] Mulcahy MF, Lewandowski RJ, Ibrahim SM, et al. Radioembolization of colorectal hepatic metastases using yttrium - 90 microspheres. Cancer 2009;115:1849 - 58. http://dx. doi. org/10. 1002/cncr. 24224.

[51] Rhee TK, Lewandowski RJ, Liu DM, et al. 90Y Radioembolization for metastatic neuroendocrine liver tumors: preliminary results from a multi - institutional experience. Ann Surg 2008;247:1029 - 35. http://dx. doi. org/10. 1097/SLA. 0b013e3181728a45.

[52] Luna - Perez P, Rodriguez - Coria DF, Arroyo B, et al. The natural history of liver metastases from colorectal cancer. Arch Med Res 1998;29:319 - 24.

[53] Kosmider S, Tan TH, Yip D, et al. Radioembolization in combination with systemic chemotherapy as first - line therapy for liver metastases from colorectal cancer. J Vasc Interv Radiol 2011;22:780 - 6. http://dx. doi. org/10. 1016/j. jvir. 2011. 02. 023.

[54] Chua TC, Bester L, Saxena A, et al. Radioembolization and systemic chemotherapy improves response and survival for unresectable colorectal liver metastases. J Cancer Res Clin Oncol 2011;137:865 - 73. http://dx. doi. org/10. 1007/s00432 - 010 - 0948 - y.

[55] Cosimelli M, Golfieri R, Cagol PP, et al. Multi - centre phase II clinical trial of yttrium - 90 resin microspheres alone in unresectable, chemotherapy refractory colorectal liver metastases. Br J Cancer 2010;103: 324 - 31. http://dx. doi. org/ 10. 1038/sj. bjc. 6605770.

[56] Nace GW, Steel JL, Amesur N, et al. Yttrium - 90 radioembolization for colorectal cancer liver metastases: a single institution experience. Int J Surg Oncol 2011; 2011:571261. http://dx. doi. org/10. 1155/2011/571261.

[57] Bester L, Meteling B, Pocock N, et al. Radioembolization versus standard care of hepatic metastases: comparative retrospective cohort study of survival outcomes and adverse events in salvage patients. J Vasc Interv Radiol 2012;23:96 - 105. http://dx. doi. org/10. 1016/j. jvir. 2011. 09. 028. pii:S1051 - 0443(11) 01344 - 3.

[58] Seidensticker R, Denecke T, Kraus P, et al. Matched - pair comparison of radioembolization plus best supportive care versus best supportive care alone for chemotherapy refractory liver - dominant colorectal metastases. Cardiovasc Intervent Radiol 2012;35:1066 - 73. http://dx. doi. org/10. 1007/s00270 - 011 - 0234 - 7.

[59] Memon K, Lewandowski RJ, Mulcahy MF, et al. Radioembolization for neuroendocrine liver metastases: safety, imaging, and long - term outcomes. Int J Radiat Oncol Biol Phys 2012;83:887 - 94. http://dx. doi. org/10. 1016/j. ijrobp. 2011. 07. 041.

[60] Kennedy AS, Dezarn WA, McNeillie P, et al. Radioembolization for unresectable neuroendocrine hepatic metastases using resin 90Y - microspheres: early results in 148 patients. Am J Clin Oncol 2008;31:271 - 9.

[61] Norton JA. Endocrine tumours of the gastrointestinal tract. Surgical treatment of neuroendocrine metasta-

ses. Best Pract Res Clin Gastroenterol 2005;19:577-83.

[62] Florman S, Toure B, Kim L, et al. Liver transplantation for neuroendocrine tumors. J Gastrointest Surg 2004;8:208-12.

[63] Berber E, Senagore A, Remzi F, et al. Laparoscopic radiofrequency ablation of liver tumors combined with colorectal procedures. Surg Laparosc Endosc Percutan Tech 2004;14:186-90.

[64] Bilchik AJ, Sarantou T, Foshag LJ, et al. Cryosurgical palliation of metastatic neuroendocrine tumors resistant to conventional therapy. Surgery 1997;122:1040-7 [discussion:1047-8]. pii:S0039-6060(97)90207-5.

[65] Nijsen F, Rook D, Brandt C, et al. Targeting of liver tumour in rats by selective delivery of holmium-166 loaded microspheres: a biodistribution study. Eur J Nucl Med 2001;28:743-9.

[66] Cao CQ, Yan TD, Bester L, et al. Radioembolization with yttrium microspheres for neuroendocrine tumour liver metastases. Br J Surg 2010;97:537-43. http://dx.doi.org/10.1002/bjs.6931.

[67] Paprottka PM, Hoffmann R-T, Haug A, et al. Radioembolization of symptomatic, unresectable neuroendocrine hepatic metastases using yttrium-90 microspheres. Cardiovasc Intervent Radiol 2012;35:334-42. http://dx.doi.org/10.1007/s00270-011-0248-1.

[68] Shaheen M, Hassanain M, Aljiffry M, et al. Predictors of response to radioembolization (TheraSphere) treatment of neuroendocrine liver metastasis. HPB (Oxford) 2012;14:60-6. http://dx.doi.org/10.1111/j.1477-2574.2011.00405.x.

[69] King J, Quinn R, Glenn DM, et al. Radioembolization with selective internal radiation microspheres for neuroendocrine liver metastases. Cancer 2008;113:921-9. http://dx.doi.org/10.1002/cncr.23685.

[70] Park J, Kim MH, Kim KP, et al. Natural history and prognostic factors of advanced cholangiocarcinoma without surgery, chemotherapy, or radiotherapy: a largescale observational study. Gut Liver 2009;3:298-305. http://dx.doi.org/10.5009/gnl.2009.3.4.298.

[71] Sagawa N, Kondo S, Morikawa T, et al. Effectiveness of radiation therapy after surgery for hilar cholangiocarcinoma. Surg Today 2005;35:548-52. http://dx.doi.org/10.1007/s00595-005-2989-4.

[72] Metz JM. The role of radiation therapy in intrahepatic cholangiocarcinoma. Cancer J 2006;12:102-4.

[73] Mouli S, Memon K, Baker T, et al. Yttrium-90 radioembolization for intrahepatic cholangiocarcinoma: safety, response, and survival analysis. J Vasc Interv Radiol 2013;24:1227-34. http://dx.doi.org/10.1016/j.jvir.2013.02.031. pii:S1051-0443(13)00719-7.

[74] Rafi S, Piduru SM, El-Rayes B, et al. Yttrium-90 radioembolization for unresectable standard-chemorefractory intrahepatic cholangiocarcinoma: survival, efficacy, and safety study. Cardiovasc Intervent Radiol 2013;36:440-8. http://dx.doi.org/10.1007/s00270-012-0463-4.

[75] Sangro B, Gil-Alzugaray B, Rodriguez J, et al. Liver disease induced by radioembolization of liver tumors: description and possible risk factors. Cancer 2008;112:1538-46. http://dx.doi.org/10.1002/cncr.23339.

[76] Kennedy AS, McNeillie P, Dezarn WA, et al. Treatment parameters and outcome in 680 treatments of internal radiation with resin 90Y-microspheres for unresectable hepatic tumors. Int J Radiat Oncol Biol Phys 2009;74:1494-500.

[77] Young JY, Rhee TK, Atassi B, et al. Radiation dose limits and liver toxicities resulting from multiple yttrium-90 radioembolization treatments for hepatocellular carcinoma. J Vasc Interv Radiol 2007;18:1375

-82. http://dx.doi.org/10.1016/j.jvir.2007.07.016. pii:18/11/1375.

[78] Atassi B, Bangash AK, Lewandowski RJ, et al. Biliary sequelae following radioembolization with Yttrium-90 microspheres. J Vasc Interv Radiol 2008;19:691-7. http://dx.doi.org/10.1016/j.jvir.2008.01.003. pii:S1051-0443(08)00092-4.

[79] Carretero C, Munoz-Navas M, Betes M, et al. Gastroduodenal injury after radioembolization of hepatic tumors. Am J Gastroenterol 2007;102:1216-20. http://dx.doi.org/10.1111/j.1572-0241.2007.01172.x. pii:AJG1172.

[80] Leung TW, Lau WY, Ho SK, et al. Radiation pneumonitis after selective internal radiation treatment with intraarterial 90yttrium-microspheres for inoperable hepatic tumors. Int J Radiat Oncol Biol Phys 1995;40:583-92.

[81] Salem R, Parikh P, Atassi B, et al. Incidence of radiation pneumonitis after hepatic intra-arterial radiotherapy with yttrium-90 microspheres assuming uniform lung distribution. Am J Clin Oncol 2008;31:431-8.

[82] Carr BI. Hepatic arterial 90Yttrium glass microspheres (Therasphere) for unresectable hepatocellular carcinoma: interim safety and survival data on 65 patients. Liver Transpl 2004;10:S107-10. http://dx.doi.org/10.1002/lt.20036.

[83] Salem R, Lewandowski RJ, Atassi B, et al. Treatment of unresectable hepatocellular carcinoma with use of 90Y microspheres (TheraSphere): safety, tumor response, and survival. J Vasc Interv Radiol 2005;16:1627-39.

第十章　肝细胞癌和胆管癌的系统性治疗

Vincent Chung, MD

【关键词】

肝细胞癌；胆管癌；化疗；分子靶向

要点

- 肝细胞癌是世界上致死率位居第二的癌症。
- 索拉非尼是系统治疗肝细胞癌最有效的药物。
- 吉西他滨和顺铂联合使用是胆管癌的标准化疗方案。
- 对致癌重要信号通路的了解已经取得了显著的进步，也引导开展了许多有意义的临床研究。

一、概述

肝癌是一个日益严重的问题。在美国，从 2006—2010 年，肝癌的发病率增长了 4%，2014 年预计新发人数为 33 190 例。肝癌可起源于肝细胞，并向肝细胞癌发展，也可起源于肝内胆管细胞，向胆管癌发展。肝癌治疗需要一个多学科团队（包括外科医生、消化科医生、放射科医生、肿瘤科医生）协作，才能达到最好的治疗效果。本文讨论了肝癌化疗方案的选择标准。

作者无其他声明。

Department of Medical Oncology and Therapeutics Research, City of Hope, 1500 East Duarte Road, Duarte, CA 91010, USA

E-mail address: vchung@coh.org

二、肝细胞癌

(一) 简介

肝细胞癌一直是一个全球性问题,每年都有超过74.5万人罹患肝癌。肝癌的致死率位居第二,仅次于肺癌,大多数肝癌患者位于东亚和撒哈拉以南非洲地区。在美国,每年有将近2.7万人被确诊为肝癌,并且人数在逐渐增长[1]。

肝癌的区域性差异很可能是由肝炎的区域性差异引起的。在亚洲,父母到孩子可垂直传播乙型肝炎。黄曲霉毒素是黄曲霉或寄生曲霉所产生的一种霉菌毒素,在发展中国家,也是一种致病的主要原因。黄曲霉毒素在湿度高的地区会污染库存的玉米、花生和黄豆。而较年轻的群体罹患肝细胞癌,则正是因为他们从小暴露在黄曲霉毒素的环境中。在美国,大多数肝癌患者是由丙型肝炎或酒精性肝硬化发展而来,并且多发生在高龄群体,与此同时,非酒精性脂肪肝致肝细胞癌比例在上升[2]。

(二) 肝细胞癌的分子靶向治疗

了解癌症的生物学是指导治疗的基础。癌症的发展是一个多步骤的过程,包括抑癌基因的突变或突变导致信号通路组成性激活。本文不对信号通路作完整的讨论,但 Ras/Raf/MAPK(丝裂原活化蛋白激酶)通路是肝癌发生机制中最重要的信号通路之一[3]。表皮生长因子、血小板衍生生长因子和血管内皮生长因子与细胞表面受体的结合通过 Ras 蛋白家族的激活触发了信号级联反应(图10-1)。因为它是调控细胞增殖的重要通路,这条信号通路通常会作为治疗的潜在靶点。

(三) 索拉非尼

索拉非尼是一种多激酶抑制剂,其靶向 Ras/MAPK 通路中 Raf-1 丝氨酸-苏氨酸激酶同时也有抗血管生成的作用。在索拉非尼的Ⅰ期临床试验中,根据 RECIST 标准,1 例患者对索拉非尼具有药物客观反应。在后续的Ⅱ期研究中,137 例未接受治疗、Child-Pugh A 级或 B 级肝癌患者进行了索拉非尼治疗。以往接受传统细胞毒性药物化疗的中位生存期是 6 个月,但此研究的中位生存期是 9.2 个月。这个研究结果使得国际Ⅲ期 SHARP 试验(索拉非尼治疗肝细胞癌随机协议)继续进行,这项试验对 602 例患有晚期肝细胞癌(不能行手术治疗或局部治疗;在手术治疗或局部治疗后疾病进展)但肝功能较好的患者进行研究,将其随机分配到索拉非尼组(400mg,每日 2 次)或安慰剂组。这项研究在欧洲、南美和澳大利亚实施。大约 20% 患者患有乙型肝炎,30% 患有丙型肝炎,25% 患有酒精性肝硬化。主要观察终点是总生存期和症状进展时间。这项试验将研究对象限于 Child-Pugh A 级肝癌患者,因其生存期更短。SHARP 试验结果表明,索拉非尼组患者的生存期为 10.7 个月,相比安慰剂组生存期(7.9 个月)有统计学意义。尽管 SHARP 试验并不是为了评估不同分组中索拉非尼的疗效,但是,通过对丙型肝炎相关肝癌患者的研究表明,索拉非尼组的总生存期是 14 个月,优于安慰剂组

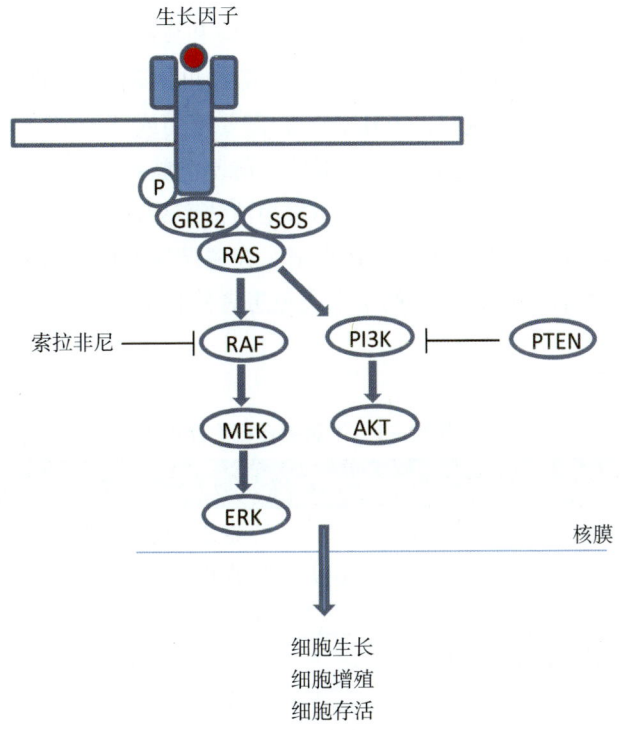

图 10-1　Ras/Raf/MAPK 信号通路。PI3K,磷脂酰肌醇-3-羟激酶

(7.9 个月)。另一个平行试验在亚洲进行。这个试验将 226 例来自中国、韩国和台湾的 Child-Pugh A 级肝硬化肝癌患者随机分配到索拉非尼组或安慰剂组。索拉非尼组的生存受益是 6.5 个月,对比安慰剂组的 4.2 个月,有统计学意义。但是,这个结果仍然比 SHARP 试验所观察到的 10.7 个月短得多。造成这种差异的可能原因是,亚洲试验中大多数患者都患有乙型肝炎,而 SHARP 试验中丙型肝炎患者更多。因为索拉非尼是 Raf-1 激酶的抑制剂,所以丙型肝炎中激活 Raf-1 信号的核心蛋白对索拉非尼更敏感。2007 年 11 月 16 日,美国食品药品监督管理局(FDA)批准了索拉非尼可用于治疗不可切除的肝细胞癌患者[4]。

1. 索拉非尼毒性的处理

(1)腹泻

在 SHARP 试验中,索拉非尼组治疗相关的副作用的发生率是 80%,安慰剂组为 52%,但两组的停药率接近。胃肠道毒性反应是最为常见的副作用,大部分患者都出现腹泻。其中酪氨酸激酶抑制剂索拉非尼诱导腹泻的一个机制是胰腺功能不全。有一项研究对粪便的脂肪含量进行检测并发现其增高,这一结果支持胰腺外分泌功能不足的假设。脂肪吸收不良导致食物经过时间过快,维生素 D 不足、继发性甲状旁腺功能亢进。油腻饮食会增加排便的次数,对这类患者而言,胰酶有助于降低排便的频率[5]。对大多数患者可使用抗动力药对症处理,如洛哌丁胺,可延缓食物经过时间,舒缓纵向平滑肌的运动,使水的吸收更为缓慢。

(2) 手足综合征

索拉非尼另一个常见的毒副作用是手足皮肤反应和皮疹,这类毒副作用足以达到停药的标准。其典型表现是皮肤干燥、黄斑/丘疹。掌跖部位可出现红斑,严重者会有水疱和脱屑。早期皮肤护理是治疗得以持续进行的基础,否则,需要停药或减少用药剂量。患者开始服用索拉非尼时需经常使用保湿乳液,尤其是手足部位。脲基润肤霜的效果很好,可预防容易引起感染的皮肤皲裂。不能接触刺激性化学物质,如家用清洁产品,穿柔软的鞋子以减少摩擦。根据索拉非尼的毒性等级,表10-1提供了剂量指南。在遵循这份指南的情况下,多数患者可以耐受索拉非尼治疗。可暂停治疗或减少剂量来避免患者停止治疗。在SHARP试验中,11%的患者因副作用停止了治疗。

表 10-1 手足综合征治疗指南

皮肤毒副作用级别	出现次数	建议调整剂量
级别1:麻木,感觉迟钝、异常,刺痛,无痛肿胀,红疹,或手足不适,但不影响正常活动	任何时间	继续使用索拉非尼治疗,考虑局部治疗以缓解症状
级别2:红疹疼痛,手脚肿胀、不适,影响患者正常活动	首次出现	继续使用索拉非尼治疗,考虑局部治疗以缓解症状
	7天内无改善或第二次、三次出现	如7天内无改善,参考下列索拉非尼中断治疗,直到毒副作用降至0~1级。当治疗继续时,将索拉非尼用量降至1级(每天400mg或隔天400mg)
	第四次出现	停止使用索拉非尼治疗
级别3:湿性蜕皮,溃疡,起疱,手足剧痛,或极度不适,无法正常工作、活动	第一、二次出现	中断索拉非尼治疗直到毒副作用降至0~1级。当治疗继续时,将索拉非尼用量降至1级(每天400mg或隔天400mg)
	第三次出现	停止使用索拉非尼治疗

(数据来自 Nexavar® (sorafenib) [package insert]. West Haven, CT: Bayer Healthcare; 2005.)

(3) 高血压

高血压是索拉非尼治疗过程中常见的不良反应之一,这是由于抑制了VEGF而导致的药效学反应。治疗开始后,一氧化氮生成减少,导致血管张力增加。血管张力的增加是可逆的,但可能会造成永久性内皮损伤,而即使治疗停止之后,高血压仍存在。高血压通常在治疗早期即会出现,多数患者的症状可用标准降压治疗控制。开始治疗后,患者最初6周需检测血压。收缩压>140mmHg和舒张压>90mmHg时,需进行药物降压治疗。如接受药物治疗后高血压仍持续,则需停药甚至考虑永久停用索拉非尼治疗[6]。

2. 治疗难点

晚期肝癌患者治疗的难点在于他们不但患有癌症,还患有肝脏疾病。大多数患者是由肝硬化发展成肝细胞癌,而且肝功能储备较少。Child-Pugh 评分最初是用于预测外科手术后的死亡率,但现已成为确定系统治疗的预后指标(表 10-2)。在决定治疗方案时应始终考虑到化疗的肝毒性。

表 10-2 Child-Pugh 分级

评分	1	2	3
胆红素(mg/dl)	<2	2~3	>3
血清白蛋白(g/dl)	>3.5	2.8~3.5	<2.8
INR	<1.7	1.7~2.3	>2.3
脑病	无	1~2 级	2~3 级
腹水	无	轻微	中度
A 级,5~6 分(1 年生存期,100%;2 年生存期,85%)			
B 级,7~9 分(1 年生存期,81%;2 年生存期,57%)			
C 级,10~15 分(1 年生存期,45%;2 年生存期,35%)			

手术是唯一的治愈手段,但是,许多患者因肝功能受损并不适合手术治疗。对那些患有晚期肝脏肿瘤,并且肝细胞癌特点符合米兰标准(单个病灶≤5cm,3 个病灶中每个病灶≤3cm)的患者,肝脏移植则是另一种可能治愈的手段,大概有 75% 患者经肝移植后痊愈[7,8]。旧金山加州大学扩充了米兰标准,允许病灶大小达到 6.5cm 的患者行肝移植术,生存期与符合米兰标准行肝移植术的患者相似。但是,肝脏供体是一种稀缺资源,许多患者只能进行姑息治疗或全身治疗。

索拉非尼是不可手术或肝脏栓塞治疗失败的标准治疗药物,并且是 CCN 指南对 Child-Pugh A 级患者的 1 类推荐药物。对 Child-Pugh B 级患者,索拉非尼是 2A 类推荐药物;对 Child-Pugh C 级患者,不建议使用索拉非尼治疗。索拉非尼的代谢依赖细胞色素 P-450 系统和 UDP-葡萄糖醛酸。Child-Pugh A 级和 B 级患者的药代动力学特征相似。为了更好地了解索拉非尼的毒性,有研究者开展了 GIDEON(肝癌治疗决策和索拉非尼治疗的全球性调查)试验。这是在非干预的真实情况下评估索拉非尼的安全性,尤其针对 Child-Pugh B 级患者。超过 3000 例患者接受了调查,结果显示,Child-Pugh B 级患者的药物相关性副作用比 Child-Pugh A 级患者更为严重(14.1% vs 8.8%),停药率更高(40% vs 25%),但两者的总体安全性类似。因为接受索拉非尼治疗的患者中超过 50% 出现了肝功能恶化,这对 Child-Pugh C 级患者的影响更大,并且由于自身肝脏病灶和全身治疗的生存获益甚小,此类患者的生存期往往较短。同时,这组患者对全身治疗的耐受性并不高,所以并不建议使用全身治疗。

3. 其他药物的试验尝试

这段时间里，在索拉非尼作为一线分子靶向治疗的标准下，多种小分子酪氨酸激酶抑制剂或 VEGF 单抗被研发，一项Ⅲ期临床试验证实，这些药物可延长生存期。在一些Ⅱ期试验中，发现贝伐单抗、舒尼替尼、布立尼布等药物有显著的作用，但没有一项治疗优于Ⅲ期试验中使用的索拉非尼（表 10-3）。本节讨论其他一些重要的药物作用分子途径和在临床试验实施时所遇到的困难。

表 10-3　关键的肝细胞癌Ⅲ期临床试验

试验	数量	总生存期
索拉非尼 vs 安慰剂		
SHARP[4]	602	10.7 vs 7.9 个月，HR = 0.69；P = 0.00058
亚太[11]	226	6.5 vs 4.2 个月，HR = 0.68；P = 0.014
索拉非尼 vs 贝伐单抗		
BRISK – FL[10]	1150	9.5 vs 9.9 个月，HR = 1.06；P = 0.31
索拉非尼 vs 舒尼替尼		
SUN[9]	1074	10.2 vs 7.2 个月，HR = 1.3；P = 0.001
索拉非尼 vs Linifanib		
LIGHT[12]	1035	9.8 vs 9.1 个月，HR = 1.05；P = NS
索拉非尼 vs 索拉非尼联合埃罗替尼		
SEARCH[13]	720	8.5 vs 9.5 个月，HR = 1.13；P = 0.91

HR：危险比；NS：无显著性差异

舒尼替尼是一种靶向血管内皮生长因子受体 1（VEGFR1）、VEGFR2、血小板衍生生长因子受体（PDGFR）-α/β、干细胞因子、类 Fms - 酪氨酸激酶 3 和转染重排（RET）的口服多激酶抑制剂，在早期临床试验中作用明显，毒性也小。但舒尼替尼治疗的预后较差，非亚洲患者的预后比索拉非尼组差很多。可能原因为，亚洲国家中引起肝癌最主要的原因是乙型肝炎，在西方国家则是丙型肝炎。被丙型肝炎感染的组织会激活 Raf-1/MEK 和胞外信号调节激酶途径，引起细胞增殖。因为索拉非尼抑制 Raf-1 激酶，但舒尼替尼不会，所以相比之下，索拉非尼对丙型肝炎患者的疗效更好[9]。Ⅲ期索拉非尼和舒尼替尼疗效对比试验因无价值而被终止。

成纤维细胞生长因子受体（FGF）也具有促进血管生成的重要作用，布立尼布是 VEGF 和 FGF 的小分子抑制剂。BRISK-FL 研究将不可切除的晚期肝癌患者随机分配到索拉非尼或布立尼布组，主要观察终点是总生存期非劣效性。虽然两种药物的抗肿瘤活性相似，但试验没有达到研究终点，并且，布立尼布的耐受性没有索拉非尼高。在索拉非尼组，与副作用相关的停药率是 33%，布立尼布组是 43%[10]。人们对许多种新药都进行研究，但迄今为止没有任何一种药物优于索拉非尼。

肝细胞生长因子(HGF)通过调节细胞的生长和运动在血管生成和肿瘤生成的过程中扮演重要的角色。HGF 与 c-met 受体结合后,激活信号级联反应,影响多个信号转导途径。在正常肝脏中,HGF/c-met 促进肝细胞的增殖和再生,但在肝癌中,c-met 的功能得到放大,激活 RAS 信号通路。磷脂酰肌醇 3 激酶(PI3K)是转录、wnt 和 Notch 通路的信号传感器和活化剂。因为这条信号通路在细胞增殖和转移中起着重要作用,许多公司针对它合成了小分子抑制剂,如卡博替尼、tivantinib、foretinib。在针对不可切除肝癌患者的Ⅱ期试验中,这些药物显示出一定的效果。在亚组分析中,免疫组化 c-met 表达阳性,与总生存期从 3.8 个月延长至 7.2 个月有关($P=0.01$)。这项将 c-met 表达阳性的肝癌患者随机分配到 tivantinib 或安慰剂组Ⅲ期临床研究正在进行中。

4. 索拉非尼相关的肝脏定向治疗

肝癌组织的供血大多数来自肝动脉,这使得有局部病灶的患者非常适于进行肝脏定向治疗。为肿瘤供血血管的选择性定位可以在血流中断时,使化疗药物直接输送到肿瘤部位。这种治疗方式可以保护正常的肝细胞。以往的研究表明,1 年和 2 年生存率分别是 82% 和 63%,中位生存时间超过 30 个月。肝动脉化疗栓塞术(TACE)只能延缓肿瘤的生长,几项 TACE 和口服索拉非尼联用的试验正在进行。在日本和韩国的试验中,458 例患有不可切除的肝癌患者在 TACE 术后被随机分配到索拉非尼组(400mg,每日 2 次)或安慰剂组。研究并没有到达疾病进展时间的主要观察终点,可能是因为 73% 患者要求减少剂量,这个比例远远高于 SHARP 试验。同时,大多数分配到索拉非尼组的患者在最初至少 2 个月都未开始治疗。试验过程中,给予索拉非尼是为了防止因 TACE 术引起缺氧而导致 VEGF 升高。还有一些临床试验正在测试索拉非尼和肝脏定向治疗结合的效果(表 10-4)。

表 10-4 索拉非尼联合肝脏定向治疗试验

试验	试验编号
索拉非尼联合放射治疗	NCT00892658
索拉非尼联合 SBRT 治疗	NCT01801163
索拉非尼 ± 质子束放疗	NCT01141478
RFA 前索拉非尼治疗	NCT00813293
索拉非尼联合 TACE 治疗	NCT01556815,NCT00768937 NCT00855218,NCT01829035

RFA:射频消融术;SBRT:体部立体定向放射治疗

(四)细胞毒化疗药物

多柔比星一直是肝癌化疗研究中受到最多关注的药物。在每隔 3 周 $75mg/m^2$ 的剂量下,有 8% 患者的肿瘤缩小了至少 25%。与最佳支持治疗相比,多柔比星还可带来生存获益。在过去,这是不可切除肝细胞癌的标准治疗药物。但是,多柔比星的毒性限制了其使用。在临床中,超过400mg/m^{2}的累积剂量会明显增加心脏损伤和心肌病的风险。也有可能发生中性粒细胞减少,这在胆道梗阻情况下会引起败血症。索拉非尼治疗失败后可应用多柔比星,也有一项临床研究将患者随机分配到索拉非尼组、索拉非尼和多柔比星联用组(NCT01015833)。

5-氟尿嘧啶具有很广泛的活性,在肝功能不全时可使用。胆红素高于5mg/dl的患者不推荐使用5-氟尿嘧啶,胆红素低于5mg/dl时可将5-氟尿嘧啶的剂量降至一半。因为当联用奥沙利铂以提高疗效时,应答率大概为20%,但生存期只有4个月[14]。在亚洲的一项研究中,371名患者被随机分配到FOLFOX组(5-氟尿嘧啶、甲酰四氢叶酸、奥沙利铂)或多柔比星组,结果表明,与多柔比星5个月的生存期相比,FOLFOX组生存期有所改善,为6.4个月($P=0.07$)[15]。一项器官功能障碍研究曾对奥沙利铂进行了测试,发现在任何程度肝功能不全的情况下,都可以使用标准剂量[16]。鉴于肝癌全身治疗手段较少,5-氟尿嘧啶或FOLFOX方案通常用于难治性疾病。现在的方向是针对c-met和VEGF通路以及免疫治疗(表10-5)。

表10-5 索拉非尼治疗失败后二线临床试验

试验编号	试验	作用机制
NCT01908426,NCT01737827	Cabozantinib(XL184),INC280	c-met
NCT01774344	Regorafenib	VEGF, Ret, Kit, PDGFR, Raf
NCT01752933	SGI-110	DNA甲基转移酶抑制剂
NCT01375569	TRC105	内皮糖蛋白(CD105)
NCT01777594	G-202	毒胡萝卜素前体药物
NCT01628640	肿瘤内注射疱疹性口炎病毒表达人β干扰素修饰的疫苗病毒	溶瘤病毒
NCT02089763	聚乙二醇重组人精氨酸酶1	精氨酸枯竭

三、胆管癌

(一)简介

胆管癌是较少见的癌症,起源于肝内胆管的上皮细胞,在胃肠道恶性肿瘤中仅占3%。在美国,每年有6600例肝内胆管癌新增病例,并且发病率在逐渐升高[1]。但是,大部分患者在诊断时已是晚期,只能接受全身治疗。

(二)细胞毒化疗

吉西他滨是对多种恶性肿瘤具有广泛作用的核苷类似物。通过在DNA复制的时候整合入链,引起链终止和细胞凋亡。吉西他滨也有核糖核苷酸还原酶抑制剂的功能,在 DNA 复制时阻止脱氧核糖核苷酸的合成。吉西他滨的毒性不大,最常见的副作用是骨髓抑制。恶心、呕吐可用药物控制,疲倦症状通常较轻微。吉西他滨作为单一药物治疗胆管癌时,副作用发生率在 7%~24%。在小样本Ⅱ期研究中,吉西他滨治疗患者的总生存期在 8~13 个月。后续的研究以吉西他滨为基础药物进行联合治疗。

一项欧洲研究的化疗方案联用了吉西他滨和顺铂(ABC-01)。86 例患者被随机分配,一组以 28 天为周期在第 1、8、15 天时给予吉西他滨 1000mg/m²,另一组以 21 天为周期在第 1、8 天时给予吉西他滨 1000mg/m² 和顺铂 25mg/m²。联用顺铂组嗜睡的发生率较高(28.6% vs 9.1%),但停药率并未增加。研究结果表明,没有完全应答的病例,只有部分应答的病例,联用顺铂组的疾病稳定率较高[17]。这个较为满意的研究结果使得Ⅲ期 ABC-02 试验得以开展,其目的是验证总生存期是否有改善。410 例局部晚期或转移性胆管癌、胆囊癌、壶腹癌患者被随机分配到两组。联用顺铂组的总生存期是 11.7 个月,吉西他滨组则为 8.1 个月(危险比 0.64,95% 可信区间 0.52~0.80;$P < 0.001$)[18]。基于这个大型Ⅲ期临床试验,吉西他滨和顺铂成为标准药物和后续临床试验的主体药物。

5-氟尿嘧啶一直是胃肠道恶性肿瘤化疗方案的主体药物。作为单一用药,5-氟尿嘧啶治疗胆道癌的疗效并不明显。但一项Ⅱ期临床试验中,治疗方案连续 14 天使用卡培他滨(650mg/m²,每日 2 次),并在第 1、8 天联用吉西他滨 1000mg/m²,结果 3 例完全应答。应答率达到 22/75,总生存期是 12.7 个月[19]。但是,并没有对吉西他滨和顺铂的疗效直接比较。

奥沙利铂在胃肠道恶性肿瘤治疗中应用广泛,除了神经病变外,耐受性良好。几项Ⅱ期试验在不同时间联用不同剂量的吉西他滨和奥沙利铂。在第 1、8、15 天给予吉西他滨,在第 1、15 天给予奥沙利铂。最大规模试验方案是每 2 周在第 1 天给予吉西他滨 1000mg/m²,第 2 天给予奥沙利铂 100mg/m²。有 73 例患者参加此试验,其中 73% 患有转移性癌症。非胆囊癌组的客观应答率是 20.5%,胆囊癌组则为 4.3%。36% 患者疾病稳定,中位生存期是 8.8 个月[20]。另一项Ⅱ期临床试验证实了奥沙利铂的化疗效果,但现在的标准方案仍然是吉西他滨联合顺铂化疗。要改变联合用药方案,需先进行奥沙利铂的毒性试验。

(三)胆管癌的分子靶向治疗

表皮生长因子受体(EGFR)对引起细胞增殖、血管生成、侵袭和转移的细胞内下游信号有重要意义。EGFR 有 4 个酪氨酸激酶受体:EGFR(ErbB-1)、HER2/c-neu(ErbB-2)、Her3(ErbB-3)、Her4(ErbB-4)。受体与配体结合后引起酪氨酸激酶受体的二聚化和随后的磷酸化。因为 50% 的胆管癌都过度表达 EGFR,对厄洛替尼的临床试验得以开展[21]。但是,一个 GEMOX 和无厄洛替尼随机临床试验并未在无进展生存期方面达到主要观察终点。联合厄洛替尼治疗的应答率更高,但仍需进一步的研究来确定应答标记物[22]。另一条正在研究的信号通路是 c-Met。c-Met 是一个编码 HGF 受体的原癌基因,对胚胎发育至关重要。但是,HGF 受体的异常激活导致肿瘤生长、血管生成和转移[23,24]。一个针对晚期胆管癌患者的卡博替尼Ⅱ期临床研究正在进行中(表 10-6)。

表 10-6　胆管癌临床试验

试验	作用机制
Cabozantinib（XL184）	c-met
Regorafenib	VEGF, Ret, Kit, PDGFR, Raf
Sunitinib	VEGF
Trametinib	MEK1/2
Pazopanib + GSK1120212	VEGF and MEK1/2
Gem/Cis + panitumumab	EGFR
Gem/Cis + bevacizumab	VEGF

四、小结

了解肝癌生成的核心信号通路,使肝细胞癌的治疗进入一个新时代。已证实索拉非尼是晚期肝癌的一线分子靶向治疗药物,并且是所有治疗的基准。迄今为止,没有任何一种药物优于索拉非尼。对胆管癌而言,细胞毒性化疗仍然是晚期肿瘤的主要治疗方案,目前为止,未有经 FDA 批准可用于胆管癌的分子靶向药物。本着个体化治疗的目标,临床试验试图研发阻断信号通路的药物及其衍生物。如果临床医生能够针对细胞的增殖机制,尽量将治疗的毒性最小化,患者的生存期和生活质量将会得到显著的改善。

参考文献

[1] American Cancer Society. Cancer facts & figures 2014. Atlanta（GA）：American Cancer Society；2014.

[2] White DL, Kanwal F, El-Serag HB. Association between nonalcoholic fatty liver disease and risk for hepatocellular cancer, based on systematic review. Clin Gastroenterol Hepatol 2012；10（12）：1342-59.e2.

[3] Llovet JM, Bruix J. Molecular targeted therapies in hepatocellular carcinoma. Hepatology 2008；48（4）：1312-27.

[4] Llovet JM, Ricci S, Mazzaferro V, et al. Sorafenib in advanced hepatocellular carcinoma. N Engl J Med 2008；359（4）：378-90.

[5] Mir O, Coriat R, Boudou-Rouquette P, et al. Sorafenib-induced diarrhea and hypophosphatemia：mechanisms and therapeutic implications. Ann Oncol 2012；23（1）：280-1.

[6] Maitland ML, Kasza KE, Karrison T, et al. Ambulatory monitoring detects sorafenibinduced blood pressure elevations on the first day of treatment. Clin Cancer Res 2009；15（19）：6250-7.

[7] Mazzaferro V, Bhoori S, Sposito C, et al. Milan criteria in liver transplantation for hepatocellular carcinoma：an evidence-based analysis of 15 years of experience. Liver Transpl 2011；17（Suppl 2）：S44-57.

[8] Lim KC, Chow PK, Allen JC, et al. Systematic review of outcomes of liver resection for early hepatocel-

lular carcinoma within the Milan criteria. Br J Surg 2012;99(12):1622-9.

[9] Cheng AL, Kang YK, Lin DY, et al. Sunitinib versus sorafenib in advanced hepatocellular cancer: results of a randomized phase III trial. J Clin Oncol 2013;31(32): 4067-75.

[10] Johnson PJ, Qin S, Park JW, et al. Brivanib versus sorafenib as first-line therapy in patients with unresectable, advanced hepatocellular carcinoma: results from the randomized phase III BRISK-FL study. J Clin Oncol 2013;31(28):3517-24.

[11] Cheng AL, Kang YK, Chen Z, et al. Efficacy and safety of sorafenib in patients in the Asia-Pacific region with advanced hepatocellular carcinoma: a phase III randomised, double-blind, placebo-controlled trial. Lancet Oncol 2009;10(1):25-34.

[12] Cainap C, Qin S, Huang W-T, et al. Phase III trial of linifanib versus sorafenib in patients with advanced hepatocellular carcinoma (HCC) [abstract 249]. J Clin Oncol 2013;30(suppl 34).

[13] Zhu A, Rosmorduc O, Evans J, et al. Search: a phase III, randomized, doubleblind, placebo-controlled trial of sorafenib plus erlotinib in patients with hepatocellular carcinoma (HCC). ESMO, [abstract 917].

[14] Tetef M, Doroshow J, Akman S, et al. 5-Fluorouracil and high-dose calcium leucovorin for hepatocellular carcinoma: a phase II trial. Cancer Invest 1995;13(5): 460-3.

[15] Qin S, Bai Y, Lim HY, et al. Randomized, multicenter, open-label study of oxaliplatin plus fluorouracil/leucovorin versus doxorubicin as palliative chemotherapy in patients with advanced hepatocellular carcinoma from Asia. J Clin Oncol 2013;31(28);3501-8.

[16] Doroshow JH, Synold TW, Gandara D, et al. Pharmacology of oxaliplatin in solid tumor patients with hepatic dysfunction: a preliminary report of the National Cancer Institute Organ Dysfunction Working Group. Semin Oncol 2003;30(4 Suppl 15):14-9.

[17] Valle JW, Wasan H, Johnson P, et al. Gemcitabine alone or in combination with cisplatin in patients with advanced or metastatic cholangiocarcinomas or other biliary tract tumours: a multicentre randomised phase II study - The UK ABC-01 Study. Br J Cancer 2009;101(4):621-7.

[18] Valle J, Wasan H, Palmer DH, et al. Cisplatin plus gemcitabine versus gemcitabine for biliary tract cancer. N Engl J Med 2010;362(14):1273-81.

[19] Knox JJ, Hedley D, Oza A, et al. Combining gemcitabine and capecitabine in patients with advanced biliary cancer: a phase II trial. J Clin Oncol 2005;23(10):2332-8.

[20] Andre T, Reyes-Vidal JM, Fartoux L, et al. Gemcitabine and oxaliplatin in advanced biliary tract carcinoma: a phase II study. Br J Cancer 2008;99(6):862-7.

[21] Philip PA, Mahoney MR, Allmer C, et al. Phase II study of erlotinib in patients with advanced biliary cancer. J Clin Oncol 2006;24(19):3069-74.

[22] Lee J, Park SH, Chang HM, et al. Gemcitabine and oxaliplatin with or without erlotinib in advanced biliary-tract cancer: a multicentre, open-label, randomised, phase 3 study. Lancet Oncol 2012;13(2):181-8.

[23] Socoteanu MP, Mott F, Alpini G, et al. c-Met targeted therapy of cholangiocarcinoma. World J Gastroenterol 2008;14(19):2990-4.

[24] Nakazawa K, Dobashi Y, Suzuki S, et al. Amplification and overexpression of cerbB-2, epidermal growth factor receptor, and c-met in biliary tract cancers. J Pathol 2005;206(3):356-65.

第十一章　全身治疗结合手术治疗转移性结直肠癌

Kaihong Mi, MD, PhD[a], Matthew F. Kalady, MD[a,b],
Cristiano Quintini, MD[c], Alok A. Khorana, MD[a,*]

【关键词】

结直肠癌；肝转移；肝脏靶向治疗；抗血管生成治疗；抗肿瘤治疗

> **要点**
> - 近年来，使用现代治疗方案治疗转移性结直肠癌的患者中位生存期大幅度增加至约30个月。
> - 所有转移性肿瘤患者都应该接受肿瘤潜在可切除性评估和/或肝脏定向疗法，它可以显著改善预后并可能治愈少数患者。
> - 除非存在禁忌证，否则，初始和后续的化疗方案应含有一个靶向药物。
> - 检查所有转移性结直肠癌患者的RAS基因。抗表皮生长因子受体的抗体应仅用于野生型RAS基因肿瘤患者。

一、简介

在所有类型的癌症中，转移性结直肠癌具有较高的致死率，给公共卫生带来沉重的负担。在美国，预计在2014年，将有136 830人被诊断出患有结直肠癌。与此同时，大约1/5的

Khorana 医生声明咨询酬金来源于 Genentech 公司。

[a] Taussig Cancer Institute, Department of Hematology and Oncology, Cleveland Clinic, 9500 Euclid Avenue, Cleveland, OH 44195, USA; [b] Digestive Disease Institute, Department of Colorectal Surgery, Cleveland Clinic, 9500 Euclid Avenue, Cleveland, OH 44195, USA; [c] Digestive Disease Institute, HPB and Liver Transplant Program, Cleveland Clinic, 9500 Euclid Avenue, Cleveland, OH 44195, USA

* Corresponding author. 9500 Euclid Avenue, R35, Cleveland, OH 44195.

E-mail address：Khorana@ccf.org

患者将出现远处转移病灶[1]。原发性结肠直肠癌可通过淋巴和血行播散,也可以经邻近器官和腹膜腔途径播散。右上腹疼痛、腹胀、早饱、锁骨上淋巴结肿大或脐周围存在结节通常是晚期转移病灶的标志。然而,考虑到浸润程度分期和监测方案,也可依据影像学诊断转移性癌。血行扩散的第一部位通常是肝,其次是肺和骨。而直肠癌则是一个例外,其最初可先转移至肺部,这是因为直肠下静脉直接汇入下腔静脉,而不是进入门静脉系统。

虽然未接受特定治疗的转移性病灶患者预后仍较差,但是在过去的20年里,研发出了多种治疗方案,现在已经用于转移性病灶的治疗。最新的大样本随机研究显示[2],其平均存活期从20世纪90年代的6个月增加至接近30个月[3]。生存期的改善已经不是由单一的"神奇药物"来推动,而是通过按需使用不同化疗药物,并结合靶向治疗药物而实现。后者包括单克隆抗体与血管内皮生长因子(VEGF,贝伐单抗)和表皮生长因子受体(EGFR,西妥昔单抗和帕尼单抗);阿柏西普,一种重组融合蛋白,也可对抗VEGF;瑞戈非尼,一种新型的多激酶抑制剂,阻断促进肿瘤生长的多种酶,是酪氨酸激酶的活性抑制剂。最后,少数孤立转移灶的患者也许可以通过手术和肝脏靶向治疗来治愈。

制定一个高效实用的治疗结直肠癌肝转移多种药物的指导策略是非常有必要的,以便最大限度地提高患者预期寿命和生活质量。确诊或转换治疗方案时,决定开始治疗的第一步都应该评估患者是否可以通过手术切除转移病灶。这个方法可指导化疗的选择和时机。治疗应答率最高的治疗方案和最大程度缩小转移病灶的治疗方案最适合有治愈可能的患者。如果患者治愈的可能性较低,则首选尽在可能长的时间内改善患者的生活质量,并且提供患者最长无进展生存期(PFS)和总生存期(OS)的治疗方案。此文着重描述转移性结直肠癌患者的系统性疗法,并补充一些肝切除手术的内容。

二、全身疗法治疗转移性结直肠癌

大部分转移性结直肠癌都是不可切除的,全身治疗着重于对肿瘤的控制,即间断性地缓解症状(姑息治疗),而非治愈性治疗。治疗目标是延长预期寿命,同时在尽可能长的时间内改善生活质量。在此条件下,与其他慢性疾病所采用的措施类似,多线化疗模式正在被摒弃,取而代之的是持续护理的治疗方式[4]。作者基于最新的临床和分子数据(图11-1),利用现有数据,提出关于治疗选择的方案。

治疗转移性结直肠癌的3种常规活性化疗药物是氟嘧啶(包括静脉5-氟尿嘧啶或其口服用药,卡培他滨)、伊立替康和奥沙利铂(表11-1)。患者明显受益于这些活性药物[4,5]。也可在整个持续性护理的不同阶段使用多种靶向治疗药剂,将其并入到常规化疗方案中(表11-2)。

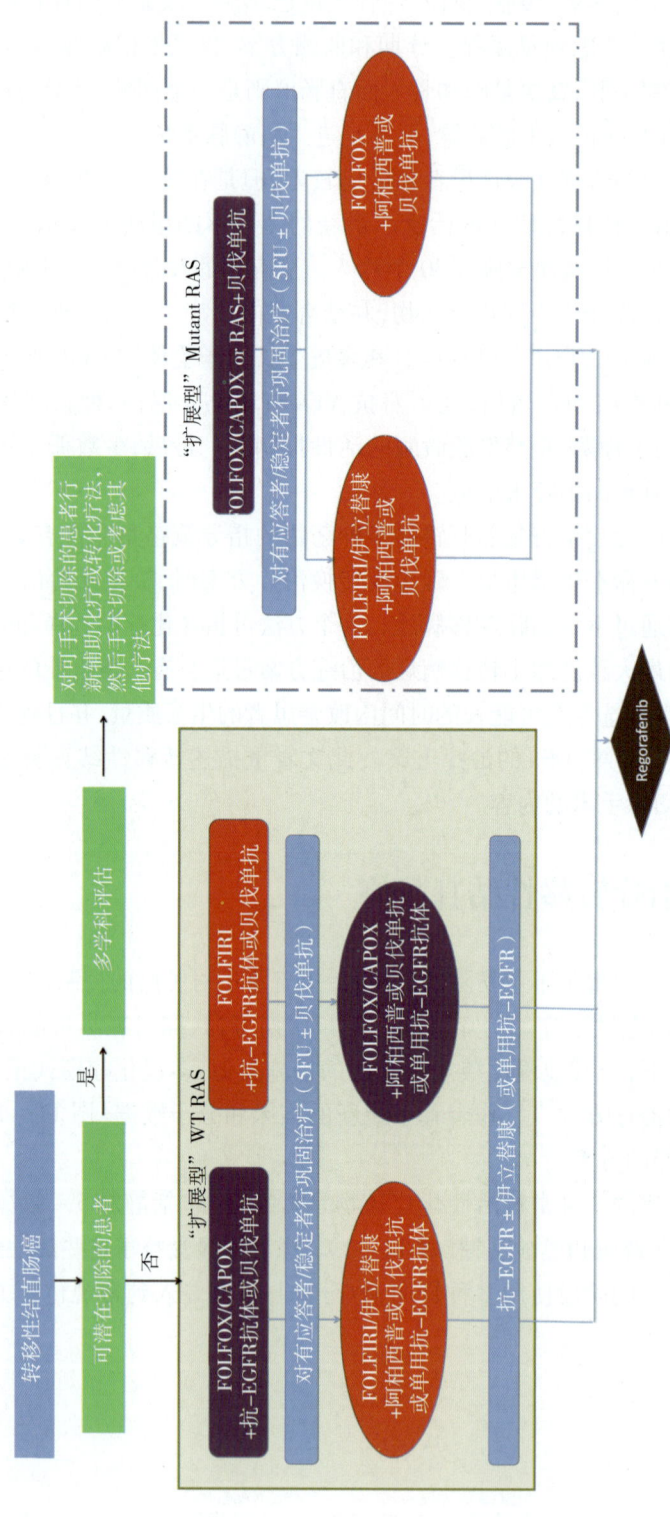

图 11-1 基于现有临床和分子数据,提出一种方案来选择进行全身治疗结合手术切除的转移性结直肠癌患者

5-FU:5-氟尿嘧啶;CAPOX:卡培他滨和奥沙利铂;FOLFIRI:伊立替康,5-氟尿嘧啶和亚叶酸;FOLFOX:奥沙利铂,5-氟尿嘧啶和亚叶酸;WT:野生型

表 11-1 传统化疗药物

药物	机制	主要不良反应
氟尿嘧啶（5-氟尿嘧啶/卡培他滨）	胸苷酸合成酶抑制剂；脱氧尿苷一磷酸作用于 DNA，导致 DNA 的合成与功能受到抑制	骨髓抑制 黏膜炎和/或腹泻 手足综合征
伊立替康	可由羧酸酯酶转化为 SN38（活性形式），为拓扑异构酶 I 抑制剂，阻止 DNA 单链断裂后的修复，干扰 DNA 复制和转录，并进一步导致双链 DNA 断裂和细胞死亡	腹泻 骨髓抑制 脱发
奥沙利铂	第三代铂类化合物，共价结合于 DNA，抑制 DNA 合成和转录	神经毒性 急性冷激发外周感觉神经病变 慢性累积性感觉神经病变

表 11-2 靶向治疗药物

药物类别	机制	主要副作用
VEGF 抑制剂（贝伐单抗，阿柏西普）	贝伐单抗：一种重组抗 VEGF-A 受体的人源化单克隆抗体； 阿柏西普：VEGF 受体诱导融合蛋白的胞外域组件中 VEGF-R1 和 VEGF-R2 与 IgG1 的 Fc 区域融合	高血压 出血倾向 胃肠道穿孔 动脉血栓栓塞 （包括中风和心肌梗死）
抗 EGFR 抗体（西妥昔单抗，帕尼单抗）	抗 EGFR 的单克隆抗体	输液反应 低镁血症 皮肤瘙痒、干燥 肺毒性 腹泻
激酶抑制剂（瑞戈非尼）	多个细胞信号激酶的一个小分子抑制剂	手足综合征 疲劳 腹泻 高血压

EGFR：表皮生长因子受体；IgG1：免疫球蛋白 G1；VEGF：血管内皮生长因子

1. 初始治疗：化疗为主

逐项对比数据表明，一线化疗药物方案奥沙利铂、5-氟尿嘧啶、亚叶酸（FOLFOX）的结果与伊立替康、5-氟尿嘧啶和亚叶酸（FOLFIRI）药物方案的结果是相似的[6]。有研究针对氟尿嘧啶口服替代药物卡培他滨，联合伊立替康（CAPIRI）和奥沙利铂（CAPOX）进行评估。CAPIRI 有较强的毒性[7]，因此并不推荐。数据也表明，CAPOX 具有相似的抗肿瘤效力，但仍有一定潜在的毒性，特别是血小板减少症、手足综合征和腹泻[8,9]，但可以考虑在患者不能接受动态输注疗法时使用。如患者不能耐受5-氟尿嘧啶,可考虑伊立替康和奥沙利铂(IROX)[10]。

治疗初始方案选择FOLFIRI联合FOLFOX还是联合CAPOX,具体要根据患者出现合并症时产生的预期治疗毒性来决定。例如,对于长期患有糖尿病或先前存在神经病变的患者,可建议使用FOLFIRI方案,而非可诱导神经系统病变的FOLFOX方案。如患者因合并症、体力活动状态或个体偏好而不适合使用强化奥沙利铂或以伊立替康为基础的化疗方案时,可以考虑单独使用氟嘧啶治疗(包含或不包含靶向治疗药)。早期研究显示,使用结合3类常规化疗药物的三联疗法(FOLFOXIRI),在一开始不可手术切除的转移性肝癌患者身上显示出较高的手术成功率和较满意的长期生存率[11,12],且该方案也可用于高度选择性的患者,直到其他附加数据可用。

在使用FOLFOX方案疾病进展后,接受FOLFIRI类方案的患者预期应答率在4%~20%,无进展生存期为2.5~7.1个月[13,14]。另一方面,对伊立替康治疗失败,接受奥沙利铂为基础治疗方案的患者进行研究,结果显示,应答率为10%左右,平均疾病进展时间为4~5个月(TTP)[14,15]。目前,治疗转移性结直肠癌的主流标准方案包括了FOLFIRI类方案治疗,疾病进展后,以奥沙利铂为基础的治疗,或以伊立替康为基础的治疗。大多数临床医生,包括作者,常以奥沙利铂为基础的方案作为首选,这是因为它有更高的应答率,表现出较轻的毒性反应,但这些观点实际上都没有通过逐项对比研究证实。在过去的1年里,既往以FOLFOX方案作为辅助治疗的患者使用FOLFIRI治疗效果较好。

2. 化疗主线:概要

(1)根据患者的个体偏好并考虑到明确的药物毒性,无论是FOLFOX或FOLFIRI,都可以作为一线用药方案。

(2)患者不能或不愿接受联合化疗的情况下,可以单独使用氟尿嘧啶类药物方案进行治疗。

(3)行积极疗法且治疗应答率较高的高度选择性的患者可以考虑使用FOLFOXIRI。

(4)条件允许的情况下,所有的化疗主线都应添加靶向治疗药物。

3. 结合抗血管内皮生长因子药物

抗VEGF单克隆抗体贝伐单抗,在治疗转移性结直肠癌的过程中,单独使用其药效并不好[16]。然而,多个临床试验表明,在持续性治疗转移性癌症患者的过程中,将贝伐单抗结合以氟嘧啶、奥沙利铂和伊立替康为基础的一线治疗,可显示出明显获益[17-19]。例如,在随机TREE-2试验中,使用奥沙利铂和5-氟尿嘧啶联合化疗方案治疗先前未经治疗的患者,一组添加贝伐单抗,另一组未添加,两者的中位总生存期分别为23.7个月和18.2个月[20]。而在二线治疗的ECOG3200试验中,将贝伐单抗加入以奥沙利铂为基础的化疗方案,在先前已经接受过治疗(通过5-氟尿嘧啶或伊立替康进行治疗)的转移性结直肠癌患者中使用,并将结果与单独FOLFOX化疗方案比较,同样发现无进展生存期(7.3 vs 4.7个月)和中位总生存期(12.9 vs 10.8个月)有所改善[16]。因此,在转移性结直肠癌的治疗方面达成共识:对个体患者进行初始或后续治疗时,应在化疗方案中添加贝伐单抗。

贝伐单抗可增加3、4级高血压及肠穿孔、伤口愈合不良、动脉血栓栓塞、出血的发生率[21]。谨慎选择患者并对药物毒性实时监测十分重要，如果要实施手术干预，要慎重考虑中断药物治疗的时机。鉴于贝伐单抗的半衰期大约3周，学者们一般建议在术前和术后继续使用4~6周的贝伐单抗，以避免术后并发症，伤口裂开。

当患者病情发生进展时，传统常规治疗是中断所有类别的药物。但是，目前尚不清楚使用生物制剂时是否应该采用类似的治疗策略，特别是使用一些具有抗血管生成活性的生物制剂。ML18147 III期试验已证实，疾病进展后继续使用贝伐单抗治疗具有一定疗效，测试结果显示无进展生存期(5.7 vs 4.1个月)和总生存期(11.2 vs 9.8个月)有较显著的改善。与一线贝伐单抗治疗方案的历史数据相比，贝伐单抗相关的不良反应并没有增加[22]。

在非细胞体系中，相比贝伐单抗，阿柏西普是一种对VEGF-A有着更高亲和力的重组融合蛋白[23]。在美国，根据VELOUR安慰剂对照试验结果，对于使用奥沙利铂化疗方案产生抵抗或疾病进展的转移性结直肠癌患者，可使用阿柏西普结合FOLFIRI来治疗[24]。使用阿柏西普治疗的患者，中位总生存期(13.5 vs 12.1个月)和中位无进展生存期(6.9 vs 4.7个月)有显著的提高。不管先前是否使用了贝伐单抗，其治疗获益是相似的(在试验中包含了约30%的患者)[25]。然而，并没有平行对照试验比较疾病进展后是继续使用贝伐单抗治疗的方案还是改成阿柏西普的方案。因此，两种治疗方案均可考虑。

4. 抗表皮生长因子受体药物：精准治疗中的关键角色

无论用单一制剂还是联合治疗方案，抗表皮生长因子受体(EGFR)药物都可改善转移性结直肠癌患者的预后。使用含EFGR抑制剂的治疗方案时，生物标志物分析对于患者选择十分重要。EGFR抑制剂是一种精准药物或个体化药物，依据个体样本中肿瘤突变基因的不同，选择不同的全身治疗方案。一旦KRAS基因激活突变，就会导致RAS-RAF-ERK通路组成成分激活，从而对抗EGFR治疗产生耐受[26]。2009年，美国临床肿瘤学会建议所有适用于抗EGFR治疗的患者进行肿瘤KRAS基因突变检测，并建议此类制剂只适用于野生型(WT) KRAS基因，表现为定性实时聚合酶链反应中，KRAS外显子2突变缺失[27]。最新数据表明，对于抗EGFR治疗产生耐受的患者，可以通过外显子2以外较低突变频率的KRAS基因和NRAS基因来调节[28-31]。2013年，PRIME研究表明，在所谓的经典野生型KRAS基因人群中(没有外显子突变)，在其他KRAS外显子(外显子3和4)或NRAS外显子(外显子2和3)发生基因突变时，将帕尼单抗加入FOLFOX治疗方案，并无生存获益。而且加入了抗EGFR治疗，这类患者无进展生存期(7.3 vs 8.0个月，$P = 0.33$)和总生存期(危险比1.39，$P = 0.12$)并不理想[28]。但是，检测出具有扩展野生型RAS基因(无外显子2、3、4突变的KRAS和无外显子突变的NRAS)的患者，在其化疗方案中加入帕尼单抗后，总生存期有显著提高[28]。其他分析已经证实了这些发现。现逐渐达成共识：所有的转移性结直肠癌患者都应接受扩展RAS基因突变的检测，对于检测出该类突变的患者不建议用抗EGFR治疗。

在CRYSTAL试验中，对未经治疗的转移性结直肠癌患者给予西妥昔单抗一线药物；患者被随机分配到含有或不含西妥昔单抗的FOLFIRI治疗方案组中。在野生型KRAS肿瘤患者的治疗中，使用西妥昔单抗应答率显著提高(57% vs 40%)，中位无进展生存期和总生存期也显著提高(23.5 vs 20 个月)[32]。EPIC 试验将 1298 例抗奥沙利铂药物的患者随机分配到伊立替康联合或不联合西妥昔单抗治疗组。试验证明,联合用药的患者无进展生存期显著提高(4 vs 2.6 个月),客观应答率(16% vs 4%)、总体疾病控制率(61% vs 46%)同样也有提高[33]。越来越多的数据证实,一线、二线和三线帕尼单抗联合以奥沙利铂或伊立替康为基础的治疗方案,对野生型 RAS 基因肿瘤患者有一定的治疗效果[28,34-39]。西妥昔单抗和帕尼单抗作为单独用药,补救治疗化疗耐受性转移性结直肠癌显示出相似的疗效[40,41]。同样,在转移性结直肠癌的初始和后续治疗中,这两种药物协同以伊立替康为主的化疗方案治疗,也可达类似疗效。抗 EGFR 药物的选择在很大程度上取决于机体对特定药物的反应、对输液的反应以及用药细则(西妥昔单抗是每周 1 次,帕尼单抗方案是 2 周 1 次)。

在个体研究中,对于野生型 KRAS 肿瘤患者的治疗,在其化疗方案中添加西妥昔单抗相比添加贝伐单抗,虽然治疗应答率较高,但两者的中位生存获益是相似的[16,20,32,33]。当患者的转移性癌症转为可切除肿瘤时,化疗应答率的改善则作为支持抗 EGFR 疗法一线用药的证据。针对 VEGF 和 EGFR 的双抗体治疗,经过测试发现可导致病情恶化,因此不推荐使用[42,43]。

在对野生型 RAS 基因肿瘤患者的治疗中,是否将贝伐单抗或抗 EGFR 治疗作为初始治疗方案添加到化疗主线中是非常重要的。两个小样本量的初始试验表明,"首先使用抗 EGFR"的治疗方法可带来生存获益[30,31]。然而,来自美国一份此类规模最大的研究,C80405,在 2014 年给出的最终结果表明,无论是西妥昔单抗还是贝伐单抗,在初始治疗方案中加入化疗,其生存期未明显改变(29.9 vs 29 个月,$P = 0.34$)[2]。因此,任何一种抗体药物都可以在初始治疗中使用,并可再根据毒性反应、个体偏好、用药细则进行选择。值得注意的是,C80405 也可能包含了扩展型 RAS 基因突变患者(经典 KRAS 突变体除外)。该亚组的分析结果在未来可能会改变最终的结论。

5. 瑞格菲尼

瑞格菲尼主要针对促进血管生成和肿瘤生长通路中涉及到的多种激酶。该药物治疗难治性转移性结直肠癌的活性在 CORRECT 试验中得以体现[44]。经多标准治疗后出现进展的患者给予瑞格菲尼后,中位生存期(6.4 vs 5 个月)和无进展生存期(1.9 vs 1.7 个月)有适度改善,且具有显著统计学意义[44]。目前,对于使用其他标准化疗和靶向治疗药物出现进展的肿瘤患者来说,瑞格菲尼是其保留药物。

6. 靶向治疗:概要

所有的化疗在初始和后续的治疗方案中都应附有一个靶向药物,除非存在具体禁忌证情况。

抗表皮生长因子受体疗法只适用于含有扩展野生型 RAS 基因的肿瘤患者。

贝伐单抗或抗表皮生长因子受体治疗可在含有扩展野生型 RAS 基因肿瘤患者的初始治疗方案中使用。

疾病进展后,贝伐单抗可以继续使用,但需调整化疗方案。

避免双重抗体治疗。

三、维持方案

大约有75%的患者由于疾病进展而停止了一线化疗,并面临是否考虑维持化疗或化疗中断的问题。OPTIMOX试验表明,在用FOLFOX方案进行6个周期化疗后,奥沙利铂可以安全停药,与维持5-氟尿嘧啶治疗相比,该化疗完全中断了对无进展生存期的负面影响[45,46]。CAIRO-3结果表明,CAPOX联合贝伐单抗6个疗程以后,用贝伐单抗联合卡培他滨维持治疗可延长无进展生存期(8.5 vs 4.1个月)[47]。至于决定维持化疗还是暂缓化疗还必须考虑到患者的选择和花费。

四、可能治愈的晚期结直肠癌

肝脏是大多数结直肠癌患者血行转移的第一站。大约有10%的患者即使有转移灶也可以存活5年以上[48]。可切除转移性病灶的定义在不断发展,并没有一个公认的标准,即使是两叶转移和肝外病灶,也不再被视为禁忌。该方案的决策需要多学科协作,一个实用的方案要求患者从医学角度适于手术,即应在确保有足够残肝的条件下,切除肝脏病灶,并且应对肝外病灶加以控制。对于肝脏转移病灶较少的患者,手术切除是较好的方案,预后良好的患者,5年生存率为50%~60%。一些试验表明,大约有1/5此类患者生存期超过10年[51],在一些特定试验中,这也适用于非肝脏转移灶。当原发肿瘤部位得以控制,并将转移性病灶限制在肺中,不向肺外转移(可切除或已切除的肝脏病灶除外),切除孤立的肺转移病灶可使5年生存率提高至40%。挑选出的最初无法切除的肝转移患者,如果化疗效果较好,可转化为可切除。这种方法被称为转换疗法,应将其与新辅助治疗区分开来。转换疗法让12%~33%最初无法切除或边缘可切除的转移灶符合转移灶切除术的条件[11,12,53]。5年平均生存率为30%~35%,这基本上是优于单纯化疗的预期[25,52]。

通常选择极有可能出现客观应答的方案,因为其与随后切除率密切相关。但是,选择方案的标准并不完善,与FOLFIRI联合贝伐单抗在Ⅲ期TRIB试验相比,三重化疗方案FOLFOXIRI联合贝伐单抗可显著提高应答率(65% vs 53%)和无疾病生存期(中位数12.2 vs 9个月)。

然而,FOLFOXIRI不能提高二次完整肝脏肿瘤切除率(15% vs 12%),并且会导致更为严重的不良反应[54]。抗EGFR抑制剂无论是与伊立替康还是奥沙利铂为基础的化疗方案结合,对含有野生型KRAS基因患者的切除率均有一定提高[55,56]。德国一个多中心随机Ⅱ期试验(CELM研究),通过使用FOLFOX添加西妥昔单抗,或者FOLFIRI添加西妥昔单抗,62%的患者出现肿瘤应答,其中野生型RAS基因肿瘤患者中有70%出现肿瘤应答,但总生存期和无进展生存期并没有改善[55]。近期的一个Ⅱ期研究结果显示,在最初不可切除的包含野生型KRAS基因的患者中,应用FOLFOX方案并结合缓慢增量的西妥昔单抗,可达到70%(14/20)的外科R0切除转化率[57]。不管是单纯的肝动脉介入化疗或与全身化疗结合,都可抑制肝转移癌进展[58,59]。并没有任何随机试验将肝动脉泵和现有系统化疗单独作对比,而且这种方法目前还没有在美国广泛应用。

对于最初可切除的肝转移癌患者,大都要接受初始系统化疗(特别是有同步转移病灶的患者),以获得预后信息,尽早治疗潜在分散的微小转移病灶,评估新转移病灶,并测试肿瘤的化疗药物敏感度。对于肝转移灶异时性出现的患者而言,可行前期手术。欧洲癌症研究与治疗组织的40983试验纳入了364例可切除性结直肠癌肝转移患者,其中最多有4处转移灶,没有预先给予奥沙利铂治疗,这些患者被随机分配到接受或者不接受围术期 FOLFOX 化疗肝脏切除术组[60]。初始化疗可改善患者可切除率。在化疗组中,术后并发症发生率显著提高(25% vs 16%),术后死亡率与单手术组基本持平(1 vs 2例)。最新数据显示,在中位时间为8.5年的随访中,发现存在支持化疗无统计学意义的趋势,该趋势体现在5年无进展生存期中(38% vs 33%),但是化疗组5年总生存率则没有显著改善(51% vs 48%)[61]。最近,一项回顾性研究表明,新辅助化疗只有利于高风险患者[62]。多于2个危险因素的患者接受了新辅助化疗后,中位生存期得到提高(38.9 vs 28.4个月);与此相反,对于低风险患者,接受或不接受新辅助化疗,其中位生存期(60 vs 60个月)和5年总生存率(64% vs 57%,$P > 0.05$)结果相差无几[62]。

肝转移癌患者行切除术后复发率高达80%,其中大约一半在肝脏复发。在满足上述肝脏切除术指征的患者中,重复肝脏切除术是安全的,且可达到与报道中首次肝脏切除术同等的生存率[63,64]。因此术后密切监测患者十分重要,以便在可切除阶段检测出肝转移癌复发。在行结直肠癌肝转移灶切除术后,关于转移性结直肠癌肝切除术后最佳随访策略的证据有限[65,66]。下列患者的监测策略是合理的:2年内每3~6个月进行癌胚抗原、肝功能检查,以及胸部、腹部和骨盆的CT扫描,随后5年内每6~12个月进行上述检查。

其他的肝脏靶向治疗

其他若干局部疗法,包括局部肿瘤切除术、区域性肝动脉灌注化疗或化疗栓塞和立体定向放射治疗,适用于不适合手术治疗的孤立性结直肠癌肝转移患者[67,68]。

这些疗法往往与最初的肝脏切除术结合使用,或者一些患者因为总体状况不适合接受切除手术,该疗法也可以作为一种选择。

五、原发性肿瘤切除术的作用

转移性结直肠癌的原发性肿瘤切除术有两个广泛适应证:症状缓解和意向治疗。其手术方式可以根据原发性肿瘤的症状和转移性病灶的可切除性来分类。

1. 有症状的原发性肿瘤合并不可切除的转移病灶

需要对原发肿瘤进行外科干预的最常见的症状是梗阻、出血与贫血、穿孔。一般在这种情况下,新辅助化疗没有明显作用。治疗的主要目的是尽量减轻症状和提高生活质量。虽然提倡肿瘤外科治疗原则,但是弥漫性病变或癌变可致使肿瘤手术无法进行。例如建立一个阻塞肿瘤分流造口或者旁路可抑制发病,并帮助患者更快地过渡到全身治疗阶段。

2. 有症状的原发性肿瘤合并可切除的转移病灶

如上所述,肿瘤出现症状后需要及时干预。如果转移性病灶可通过手术治疗,那就要看准时机作出决定。主要目的是缓解症状,并依照肿瘤外科的治疗原则处理原发性肿瘤,如血管的高位结扎、适当的淋巴结摘除,以及保留足够的边界。如果出现急性肠梗阻或肠穿孔,且患者需要急诊手术,则仅对原发性肿瘤进行手术。在择期手术中,是否将肝转移病灶切除取决于疾病的严重程度和手术的切除范围。一般情况下,如果只需行简单的楔形切除术或肝转移瘤切除术,那么此类手术可与结肠切除术同时进行,如需行更广泛的肝脏切除术,则应该单独处理原发性肿瘤,并制定计划进行化疗和阶段性肝转移病灶切除术。

3. 无症状的原发性肿瘤合并不可切除的转移病灶

在有不可切除的远处转移灶情况下,切除无症状的原发性肿瘤所起到的作用是有争议的。虽然回顾性资料显示切除原发性肿瘤有一定的生存获益,并且一个前瞻性研究表明,在一个亚组患者分析中,未切除的原发性肿瘤可造成一些主要并发症(n = 12 of 86)[69],但是临床证据仍不够明确。支持切除术的人认为,切除术后,患者对化疗药物应答率更高,并具有较低肿瘤负荷,进一步降低化疗期间产生并发症的风险,如肠梗阻和肠穿孔。反对切除术的论点是基于可能出现术后并发症,术后并发症的出现可能会推迟甚至阻碍化疗方案的应用[70]。改善生存率的相关因素包括年龄小于70岁、没有肝外病灶、整体功能状态良好,并且肝脏负担低于50%[70]。

4. 无症状的原发性肿瘤合并可切除的转移病灶

切除原发性肿瘤是治疗可切除转移病灶的根本。关于肝脏切除术的时间选择和化疗仍然是一个有争议的问题,各种治疗手段都有各自的特点。

经典的治疗方式包括原发性肿瘤的切除,其次是辅助化疗,然后是转移病灶切除术。某些研究团队支持新辅助治疗,它可以优先治疗全身性疾病,因为远处转移灶对生存率影响较大。这种方法通过对治疗的反应可以让肿瘤进行自身生物学表达。进展为不可切除肿瘤的患者,可以免于原发性肿瘤切除术的术后并发症。对药物作出应答的患者将继续行原发肿瘤和肝脏病灶的切除术。对同期切除术和分期切除术都进行了描述。有些治疗团队偏好于肝脏肿瘤优先的分期切除术,但其成功率不稳定[71]。多学科团队的学术讨论可为此类病例提供最好的疾病管理方法,涉及肝胆外科、结直肠外科和肿瘤科。

六、小结和未来的发展方向

在过去的10年中,转移性结直肠癌患者的预后得到质的提升。如今,在临床上已经可以讨论以"年"为单位来计算患者长短不等的预期生存期。甚至"治愈"一词开始在关于转移癌的讨论中出现。显著提高的医疗效果不仅仅来自单一的"神奇药物",更是由一股汇聚的力量来实现:我们可以循序地利用新的药物和治疗方案来保证患者的生活质量,并延长其预期寿命;不断改进外科技术,得到更有利的数据,来展示外科切除术和肝脏靶向治疗的巨大价值。

在结直肠癌患者的护理中集成个体化治疗是下一步发展的方向。分子表达谱可以显著改善野生型 RAS 基因肿瘤患者的治疗效果,其中一个例子就是不断发展的生物标记物可以预测个体对于抗 EGFR 疗法的应答,并且,分子表达谱检测还可以为 RAS 突变的肿瘤患者降低药物毒性反应,节省医疗费用。医疗供应商已经开始提供下一代的临床基因组测序技术。本文作者和其他学者参与了一项新颖的实验,该实验通过使用基因组测序测定出突变的基因,并提供针对性的靶向药物。随着对附加数据的利用变得更加有效,在不久的将来,更大型的个体化治疗将可能实现。近期,对 1290 例结直肠癌病例进行基因表达分析,6 种不同临床亚型基因被识别出来,产生不同程度的 Wnt 信号和细胞"干性"激活,在抗 EGFR 疗法和以伊立替康为基础的化疗中,产生不同程度的应答,在治疗转移病灶和辅助化疗下有不同程度的存活[72]。这样的研究将加快新药开发和测试,并让临床医生不断地对治疗方案进行完善和个性化定制。过去十年的成果已经带来了希望,对大多数患者来说,将转移性结直肠癌从一个致命性疾病转化为可持续缓解甚至可治愈的慢性疾病,可望成为现实。

参考文献

[1] Siegel R, Ma J, Zou Z, et al. Cancer statistics, 2014. CA Cancer J Clin 2014;64(1):9-29.

[2] Venook AP, Niedzwiecki D, Lenz HJ, et al. CALGB/SWOG 80405: phase III trial of irinotecan/5-FU/leucovorin (FOLFIRI) or oxaliplatin/5-FU/leucovorin (mFOLFOX6) Metastatic Colorectal Cancer 209 with bevacizumab (BV) or cetuximab (CET) for patients (pts) with KRAS wild-type (wt) untreated metastatic adenocarcinoma of the colon or rectum (MCRC). J Clin Oncol 2014;32:5s.

[3] Scheithauer W, Rosen H, Kornek GV, et al. Randomised comparison of combination chemotherapy plus supportive care with supportive care alone in patients with metastatic colorectal cancer. BMJ 1993;306(6880):752-5.

[4] Goldberg RM, Rothenberg ML, Van Cutsem E, et al. The continuum of care: a paradigm for the management of metastatic colorectal cancer. Oncologist 2007;12(1):38-50.

[5] Grothey A, Sargent D. Overall survival of patients with advanced colorectal cancer correlates with availability of fluorouracil, irinotecan, and oxaliplatin regardless of whether doublet or single-agent therapy is used first line. J Clin Oncol 2005;23(36):9441-2.

[6] Colucci G, Gebbia V, Paoletti G, et al. Phase III randomized trial of FOLFIRI versus FOLFOX4 in the treatment of advanced colorectal cancer: a multicenter study of the Gruppo Oncologico Dell'Italia Meridionale. J Clin Oncol 2005;23(22):4866-75.

[7] Patt YZ, Lee FC, Liebmann JE, et al. Capecitabine plus 3-weekly irinotecan (XELIRI regimen) as first-line chemotherapy for metastatic colorectal cancer: phase II trial results. Am J Clin Oncol 2007;30(4):350-7.

[8] Diaz-Rubio E, Tabernero J, Gomez-Espana A, et al. Phase III study of capecitabine plus oxaliplatin compared with continuous-infusion fluorouracil plus oxaliplatin as first-line therapy in metastatic colorectal cancer: final report of the Spanish Cooperative Group for the treatment of digestive tumors trial. J Clin Oncol 2007;25(27):4224-30.

[9] Porschen R, Arkenau HT, Kubicka S, et al. Phase III study of capecitabine plus oxaliplatin compared with fluorouracil and leucovorin plus oxaliplatin in metastatic colorectal cancer: a final report of the AIO Colorectal Study Group. J Clin Oncol 2007;25(27):4217-23.

[10] Sanoff HK, Sargent DJ, Campbell ME, et al. Five-year data and prognostic factor analysis of oxaliplatin and irinotecan combinations for advanced colorectal cancer: N9741. J Clin Oncol 2008;26(35):5721-7.

[11] Falcone A, Ricci S, Brunetti I, et al. Phase III trial of infusional fluorouracil, leucovorin, oxaliplatin, and irinotecan (FOLFOXIRI) compared with infusional fluorouracil, leucovorin, and irinotecan (FOLFIRI) as first-line treatment for metastatic colorectal cancer: the Gruppo Oncologico Nord Ovest. J Clin Oncol 2007;25(13):1670-6.

[12] Masi G, Loupakis F, Pollina L, et al. Long-term outcome of initially unresectable metastatic colorectal cancer patients treated with 5-fluorouracil/leucovorin, oxaliplatin, and irinotecan (FOLFOXIRI) followed by radical surgery of metastases. Ann Surg 2009;249(3):420-5.

[13] Bidard FC, Tournigand C, Andre T, et al. Efficacy of FOLFIRI-3 (irinotecan D1,D3 combined with LV5-FU) or other irinotecan-based regimens in oxaliplatinpretreated metastatic colorectal cancer in the GERCOR OPTIMOX1 study. Ann Oncol 2009;20(6):1042-7.

[14] Tournigand C, Andre T, Achille E, et al. FOLFIRI followed by FOLFOX6 or the reverse sequence in advanced colorectal cancer: a randomized GERCOR study. J Clin Oncol 2004;22(2):229-37.

[15] Rothenberg ML, Oza AM, Bigelow RH, et al. Superiority of oxaliplatin and fluorouracil-leucovorin compared with either therapy alone in patients with progressive colorectal cancer after irinotecan and fluorouracil-leucovorin: interim results of a phase III trial. J Clin Oncol 2003;21(11):2059-69.

[16] Giantonio BJ, Catalano PJ, Meropol NJ, et al. Bevacizumab in combination with oxaliplatin, fluorouracil, and leucovorin (FOLFOX4) for previously treated metastatic colorectal cancer: results from the Eastern Cooperative Oncology Group Study E3200. J Clin Oncol 2007;25(12):1539-44.

[17] Hurwitz H, Fehrenbacher L, Hainsworth JD, et al. Bevacizumab in combination with fluorouracil and leucovorin: an active regimen for first-line metastatic colorectal cancer. J Clin Oncol 2005;23(15):3502-8.

[18] Kabbinavar FF, Hambleton J, Mass RD, et al. Combined analysis of efficacy: the addition of bevacizumab to fluorouracil/leucovorin improves survival for patients with metastatic colorectal cancer. J Clin Oncol 2005;23(16):3706-12.

[19] Vincenzi B, Santini D, Russo A, et al. Bevacizumab in association with de Gramont 5-fluorouracil/folinic acid in patients with oxaliplatin-, irinotecan-, and cetuximab-refractory colorectal cancer: a single-center phase 2 trial. Cancer 2009;115(20):4849-56.

[20] Hochster HS, Hart LL, Ramanathan RK, et al. Safety and efficacy of oxaliplatin and fluoropyrimidine regimens with or without bevacizumab as first-line treatment of metastatic colorectal cancer: results of the TREE Study. J Clin Oncol 2008; 26(21):3523-9.

[21] Scappaticci FA, Skillings JR, Holden SN, et al. Arterial thromboembolic events in patients with metastatic carcinoma treated with chemotherapy and bevacizumab. J Natl Cancer Inst 2007;99(16):1232-9.

[22] Bennouna J, Sastre J, Arnold D, et al. Continuation of bevacizumab after first progression in metastatic colorectal cancer (ML18147): a randomised phase 3 trial. Lancet Oncol 2013;14(1):29-37.

[23] Holash J, Davis S, Papadopoulos N, et al. VEGF-Trap: a VEGF blocker with potent antitumor effects.

Proc Natl Acad Sci U S A 2002;99(17):11393-8.

[24] Joulain F, Van Cutsem E, Iqbal SU, et al. Aflibercept versus placebo in combination with FOLFIRI in previously treated metastatic colorectal cancer (mCRC): mean overall survival (OS) estimation from a phase III trial (VELOUR). J Clin Oncol 2012;30(15). Abstract: 3602.

[25] Allegra CJ, Lakomy R, Tabernero J, et al. Effects of prior bevacizumab (B) use on outcomes from the VELOUR study: a phase III study of aflibercept (Afl) and FOLFIRI in patients (pts) with metastatic colorectal cancer (mCRC) after failure of an oxaliplatin regimen. J Clin Oncol 2012;30(15). Abstract: 3505.

[26] Dahabreh IJ, Terasawa T, Castaldi PJ, et al. Systematic review: anti-epidermal growth factor receptor treatment effect modification by KRAS mutations in advanced colorectal cancer. Ann Intern Med 2011;154(1):37-49.

[27] Allegra CJ, Jessup JM, Somerfield MR, et al. American Society of Clinical Oncology provisional clinical opinion: testing for KRAS gene mutations in patients with metastatic colorectal carcinoma to predict response to anti-epidermal growth factor receptor monoclonal antibody therapy. J Clin Oncol 2009;27(12):2091-6.

[28] Douillard JY, Oliner KS, Siena S, et al. Panitumumab-FOLFOX4 treatment and RAS mutations in colorectal cancer. N Engl J Med 2013;369(11):1023-34.

[29] Loupakis F, Ruzzo A, Cremolini C, et al. KRAS codon 61, 146 and BRAF mutations predict resistance to cetuximab plus irinotecan in KRAS codon 12 and 13 wildtype metastatic colorectal cancer. Br J Cancer 2009;101(4):715-21.

[30] Schwartzberg LS, Rivera F, Karthaus M, et al. Analysis of KRAS/NRAS mutations in PEAK: A randomized phase II study of FOLFOX6 plus panitumumab (pmab) or bevacizumab (bev) as first-line treatment (tx) for wild-type (WT) KRAS (exon 2) metastatic colorectal cancer (mCRC). J Clin Oncol 2013;31(15). Abstract: 3631.

[31] Stintzing S, Jung A, Rossius L, et al. Analysis of KRAS/NRAS and BRAF mutations in FIRE-3: a randomized phase III study of FOLFIRI plus cetuximab or bevacizumab as first-line treatment for wild-type (WT) KRAS (exon 2) metastatic colorectal cancer (mCRC) patients. Data presented at the 13th annual European Cancer Congress (ECC), Amsterdam, The Netherlands. September 28, 2013.

[32] Van Cutsem E, Kohne CH, Lang I, et al. Cetuximab plus irinotecan, fluorouracil, and leucovorin as first-line treatment for metastatic colorectal cancer: updated analysis of overall survival according to tumor KRAS and BRAF mutation status. J Clin Oncol 2011;29(15):2011-9.

[33] Sobrero AF, Maurel J, Fehrenbacher L, et al. EPIC: phase III trial of cetuximab plus irinotecan after fluoropyrimidine and oxaliplatin failure in patients with metastatic colorectal cancer. J Clin Oncol 2008;26(14):2311-9.

[34] Andre T, Blons H, Mabro M, et al. Panitumumab combined with irinotecan for patients with KRAS wild-type metastatic colorectal cancer refractory to standard chemotherapy: a GERCOR efficacy, tolerance, and translational molecular study. Ann Oncol 2013;24(2):412-9.

[35] Cohn AL, Shumaker GC, Khandelwal P, et al. An open-label, single-arm, phase 2 trial of panitumumab plus FOLFIRI as second-line therapy in patients with metastatic colorectal cancer. Clin Colorectal Cancer 2011;10(3):171-7.

[36] Douillard JY, Siena S, Cassidy J, et al. Randomized, phase III trial of panitumumab with infusional flu-

orouracil, leucovorin, and oxaliplatin (FOLFOX4) versus FOLFOX4 alone as first-line treatment in patients with previously untreated metastatic colorectal cancer: the PRIME study. J Clin Oncol 2010;28(31):4697-705.

[37] Kohne CH, Hofheinz R, Mineur L, et al. First-line panitumumab plus irinotecan/5-fluorouracil/leucovorin treatment in patients with metastatic colorectal cancer. J Cancer Res Clin Oncol 2012;138(1):65-72.

[38] Peeters M, Price TJ, Cervantes A, et al. Final results from a randomized phase 3 study of FOLFIRI {1/-} panitumumab for second-line treatment of metastatic colorectal cancer. Ann Oncol 2014;25(1):107-16.

[39] Seymour MT, Brown SR, Middleton G, et al. Panitumumab and irinotecan versus irinotecan alone for patients with KRAS wild-type, fluorouracil-resistant advanced colorectal cancer (PICCOLO): a prospectively stratified randomised trial. Lancet Oncol 2013;14(8):749-59.

[40] Price T, Peeters M, Kim TW, et al. ASPECCT: a randomized, multicenter, openlabel, phase 3 study of panitumumab (pmab) vs cetuximab (cmab) for previously treated wild-type (WT) KRAS metastatic colorectal cancer (mCRC). Data presented at the 2013 annual European Cancer Congress (ECC), Amsterdam, The Netherlands. September 29, 2013.

[41] Van Cutsem E, Peeters M, Siena S, et al. Open-label phase III trial of panitumumab plus best supportive care compared with best supportive care alone in patients with chemotherapy-refractory metastatic colorectal cancer. J Clin Oncol 2007;25(13):1658-64.

[42] Hecht JR, Mitchell E, Chidiac T, et al. A randomized phase IIIB trial of chemotherapy, bevacizumab, and panitumumab compared with chemotherapy and bevacizumab alone for metastatic colorectal cancer. J Clin Oncol 2009;27(5):672-80.

[43] Tol J, Koopman M, Cats A, et al. Chemotherapy, bevacizumab, and cetuximab in metastatic colorectal cancer. N Engl J Med 2009;360(6):563-72.

[44] Grothey A, Van Cutsem E, Sobrero A, et al. Regorafenib monotherapy for previously treated metastatic colorectal cancer (CORRECT): an international, multicentre, randomised, placebo-controlled, phase 3 trial. Lancet 2013;381(9863):303-12.

[45] Chibaudel B, Maindrault-Goebel F, Lledo G, et al. Can chemotherapy be discontinued in unresectable metastatic colorectal cancer? The GERCOR OPTIMOX2 Study. J Clin Oncol 2009;27(34):5727-33.

[46] Tournigand C, Cervantes A, Figer A, et al. OPTIMOX1: a randomized study of FOLFOX4 or FOLFOX7 with oxaliplatin in a stop-and-go fashion in advanced colorectal cancer – a GERCOR study. J Clin Oncol 2006;24(3):394-400.

[47] Koopman M, Simkens L, May A, et al. Final results and subgroup analyses of the phase 3 CAIRO3 study: maintenance treatment with capecitabine and bevacizumab versus observation after induction treatment with chemotherapy and bevacizumab in metastatic colorectal cancer (mCRC). J Clin Oncol 2014;32(3). Abstract: LBA388.

[48] Ferrarotto R, Pathak P, Maru D, et al. Durable complete responses in metastatic colorectal cancer treated with chemotherapy alone. Clin Colorectal Cancer 2011;10(3):178-82.

[49] Rees M, Tekkis PP, Welsh FK, et al. Evaluation of long-term survival after hepatic resection for metastatic colorectal cancer: a multifactorial model of 929 patients. Ann Surg 2008;247(1):125-35.

[50] Fong Y, Fortner J, Sun RL, et al. Clinical score for predicting recurrence after hepatic resection for metastatic colorectal cancer: analysis of 1001 consecutive cases. Ann Surg 1999;230(3):309-18 [discussion: 318-21].

[51] Tomlinson JS, Jarnagin WR, DeMatteo RP, et al. Actual 10-year survival after resection of colorectal liver metastases defines cure. J Clin Oncol 2007;25(29):4575-80.

[52] Pfannschmidt J, Dienemann H, Hoffmann H. Surgical resection of pulmonary metastases from colorectal cancer: a systematic review of published series. Ann Thorac Surg 2007;84(1):324-38.

[53] Adam R, Wicherts DA, de Haas RJ, et al. Patients with initially unresectable colorectal liver metastases: is there a possibility of cure? J Clin Oncol 2009;27(11): 1829-35.

[54] Falcone A, Cremolini C, Masi G, et al. FOLFOXIRI/bevacizumab (bev) versus FOLFIRI/bev as first-line treatment in unresectable metastatic colorectal cancer (mCRC) patients (pts): results of the phase III TRIBE trial by GONO group. J Clin Oncol 2013;31(15). Abstract: 3505.

[55] Folprecht G, Gruenberger T, Bechstein W, et al. Survival of patients with initially unresectable colorectal liver metastases treated with FOLFOX/cetuximab or FOLFIRI/cetuximab in a multidisciplinary concept (CELIM study). Ann Oncol 2014;25(5):1018-25.

[56] Ye LC, Liu TS, Ren L, et al. Randomized controlled trial of cetuximab plus chemotherapy for patients with KRAS wild-type unresectable colorectal liver-limited metastases. J Clin Oncol 2013;31(16):1931-8.

[57] Wagman LD, Geller DA, Jacobs SA, et al. NSABP FC-6: phase II study to determine surgical conversion rate in patients (pts) receiving neoadjuvant (NA) mFOLFOX7 plus dose-escalating cetuximab (C) for unresectable K-RAS wild-type (WT) colorectal cancer with metastases (mCRC) confined to the liver. Ann Surg Oncol 2014;21:S13.

[58] Goere D, Deshaies I, de Baere T, et al. Prolonged survival of initially unresectable hepatic colorectal cancer patients treated with hepatic arterial infusion of oxaliplatin followed by radical surgery of metastases. Ann Surg 2010;251(4):686-91.

[59] Kemeny NE, Melendez FD, Capanu M, et al. Conversion to resectability using hepatic artery infusion plus systemic chemotherapy for the treatment of unresectable liver metastases from colorectal carcinoma. J Clin Oncol 2009;27(21):3465-71.

[60] Nordlinger B, Sorbye H, Glimelius B, et al. Perioperative chemotherapy with FOLFOX4 and surgery versus surgery alone for resectable liver metastases from colorectal cancer (EORTC Intergroup trial 40983): a randomised controlled trial. Lancet 2008;371(9617):1007-16.

[61] Nordlinger B, Sorbye H, Glimelius B, et al. Perioperative FOLFOX4 chemotherapy and surgery versus surgery alone for resectable liver metastases from colorectal cancer (EORTC 40983): long-term results of a randomised, controlled, phase 3 trial. Lancet Oncol 2013;14(12):1208-15.

[62] Zhu D, Zhong Y, Wei Y, et al. Effect of neoadjuvant chemotherapy in patients with resectable colorectal liver metastases. PLoS One 2014;9(1):e86543.

[63] Adam R, Bismuth H, Castaing D, et al. Repeat hepatectomy for colorectal liver metastases. Ann Surg 1997;225(1):51-60 [discussion: 60-2].

[64] Kulik U, Bektas H, Klempnauer J, et al. Repeat liver resection for colorectal metastases. Br J Surg 2013;100(7):926-32.

[65] Jones RP, Jackson R, Dunne DF, et al. Systematic review and meta-analysis of follow-up after hepatectomy for colorectal liver metastases. Br J Surg 2012; 99(4):477-86.

[66] Verberne CJ, Wiggers T, Vermeulen KM, et al. Detection of recurrences during follow-up after liver surgery for colorectal metastases: both carcinoembryonic antigen (CEA) and imaging are important. Ann Surg Oncol 2013;20(2):457-63.

[67] Fiorentini G, Aliberti C, Tilli M, et al. Intra-arterial infusion of irinotecan-loaded drug-eluting beads (DEBIRI) versus intravenous therapy (FOLFIRI) for hepatic metastases from colorectal cancer: final results of a phase III study. Anticancer Res 2012;32(4):1387-95.

[68] Wong SL, Mangu PB, Choti MA, et al. American Society of Clinical Oncology 2009 clinical evidence review on radiofrequency ablation of hepatic metastases from colorectal cancer. J Clin Oncol 2010;28(3):493-508.

[69] McCahill LE, Yothers G, Sharif S, et al. Primary mFOLFOX6 plus bevacizumab without resection of the primary tumor for patients presenting with surgically unresectable metastatic colon cancer and an intact asymptomatic colon cancer: definitive analysis of NSABP trial C-10. J Clin Oncol 2012;30(26):3223-8.

[70] de Mestier L, Manceau G, Neuzillet C, et al. Primary tumor resection in colorectal cancer with unresectable synchronous metastases: a review. World J Gastrointest Oncol 2014;6(6):156-69.

[71] Jegatheeswaran S, Mason JM, Hancock HC, et al. The liver-first approach to the management of colorectal cancer with synchronous hepatic metastases: a systematic review. JAMA Surg 2013;148(4):385-91.

[72] Sadanandam A, Lyssiotis CA, Homicsko K, et al. A colorectal cancer classification system that associates cellular phenotype and responses to therapy. Nat Med 2013;19(5):619-25.